Your *Clinics* subscripti...

**You can now access the FULL TEXT of this p...
online at no additional cost! Activate your o...
subscription today and receive...**

- Full text of all issues from 2002 to the present
- Photographs, tables, illustrations, and references
- Comprehensive search capabilities
- Links to MEDLINE and Elsevier journals

Activate Your Online Access Today!

Plus, you can also sign up for E-alerts of upcoming issues or articles that interest you, and take advantage of exclusive access to bonus features!

To activate your individual online subscription:

1. Visit our website at **www.TheClinics.com**.

2. Click on "Register" at the top of the page, and follow the instructions

3. To activate your account, you will need your subscriber account number, which you can find on your mailing label (note: the number of digits in your subscriber account number varies from six to ten digits). See the sample below where the subscriber account number has been circled.

This is your subscriber account number

```
************************************************3-DIGIT 001
FEB00   J0167   C7   123456-89   10//

J.H. DOE, MD
531 MAIN ST
CENTER CITY, NY  10001-001
```

D1522189

4. That's it! Your online access to the most trusted
   is now available.

the**clinics**.com

theclinics.com

JAN   2006

VETERINARY CLINICS

OF NORTH AMERICA

Small Animal Practice

Geriatrics

GUEST EDITOR
William D. Fortney,

May 2005   •   V

SAUNDERS

An Imprint of Elsevier, Inc.
PHILADELPHIA   LONDON   TO

W.B. SAUNDERS COMPANY
A Division of Elsevier Inc.

Elsevier, Inc., 1600 John F. Kennedy Blvd., Suite 1800, Philadelphia, PA 19103-2899.

http://www.vetsmall.theclinics.com

VETERINARY CLINICS OF NORTH AMERICA:
SMALL ANIMAL PRACTICE
May 2005
Editor: John Vassallo

Volume 35, Number
ISSN 0195-561
ISBN 1-4160-2845-

The ideas and opinions expressed in *Veterinary Clinics of North America: Small Animal Practice* do not necessarily refle
those of the Publisher. The Publisher does not assume any responsibility for any injury and/or damage to persons c
property arising out of or related to any use of the material contained in this periodical. The reader is advised to chec
the appropriate medical literature and the product information currently provided by the manufacturer of each drug t
be administered to verify the dosage, the method and duration of administration, or contraindications. It is the respor
sibility of the treating physician or other health care professional, relying on independent experience and knowledge (
the patient, to determine drug dosages and the best treatment for the patient. Mention of any product in this issue shoul
not be construed as endorsement by the contributors, editors, or the Publisher of the product or manufacturers' claim

Veterinary Clinics of North America: Small Animal Practice (ISSN 0195-5616) is published bimonthly (For Post Office us
only: volume 35 issue 3 of 6) by Elsevier, Inc. Corporate and editorial offices: Elsevier, Inc., 1600 John F. Kenned
Blvd., Suite 1800, Philadelphia, PA 19103-2899. Accounting and circulation offices: 6277 Sea Harbor Drive, Orland
FL 32887-4800. Periodicals postage paid at Orlando, FL 32862, and additional mailing offices. Subscription prices a
$170.00 per year for US individuals, $260.00 per year for US institutions, $85.00 per year for US students and res
dents, $215.00 per year for Canadian individuals, $325.00 per year for Canadian institutions, $225.00 per year fc
international individuals, $325.00 per year for international institutions and $113.00 per year for Canadian and fo
eign students/residents. To receive student/resident rate, orders must be accompanied by name of affiliated inst
tution, date of term, and the *signature* of program/residency coordinator on institution letterhead. Orders will b
billed at individual rate until proof of status is received. Foreign air speed delivery is included in all *Clinics* subscri
tion prices. All prices are subject to change without notice. POSTMASTER: Send address changes to *Veterinary Clinic
of North America: Small Animal Practice*, Elsevier, Customer Service Department, 6277 Sea Harbor Drive, Orland
FL 32887-4800, USA; phone: (+1)(877) 8397126 [toll free number for US customers], or (+1)(407) 3454020 [customer
outside US]; fax: (+1)(407) 3631354; email: usjcs@elsevier.com

Veterinary Clinics of North America: Small Animal Practice is also published in Japanese by Gakusosha Company Ltd., 2
16-28 Nishikata, Bunkyo-ku, Tokyo 113, Japan.

Reprints. For copies of 100 or more, of articles in this publication, please contact the Commercial Reprints Depar
ment, Elsevier Inc., 360 Park Avenue South, New York, New York 10010-1710. Tel. (212) 633-3813 Fax: (212) 462
1935, email: reprints@elsevier.com

Veterinary Clinics of North America: Small Animal Practice is covered in *Current Contents/Agriculture, Biology an
Environmental Sciences, Science Citation Index, ASCA, Index Medicus, Excerpta Medica, and BIOSIS*.

Printed in the United States of America.

GUEST EDITOR

WILLIAM D. FORTNEY, DVM, Assistant Professor, Department of Diagnostic Medicine/ Pathobiology, Kansas State University College of Veterinary Medicine, Manhattan, Kansas

CONTRIBUTORS

A. RICK ALLEMAN, DVM, PhD, Diplomate, American Board of Veterinary Practitioners; Diplomate, American College of Veterinary Pathologists; Associate Professor, Clinical Pathology, Department of Physiological Sciences, College of Veterinary Medicine, University of Florida, Gainesville, Florida

JOSEPH A. ARAUJO, BSc, Graduate Student, Department of Pharmacology, University of Toronto, Toronto; CanCog Technologies, Toronto, Ontario, Canada

BRIAN S. BEALE, DVM, Diplomate, American College of Veterinary Surgeons; Gulf Coast Veterinary Specialists, Houston, Texas

RACHAEL E. CARPENTER, DVM, Clinical Assistant Professor, Anesthesia and Pain Management, Department of Veterinary Clinical Medicine, University of Illinois, Urbana, Illinois

PATRICIA M. DOWLING, DVM, MSc, Diplomate, American College of Veterinary Internal Medicine; Diplomate, American College of Veterinary Clinical Pharmacology; Professor, Department of Veterinary Biomedical Sciences, Western College of Veterinary Medicine, University of Saskatchewan, Saskatoon, Saskatchewan, Canada

GREGORY F. GRAUER, DVM, MS, Diplomate, American College of Veterinary Internal Medicine (Internal Medicine); Professor and Head, Department of Clinical Sciences, College of Veterinary Medicine, Kansas State University, Manhattan, Kansas

REBEKAH G. GUNN, DVM, Resident, Clinical Pathology Service, Department of Physiological Sciences, College of Veterinary Medicine, University of Florida, Gainesville, Florida

ROBERT L. HAMLIN, DVM, PhD, Diplomate, American College of Veterinary Internal Medicine (Cardiology/Internal Medicine); Professor, Department of Veterinary Biosciences, The Ohio State University College of Veterinary Medicine, Columbus, Ohio

STEVEN E. HOLMSTROM, DVM, Diplomate, American Veterinary Dental College, Animal Dental Clinic, San Carlos, California

JOHNNY D. HOSKINS, DVM, PhD, Small Animal Consultant, DocuTech Services, Inc., Choudrant, Louisiana

DOROTHY P. LAFLAMME, DVM, PhD, Nestle Purina PetCare Research, St. Louis, Missouri

GARY LANDSBERG, DVM, Diplomate, American College of Veterinary Behaviorists; Doncaster Animal Clinic, Thornhill, Ontario, Canada

SUSAN A. MEEKING, DVM, Resident in Internal Medicine and Emergency/Critical Care, Animal Medical Center, New York, New York

FRED L. METZGER, DVM, Diplomate, American Board of Veterinary Practitioners (Canine/Feline); Metzger Animal Hospital, State College, Pennsylvania

GLENN R. PETTIFER, DVM, DVSc, Diplomate, American College of Veterinary Anesthesiologists; Associate Professor of Veterinary Anesthesiology, Department of Veterinary Clinical Sciences, School of Veterinary Medicine, Louisiana State University, Baton Rouge, Louisiana

WILLIAM J. TRANQUILLI, DVM, MS, Diplomate, American College of Veterinary Anesthesiologists; Professor, Anesthesia and Pain Management, Department of Veterinary Clinical Medicine, University of Illinois, Urbana, Illinois

CONTENTS

Preface   xi
William D. Fortney

Clinical Pathology in Veterinary Geriatrics   537
Rebekah G. Gunn and A. Rick Alleman

> Geriatric "care packages" that include senior wellness or biochem-
> ical screening panels are a routine offering at most veterinary
> clinics. Interpretation of abnormal results may be ambiguous, how-
> ever, especially because a variety of factors involving the animal,
> sample, and methodology used can affect results. A thorough
> understanding of these factors and their interrelations to one
> another can help the clinician become better able to address
> abnormalities revealed through blood work. When additional
> laboratory profiling is deemed appropriate, knowledge of organ-
> specific biochemical profiling helps the clinician attain more
> fruitful diagnostic results.

Geriatric Pharmacology   557
Patricia M. Dowling

> The process of aging causes changes in pharmacokinetics (altered
> drug concentration at the site of action) and pharmacodynamics
> (altered drug action). Many geriatric patients have dysfunction of
> more than one major organ system, which affects drug therapy.
> This article reviews the effects of renal, hepatic, and cardiac disease
> on drug disposition in geriatrics. Dosage adjustment can be made
> by the interval-extension method, the dose-reduction method, or a
> combination of the two. General adjustment guidelines are given
> for commonly used drugs in geriatric veterinary patients.

Anesthesia for Geriatric Patients
Rachael E. Carpenter, Glenn R. Pettifer, and
William J. Tranquilli

571

Choosing the best anesthetic agents for each geriatric animal does
not in itself ensure a successful outcome. Aggressive, careful, vigilant monitoring during the anesthetic and recovery periods is
required to detect and correct alterations in homeostasis that may
develop during the perianesthetic period. With appropriate preoperative screening, informed choice and judicious dosing of anesthetics, and careful monitoring and supportive care, the risk of
anesthesia in geriatric animals can be greatly reduced.

Early Detection of Renal Damage and Disease in Dogs
and Cats
Gregory F. Grauer

581

Renal damage and disease can be caused by acute or chronic
insults to the kidney. Acute renal damage often results from
ischemic or toxic insults and usually affects the tubular portion
of the nephron. In contrast, chronic renal disease can be caused
by diseases and/or disorders that affect any portion of the
nephron, including its blood supply and supporting interstitium.
Early detection of acute renal disease facilitates appropriate intervention that can arrest or at least attenuate tubular cell damage
and the development of established acute renal failure. Similarly,
early detection of chronic renal disease, before the onset of renal
azotemia and chronic renal failure, should facilitate appropriate
intervention that stabilizes renal function or at least slows its progressive decline.

Geriatric Heart Diseases in Dogs
Robert L. Hamlin

597

A discussion of the diagnosis and therapy of heart disease in an
aged pet does not differ significantly from that in a pet of any
age. Mitral regurgitation constitutes by far the most important geriatric heart disease, and the selection of drugs to treat heart disease
of aging pets is based on identification of specific pathologic features (eg, atrial fibrillation, left atrial enlargement) for which each
aspect of treatment (eg, diuretics, angiotensin-converting enzyme
inhibitors, spironolactone) is specific.

Liver Disease in the Geriatric Patient
Johnny D. Hoskins

617

Older dogs and cats are at great risk for the development of liver
disease. The diagnosis of liver disease is initiated by the veterinarian's suspicion that liver disease might be present, followed by the
case history and a physical examination. The initial workup for the
older dog or cat with suspected liver disease should begin with a

complete blood cell count, serum chemistry profile, and urinalysis. This may be followed by serum bile acid determinations, radiographic or ultrasonographic imaging studies, hepatic fine-needle aspiration, and, ultimately, liver biopsy.

Thyroid Disorders in the Geriatric Patient 635
Susan A. Meeking

Thyroid disorders are common in geriatric veterinary patients. These disorders can manifest in many different ways because of the multisystemic effects of thyroid hormones in the body. This article reviews the clinical presentation, diagnosis, and treatment options for feline hyperthyroidism, canine hypothyroidism, and canine thyroid tumors.

Orthopedic Problems in Geriatric Dogs and Cats 655
Brian S. Beale

Senior dogs and cats with orthopedic injuries and diseases often require a treatment plan that differs from that of younger patients. Injured bone and soft tissues tend to heal more slowly in the geriatric patient. The older animal is likely to have a less competent immune system and may have compromised metabolic and endocrine function. Pre-existing musculoskeletal problems may make ambulation difficult for an animal convalescing from a new orthopedic problem. Special attention is often needed when treating these patients for fractures, joint instability, infection, and neoplasia. In general, issues that should be addressed in the geriatric patient include reducing intraoperative and anesthesia time, enhancing bone and soft tissue healing, return to early function, control of postoperative pain, physical therapy, and proper nutrition.

Behavior Problems in Geriatric Pets 675
Gary Landsberg and Joseph A. Araujo

Aging pets often suffer a decline in cognitive function (eg, memory, learning, perception, awareness) likely associated with age-dependent brain alterations. Clinically, cognitive dysfunction may result in various behavioral signs, including disorientation; forgetting of previously learned behaviors, such as house training; alterations in the manner in which the pet interacts with people or other pets; onset of new fears and anxiety; decreased recognition of people, places, or pets; and other signs of deteriorating memory and learning ability. Many medical problems, including other forms of brain pathologic conditions, can contribute to these signs. The practitioner must first determine the cause of the behavioral signs and then determine an appropriate course of treatment, bearing in mind the constraints of the aging process. A diagnosis of cognitive dysfunction syndrome is made once other medical and behavioral causes are ruled out.

**Geriatric Veterinary Dentistry: Medical and Client
Relations and Challenges**   **699**
Steven E. Holmstrom

> Quality of life is an important issue for geriatric patients. Allowing
> periodontal disease, fractured teeth, and neoplasia to remain
> untreated decreases this quality of life. Age itself should be recog-
> nized; however, it should not be a deterrent to successful veterinary
> dental care.

**Nutrition for Aging Cats and Dogs and the Importance of
Body Condition**   **713**
Dorothy P. Laflamme

> A thorough geriatric evaluation and management plan should
> include a comprehensive dietary evaluation, with consideration
> for changing nutritional needs of the older pet. The most common
> nutrition-related problem in pet dogs and cats is obesity. Con-
> versely, many geriatric pets are underweight or losing weight. This
> article addresses these topics as well as other obesity-related condi-
> tions that may benefit from dietary management.

Senior and Geriatric Care Programs for Veterinarians   **743**
Fred L. Metzger

> Senior care has emerged as one of the most important medical and
> financial components of the modern successful veterinary practice.
> Advances in diagnostics, therapeutics, and nutrition coupled with
> increasing client awareness via increased advertising and media
> attention put senior care at the forefront of veterinary medicine
> in the twenty-first century. Follow a successful practice's senior
> and geriatric care blueprint to increase your practice's senior care
> compliance.

Index   **755**

GOAL STATEMENT

The goal of the *Veterinary Clinics of North America: Small Animal Practice* is to keep practicing veterinarians up-to-date with current clinical practice in small animal medicine by providing timely articles reviewing the state of the art in small animal care.

ACCREDITATION

The *Veterinary Clinics of North America: Small Animal Practice* will be offering continuing education credits, to be awarded by a school of veterinary medicine, contract pending.

The aforementioned school of veterinary medicine is a designated provider of continuing veterinary education. Veterinarians participating in this learning activity may earn up to 6 credits per issue up to a maximum of 36 credits per year. Credits awarded may not apply toward license renewal in all states. It is the responsibility of each participant to verify the requirements of their state licensing board.

Credit can be earned by reading the text material, taking the examination online at *http:// www.theclinics.com/home/cme*, and completing the program evaluation. Each test question must be answered correctly; you will have the opportunity to retake any questions answered incorrectly. Following successful completion of the test and the program evaluation, you may print your certificate.

TO ENROLL

To enroll in the *Veterinary Clinics of North America: Small Animal Practice* Continuing Education program, call customer service at 1-800-654-2452 or sign up online at http://www.theclinics.com/home/cme. The CME program is available to subscribers for an additional annual fee of $99.95.

FORTHCOMING ISSUES

July 2005
   Dentistry
   Steven E. Holmstrom, DVM, *Guest Editor*

September 2005
   General Orthopedics
   Walter C. Renberg, DVM, MS and
   James K. Roush, DVM, MS, *Guest Editors*

November 2005
   Veterinary Rehabilitation and Therapy
   David Levine, PhD, PT, Darryl L. Millis, MS,
   DVM, Denis J. Marcellin-Little, DEDV, and
   Robert Taylor, MS, DVM, *Guest Editors*

RECENT ISSUES

March 2005
   Emergency Medicine
   Kenneth J. Drobatz, DVM, MSCE
   Guest Editor

January 2005
   Advances in Feline Medicine
   James R. Richards, DVM, *Guest Editor*

November 2004
   Neuromuscular Diseases II
   G. Diane Shelton, DVM, PhD, *Guest Editor*

The Clinics are now available online!

Access your subscription at:
www.theclinics.com

VETERINARY
CLINICS
Small Animal Practice

Vet Clin Small Anim
35 (2005) xi–xii

Preface

Geriatrics

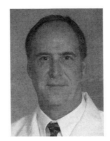

William D. Fortney, DVM
Guest Editor

Geriatric patients can represent major challenges to the owner as well as the veterinarian. Within the past decade, the improved knowledge base, newer technologies, and additional therapeutic options have allowed today's veterinarians to meet the medical and behavioral challenges of age-related disease better. These significant medical advances have been driven, in part, by increased human-animal bonding; the practitioner's desire to provide better care to the aging pet; and industry support in the form of age-specific medications, diets, continuing education, and client awareness campaigns.

In addition to raising the "standard of care" that we can now provide our senior patients, the hospital emphasis is rapidly shifting from the traditional reactive and/or overt disease management to a more proactive health maintenance and/or early detection strategy. Practices are also becoming more cognizant that with increasing veterinary competition and decreases in preventative health-related income, addressing the needs of the aging patient can also be considered a profit center.

This issue represents a "systems-based" approach to the common age-related problems seen in older dogs and cats. Each article was designed to be a "stand-alone" reference on the subject matter, including the latest and most pertinent clinical information on each topic. The authors were selected on the basis of their expertise and ability to convey practical knowledge to the reader. Their work has exceeded my expectations.

I would like to dedicate this book to the acknowledged father of veterinary geriatrics and my mentor, the late Dr. Jacob (Jake) Mosier, and to Drs. Johnny Hoskins and Richard Goldston for taking the discipline to the

doi:10.1016/j.cvsm.2005.01.002

next level. Without John Vassallo's leadership, editorial genius, and patience, this issue would not have been possible. Lastly, thanks to my dear departed senior friends (Peekie, Shadow, Faith, and B.G.), who were such an integral part of my life for so long and instrumental in my first-hand geriatric education.

My hope is that this edition helps to provide a higher standard of care to your older patients.

William D. Fortney, DVM
Diagnostic Medicine/Pathology
College of Veterinary Medicine
Kansas State University
Manhattan, KS 66506, USA

E-mail address: wfortney@vet.k-state.edu

ELSEVIER
SAUNDERS

Vet Clin Small Anim
35 (2005) 537–556

VETERINARY
CLINICS
Small Animal Practice

Clinical Pathology in Veterinary Geriatrics

Rebekah G. Gunn, DVM*,
A. Rick Alleman, DVM, PhD

*Clinical Pathology Service, Department of Physiological Sciences,
University of Florida, College of Veterinary Medicine,
PO Box 100103C, Gainesville, FL 32610–0103, USA*

In the past decade, a focus on the health and well-being of the geriatric companion animal has become a growing trend. Special needs of senior animals are becoming better recognized, as evidenced by the increasing availability of specially formulated diets, nutraceutical agents, and other products intended for the elderly animal. Not surprisingly, geriatric medicine has gained increasing attention, with the objective of maximizing quality of life through preventative medicine, early disease detection, and therapeutic intervention. To this end, geriatric "care packages" that include senior wellness or biochemical screening panels are a routine offering at most veterinary clinics.

When offering diagnostics of any type, the practitioner assumes the responsibility of interpreting the results correctly and taking appropriate action. Unfortunately, there is a dearth of information regarding biochemical testing in older animals, because little research has been performed on this age group. Age-related but clinically insignificant changes are to be expected; however, we are not aware of the existence of reference ranges specifically targeted for geriatric patients. Thus, biochemical abnormalities (defined as values that lie outside the reference range for clinically healthy adult animals) revealed by blood work performed during a wellness examination may be obscure as to their clinical significance. An 11-year-old Labrador Retriever would not be expected to have the same physiologic function as a 2-year-old, even if both dogs are clinically healthy. It is possible, and even probable, to find abnormalities on the blood work of

---

* Corresponding author.
E-mail address: gunnr@mail.vetmed.ufl.edu (R.G. Gunn).

doi:10.1016/j.cvsm.2004.12.004   *vetsmall.theclinics.com*

either animal; however, a plethora of reasons exist to explain the potential source of these abnormalities, many of which may not be related to the presence of a primary disease.

This article reviews biochemical testing of the geriatric patient, such as might be performed during an annual wellness examination. Performing biochemical profiles and complete blood cell counts (CBCs) on geriatric clinically healthy patients often results in abnormal laboratory findings. These findings could be classified as "unexpected" in the sense that most animals tested are apparently healthy. Some of these "abnormal" results are truly the result of occult disease that may require further investigation by the clinician and possible therapeutic intervention. Abnormal test results also occur because of multiple extraneous factors that have nothing to do with actual physiologic function in the patient, however. This article addresses various factors that can cause unexpected laboratory results and aims to assist the clinician in recognizing which abnormalities indicate an actual underlying disease process and which ones may not. This article also includes a discussion of organ-specific biochemical analytes useful in evaluating particular organ systems when further investigation through additional diagnostic testing is deemed appropriate.

Establishing reference intervals

Before a test can be used as a diagnostic tool, reference intervals must be established. A basic comprehension of this process allows a more thorough understanding of what a normal test result actually means. Not all abnormal test results actually reflect a pathologic condition in the organ system that they are being used to evaluate. Conversely, disease in a specific organ system may not always be reflected by a test result outside the reference range. When discrepancies exist between clinical findings and laboratory results, knowledge of how reference intervals are determined may help to prevent potential confusion.

The first step in establishing the reference interval for any test is to sample a group of apparently healthy normal animals that meet specific selection criteria based on various population parameters, such as species, breed, age, and gender. Environmental and physiologic conditions, such as diet, fasting, and pregnancy status, could also be invoked when defining the selection criteria. The more selection parameters that are used, the narrower the resulting reference intervals are likely to be and the greater the test's sensitivity for disease detection. The actual population on which a diagnostic test is used in practice is likely to exhibit much more heterogeneity than the sample population, however, even when only a few selection criteria are used [1]. As a consequence of applying reference ranges to a population with more inherent diversity than the sample population, many healthy animals are likely to have results deemed as abnormal because they are outside the narrow reference range. To avoid such an untoward outcome, most reference intervals are simply based on a mixed-gender sample of normal adult animals of a particular species. Although acceptable precision mandates that at least 120 samples be analyzed, availability of animals meeting the selection criteria as well as economic constraints often limits the number actually sampled for each analyzer in a particular laboratory. Fortunately, only 40 samples are necessary to determine a reliable reference interval [2].

After a set of test values is obtained, their distribution is examined and the range that encompasses the values from the middle 95% of the sample population is established. Typically, this is determined by calculating the mean of the results and including 2 SDs on either side of the mean. The method used to calculate the reference interval may vary, however, depending on the whether or not the data obtained have a normal bell-shaped (Gaussian) distribution. By definition, 5% of all healthy animals have a value that is outside the reference interval of any particular analyte. The statistical ramifications of omitting these outliers from the reference interval are striking: if a biochemical profile comprises 20 individual tests, each with a specificity of 95%, only 36% of truly normal animals have normal values in all 20 tests [3]. Abnormal results of this type are usually only slightly above or below the reference interval, however, a key feature that may help to prevent the clinician from overinterpreting minor abnormalities.

Laboratory-specific variables

Reference intervals for each analyte are often different between diagnostic laboratories. This may be a reflection of regional differences in populations of animals tested when establishing the reference ranges, or it may be a reflection of differences in analyzers or methodology used. Ideally, each laboratory should establish its own reference ranges, and new reference ranges should be generated whenever reagents or methodologies are changed. In practice, this process is usually restricted to academia and commercial diagnostic laboratories because it may not be practical for small hospitals using in-house analyzers. Because of the uniqueness of reference ranges, each commercial laboratory should include its own reference ranges with the results so as to ensure meaningful interpretation.

If blood samples are sent to a human laboratory, animal-specific reference ranges may not have been established, thus negatively influencing the interpretation of test results. Other significant drawbacks to using human diagnostic laboratories include a lack of methodology or reagents specific for nonhuman species, inadequate knowledge of species-specific hematologic and biochemical variables, and absence of a readily available clinical pathologist for consultation. Because of these reasons, extreme caution should be exercised if human laboratories are to be used for veterinary diagnostics.

Group-specific variables

In the diverse field of veterinary medicine, there are many well-documented biochemical and hematologic differences between groups and subgroups of animals based on such parameters as species, breed, age, and fasting status. These factors must also be considered to interpret test results accurately.

Interpretation of liver enzyme alkaline phosphatase (ALP) and alanine aminotransferase (ALT) is markedly different in the dog versus the cat. The half-life ($T_{1/2}$) of ALP and ALT is approximately 72 hours in the dog but only 7 hours in the cat. Furthermore, marked elevations can be seen in the dog with certain extrahepatic diseases, especially those in which endogenous or exogenous glucocorticoids are involved. Cats lack the corticosteroid-induced isoenzyme of ALP found in the dog, however. When interpreting ALP and ALT activities, elevations may bear no specific clinical significance in the dog; however, even minor elevations of feline liver enzymes are quite significant, and ALP is a specific indicator of feline cholestatic liver disease [4].

Pertaining to breed-associated discrepancies, Greyhounds are noted as having a physiologically normal packed cell volume (PCV) higher than that of most other breeds of dogs, and mild elevations should not be automatically interpreted as an abnormality, such as dehydration. Some Japanese dog breeds, such as the Akita and Shiba, have erythrocytes with an unusually high intraerythrocytic potassium concentration. In these breeds, in vitro hemolysis or delayed removal of serum or plasma from erythrocytes with subsequent leakage of potassium may result in a pseudohyperkalemia noted on blood work.

With regard to age, maturity is attained by 6 to 8 months in the dog and by 4 to 6 months in the cat. In young growing animals, the bone isoenzyme of ALP activity is normally increased in all species. This elevation can be of particular significance in large and giant breeds of dogs, however, in which values may reach 2 to 10 times those of the adult. In these animals, values begin to decline by 3 months of age but may not fall within the normal adult reference range until 15 months of age.

Some analytes, such as glucose and lipids, can be affected by the fasting status of the patient. Hyperglycemia and hyperlipidemia are normal postprandial phenomena; however, they may indicate pathologic conditions if noted on fasting samples. To rule out normal physiologic causes, fasting samples are recommended.

Laboratory methodology and substance interference

Most laboratory results on a biochemical profile are obtained through spectrophotometric methodology. In this process, a beam of light is split into different wavelengths by a prism. This light is directed into a slit-like opening that directs a selected range of wavelengths toward a cuvette containing an absorbing substance. In general terms, this substance is composed of a biologic sample (usually serum) to which one or more reagents have been added. These reagents cause a chemical reaction with the analyte of interest, resulting in a color change. The intensity of the color change is directly proportional to the concentration of the analyte. On the opposite side of the cuvette, a light detector measures the amount of light that is capable of passing through the reaction mixture. The amount of light absorbed by the liquid is proportional to the concentration of the analyte in the reaction mixture. The absorbance is described mathematically as Beer's law, the basis of spectrophotometry ($A = abc$), where A is absorbance, a is absorptivity, b is the light path length of the solution (measured in centimeters), and c is concentration of the analyte.

Absorbance spectrophotometry is typically performed using one of two types of assays: end point and kinetic. Both assays are based on the same fundamental principles of absorbance spectrophotometry but use slightly different methodologies. In an end point assay, the absorbance reading is taken at a single point near the end of the reaction time and the concentration of the analyte is based on the absorbance of light at this time. Assays of this type are generally used to measure the concentration of a preexisting substance. In contrast, absorbance readings are taken twice in a kinetic assay: once at the beginning and again before the end of the linear phase of the chemical reaction occurring in the cuvette. The change in absorbance between the beginning and end of the reaction is used to calculate the concentration of the analyte. Kinetic assays are often used to measure enzyme activities, although they may also be used to measure a preexisting substance [4].

Any interfering substance in the patient's serum that can increase the absorptivity or scatter light so that it is deflected from the light detector alters the recorded concentration of the measured analyte. In end point assays, the absorbance is falsely increased, resulting in an erroneously elevated analyte concentration. If the concentration of an interfering substance is of sufficient quantity in a kinetic assay, the change in absorbance between the first and second readings is not detected as easily and the concentration of the analyte may be falsely reduced. Three common sample conditions can dramatically affect assays in this manner: lipemia, hemolysis, and hyperbilirubinemia. In addition to skewing spectrophotometric measurements by absorbing or scattering light, the presence of hemolysis or lipemia may result in the addition or dilution of specific analytes in the patient's serum, as discussed elsewhere in this article.

Hemolysis

Although in vivo hemolysis may occur, it is more frequently encountered as an in vitro event during or after blood collection. The leakage of intracellular constituents from erythrocytes can significantly interfere with laboratory results in a number of ways. First, hemolysis may result in direct color interference because of light absorbance, as described previously. Hemolysis can have a variable effect on the measurement of an analyte, but the magnitude of this effect depends on the instrumentation and specific assay used. In general, end point assays, including total protein, total bilirubin, albumin, calcium, creatinine, and bile acids, are routinely elevated. Many enzyme assays are kinetic assays, and they may be falsely reduced by interfering substances that absorb light within the wavelength of the reaction. Aspartate aminotransferase (AST), ALP, creatine phosphokinase (CPK), and lipase results thus may be artificially lowered.

Hemolysis also can result in the release of red cell constituents into the serum, which are subsequently measured. Intracellular molecules, such as lactate dehydrogenase (LDH), AST, ALT, CPK, folate, and phosphorus, may be falsely increased depending on the severity of the hemolysis. A specific consideration relates to many Japanese Akita and Shiba dogs because their erythrocytes have a higher intracellular potassium concentration than those of other breeds. Hemolysis can consequently cause an in vitro or pseudohyperkalemia.

Finally, hemolysis may result in the dilution of substances normally found in the serum. This decrease is negligible, however, and usually considered insignificant as compared with the first two adverse effects described.

Lipemia

Lipemia causes light scattering as a result of excess chylomicrons or very low density lipoproteins (VLDLs) in the serum. Red cell fragility and subsequent hemolysis with release of intracellular constituents can also be increased in lipemic samples. As with hemolysis, whether an assay is falsely increased or decreased depends on the instrumentation used and the type of assay. End point assays that are often falsely increased by the presence of lipemia include those for total protein, total bilirubin, albumin, globulins, glucose, calcium, phosphorus, and bile acids. Kinetic assays that may be falsely decreased are those for ALT, AST, ALP, amylase, and lipase.

Icterus (hyperbilirubinemia)

High levels of bilirubin present in an icteric sample can also interfere with the absorbance of light in spectrophotometry. The presence of bilirubin may falsely increase measurements of total protein, ALP, and chloride; it may also falsely lower concentrations of creatinine, triglyceride, phosphorus, and magnesium. The effect of bilirubin on albumin, glucose, cholesterol, and lipase is variable and depends on the laboratory methodology used.

Blood substitutes (Oxyglobin)

Evaluation of the effects of a therapeutic dose of hemoglobin glutamer-200 (bovine) (Oxyglobin) was performed by the University of Florida College of Veterinary Medicine using a biochemical analyzer, the Hitachi 911 (Boehringer Mannheim, Indianapolis, IN). Oxyglobin therapy has experimentally been shown to result in spurious increases in total bilirubin, total protein, albumin, globulin, cholesterol, and magnesium. Decreases were observed in measurements of calcium, glucose, and carbon dioxide. Decreased and erroneous values were also obtained when measuring ALP, AST, ALT, phosphorus, and creatinine (A. Rick Alleman, DVM, PhD, Gainesville, FL, personal communication, 2004). The manufacturer's web site openly addresses the likelihood that some biochemical values may be altered and includes a table of analytes, categorized by analyzer, that would be unaffected by Oxyglobin immediately after a dose of 30 mL/kg [5]. Despite the inclusion of calcium, glucose, AST, ALP, and creatinine in the table of analytes whose values would be unaffected when obtained by means of a Hitachi 911 biochemical analyzer, the University of Florida study noted decreases or erroneous values in these analytes. The decreases in end point assays and erroneous values were attributed to a dilution effect on the analyte or to the creation of absorbance levels outside the range of the analyzer (A. Rick Alleman, DVM, PhD, Gainesville, FL, unpublished data, 2002).

Solutions to interfering substances

Some problems associated with interfering substances can be easily rectified. When possible, the use of samples containing the aforementioned substances should be avoided. Atraumatic venipuncture and careful sample handling can help to reduce iatrogenic hemolysis. An 8- to 12-hour fast is generally recommended to decrease lipemia in samples. Finally, biochemical profiles should be obtained on all patients before administration of blood substitute products, and a sample of this serum should be frozen and banked for potential diagnostic use later. Additional remedies include the use of alternate methodologies that are more impervious to interfering substances and retesting questionable values using dry reagent analyzers that filter out many interfering substances.

In practice, it is not always possible to use samples without interfering substances. For instance, animals with intravascular hemolysis inevitably have hemoglobinemia, and many hypothyroid animals experience a fasting hyperlipidemia. Unfortunately, alternate methodologies are not always readily available to the small animal practitioner in private practice. In these circumstances, a thorough understanding of the methodologies used and the specific analytes that may be skewed aids in accurate interpretation of results. As mentioned previously, laboratory results that are unexpected or do not correlate with the clinical presentation of a patient need to be carefully scrutinized to interpret their significance accurately.

Organ system–oriented biochemical profiling

A full biochemical profile is often run as part of a wellness check or diagnostic workup, but it is sometimes more convenient to organize the constituent assays according to their use in evaluating specific organs or systems. As with a full chemistry panel, the individual results must be evaluated in conjunction with patient variables, such as species and age, along with clinical findings to determine the relevance and credibility of any apparent abnormalities. In addition to localizing pathologic processes, diagnostic testing can be used to track disease progression and to monitor response to therapy. The following discussion of organ system–oriented biochemical profiling is intended to be a starting point rather than an all-inclusive "laundry list" of diagnostic tests.

Urinary system

A list of core tests for the urinary system is provided in Box 1. Collectively, this battery of tests assesses the function of the urinary system, especially the kidneys. If any of these assays yields abnormal results, concurrent urinalysis is required to determine the significance of the abnormality. Proteinuria or renal tubular casts may occur before serum biochemical abnormalities, thus providing additional justification for quantitative and qualitative assessments of urine if kidney disease is suspected.

Azotemia, denoted by elevations in BUN and creatinine, indicates decreased renal clearance of waste products, although the actual cause may

---

Box 1. Urinary system

Core tests
    Blood urea nitrogen (BUN)
    Creatinine
    Electrolytes: sodium, potassium, chloride
    Total carbon dioxide (TCO_2)
    Anion gap: $(Na + K) - (Cl + HCO_3)$
    Phosphorus and calcium
    Albumin
    Cholesterol
Ancillary test
    Urine electrolytes

be prerenal, renal, postrenal, or a combination of these factors. Differentiation between these causes is made through evaluation of clinical signs, hydration status, urine specific gravity, and serum electrolytes. Clinical signs, such as vomiting or diarrhea, and physical examination findings, such as decreased skin turgor or enophthalmos, may suggest dehydration and a resultant prerenal component. An isosthenuric specific gravity in the face of dehydration strongly suggests azotemia of a renal origin. Conversely, hypersthenuria with evidence of dehydration confirms that the kidneys have adequate concentrating ability. Although the combination of azotemia and isosthenuric urine is relatively specific for renal disease, at least three quarters of renal function must be lost before an elevated BUN level is apparent because of the extensive functional reserve of the kidneys. Therefore, azotemia is not a sensitive indicator of renal disease.

The electrolytes sodium, potassium, and chloride as well as their relative ratios may also help to determine the cause of azotemia. Sodium and chloride are often elevated in the case of prerenal azotemia but decreased when the kidneys are not capable of preventing urinary loss. Potassium tends to be elevated in animals with postrenal azotemia, such as urinary obstruction or uroabdomen, because of reabsorption along the concentration gradient of a substance normally excreted in high concentrations in the urine.

TCO_2 may help to pinpoint the disease process to the kidneys, because animals with renal pathologic changes often become acidotic. This acidosis occurs through two general mechanisms: renal loss of bicarbonate and accumulation of organic acid wastes. Calculation of the anion gap is quite useful when the TCO_2 is abnormal because it helps to clarify the electrolyte and acid-base abnormalities. If acidosis is the result of bicarbonate loss, chloride is often elevated as a compensatory mechanism, and the anion gap is subsequently normal. Therefore, a hyperchloremic metabolic acidosis is a common finding in animals with renal disease. If the acidosis is caused by build-up of organic acid waste or of compounds not normally measured, such as ethylene glycol, the anion gap is elevated.

Phosphorus elevations often occur in animals with renal disease because of decreased urinary excretion as well as renal secondary hyperparathyroidism. Hypercalcemia as a result of renal disease is unusual in dogs and cats, because calcium is more closely regulated than phosphorous. Elevations in calcium tend to be an initiating cause rather than an effect of renal disease and should be diagnostically pursued as such. In rare cases, renal disease may cause mild hypercalcemia that is diagnostically confirmed by decreased fractional urinary excretion of calcium. Much more commonly, a low-normal or mild hypocalcemia is noted with renal failure, resulting from decreased renal mass and subsequent reduced formation of 1,25-DHCC [6].

Other assays of considerable diagnostic utility are those for albumin and cholesterol. Dehydration with prerenal azotemia can lead to increases in albumin, whereas protein-losing nephropathies, particularly those in which the glomeruli are affected, tend to result in hypoalbuminemia. Markedly decreased albumin can lead to a finding of hypocalcemia on the laboratory results, because a large percentage of total calcium is protein bound. The physiologically active unbound fraction of calcium is usually within normal limits, however. Decreased albumin with a high BUN level warrants urinalysis with a protein/creatinine ratio (UP/UC) for further evaluation. The UP/UC ratio is normally less than 0.5, and a ratio greater than 1.0 confirms renal proteinuria. Questionable results occur between these numbers. Cholesterol is also important, because hypoalbuminemia may lead to a compensatory hypercholesterolemia in an effort to maintain an appropriate vascular colloidal osmotic pressure.

Hepatic system

A list of core tests for the hepatic system is provided in Box 2. This combination of core tests assists in evaluating a patient for evidence of liver disease. Four main categories of disorders affect the liver: hepatocellular injury or necrosis, alterations in synthetic or excretory functions, cholestasis, and altered portal circulation. Liver enzymes (ALT, ALP, AST, and GGT) are not specific indicators of liver disease or liver function, however, because they can become elevated in association with many other problems, especially in dogs. Thus, evaluation of these enzymes in the context of the other proposed assays for hepatic system evaluation is critical to the assessment of the patient.

ALT and ALP are enzymes that indicate hepatocellular leakage and cholestasis, respectively. As noted in the elsewhere in this article, several

---

Box 2. Hepatic system

Core tests
  ALT
  ALP
  AST
  γ-Glutamyltransferase (GGT)
  Albumin
  Cholesterol
  Triglycerides
  Glucose
  BUN
  Total bilirubin
Ancillary tests
  Bile acids
  Ammonia

noteworthy differences exist between canine and feline species. In the dog, these enzymes are not specific for primary hepatic disease, because numerous conditions, many of which are not of primary hepatic origin, can lead to marked elevations. The magnitude of response of ALP versus ALT may help to differentiate corticosteroid-induced enzyme elevations in dogs, because corticosteroids tend to cause a markedly elevated ALP with a moderate to marked elevation in ALT. Furthermore, bilirubin is usually normal or near normal in such animals. A much stronger indication for primary liver disease is indicated when bilirubin, ALP, and ALT are all elevated. True liver pathologic findings may still be a secondary condition, however, such as in patients with pancreatitis. In contrast, even slight elevations are quite significant in the cat because of the substantially shorter half-life and lack of corticosteroid-induced isoenzyme.

ALT is a cytosolic enzyme that is released into the blood with cellular death and subsequent lysis as well as with sublethal insult and accompanying increased membrane permeability. The sensitivity of ALT is much poorer than its specificity, because animals with end-stage liver disease may have normal values. This enzyme is relatively liver specific, although erythrocytes and striated myocytes contain low concentrations of ALT. Elevations may be seen in animals with hemolysis, myopathies, or hepatic disease; further diagnostic testing may thus be needed. ALP is an inducible enzyme, and elevations are not seen as rapidly in response to hepatic injury as with leakage enzymes. Several clinically significant isoenzymes of ALP exist, including corticosteroid and bone, thus potentially complicating interpretation of elevated values.

AST and GGT are similar to ALT and ALP to the extent that they are also leakage and cholestatic enzymes, respectively. AST is a mitochondrial enzyme, however, and elevations may reflect more severe hepatic pathologic changes. Thus, elevations in both ALT and AST may indicate a more severe disease than would elevations in ALT alone. Concurrent elevations in ALT and AST also are highly suggestive of primary liver pathologic findings.

GGT may be slightly more specific than ALP for cholestasis in the dog, because corticosteroids do not seem to have as dramatic an influence on GGT levels. Measurement of GGT may be indicated more often in cats because of the slightly higher sensitivity and possibly higher specificity for feline hepatic diseases other than hepatic lipidosis. This decreased sensitivity relating to hepatic lipidosis can also be exploited as a diagnostic tool: cholangiohepatitis results in elevations in ALP and GGT of a similar magnitude, whereas hepatic lipidosis classically has markedly elevated ALP but normal to slightly elevated GGT.

As with renal disease, some patients with liver disease have hypoalbuminemia and hypercholesterolemia. Decreased albumin is seen with chronic liver failure as a result of depressed production, and cholestatic disease leads to decreased excretion of cholesterol. Triglycerides may be elevated because of altered lipid metabolism, especially in cats with hepatic lipidosis. Patients with severe liver disease and failure may have low glucose and BUN values because of decreased gluconeogenesis or decreased protein catabolism, respectively.

Generally speaking, hyperbilirubinemia is indicative of hemolytic disease or hepatobiliary disease. If the CBC indicates a massive rapid decrease in erythrocyte numbers or evidence of regenerative anemia, hemolysis is the more likely cause. If hemolysis is not supported by the CBC, however, hepatobiliary disease is more likely. Hyperbilirubinemia in conjunction with elevations in GGT or ALP is even better verification that hepatic disease is present. Hyperbilirubinemia is not a sensitive indicator for hepatic disease, however, nor is it specific for primary liver dysfunction, because secondary or reactive liver disease may also cause elevations.

A concurrent urinalysis may yield additional information, because similar biochemical abnormalities may be found with disease processes not originating from the liver. Hypoalbuminemia and hypercholesterolemia are features of hepatic and renal disease, but a finding of proteinuria on urinalysis suggests renal loss rather than decreased hepatic production. Furthermore, bilirubin spills into the urine before serum or tissue accumulation occurs. A finding of bilirubinuria may facilitate earlier detection of hepatic disease. Although 1+ bilirubin may be normal in extremely concentrated urine from male dogs, this finding is never normal in cats, and moderate to marked increases should be investigated in dogs.

If the initial diagnostic workup of hepatic function is ambiguous, it may be necessary to perform tests of hepatic function, such as ammonia and bile acid concentrations. Elevated ammonia levels arise from a decreased functional hepatic mass or portosystemic shunts, thus making this test highly specific for liver disease. The sensitivity of this test is generally low, because a significant amount of hepatic involvement is necessary before elevations are apparent. Measurements of bile acid levels analyze liver function by testing hepatocellular ability to confine bile salts to the enterohepatic circulation. If cellular function or blood supply is compromised, as with hepatobiliary disease or portosystemic shunts, respectively, elevations in preprandial and postprandial bile acid levels are common. Measuring both pre- and postprandial serum bile acid levels greatly increases the sensitivity of this test. Performing a bile acid test on an icteric patient with hepatic or extrahepatic biliary tract disease does not yield any additional information, however. This test is somewhat specific for primary liver disease, because secondary hepatic disease usually does not elevate bile acids. As compared with resting blood ammonia concentrations, fasting serum bile acid concentrations are also likely to have a higher sensitivity [7].

The assays used to evaluate a patient for liver disease only occasionally provide an indication of the cause, extent of damage, or reversibility. Chronic hepatic disease in which many hepatocytes have been undergoing continuous insult may manifest the same enzyme elevations as an acute severe lesion in which only a few hepatocytes are affected. Ultimately, fine-needle aspiration or hepatic biopsy is usually needed for a definitive diagnosis.

Exocrine pancreas and/or pancreatitis

A list of core tests for the exocrine pancreas and/or pancreatitis is provided in Box 3. Pathologic findings of the exocrine pancreas are classified into two main processes: inflammatory conditions, which are often accompanied by necrosis, and exocrine pancreas insufficiency (EPI). The most important diagnostic assays for the exocrine pancreas are amylase, lipase, and TLI. Other core tests are included in the diagnostic workup for their utility in excluding other diseases that may mimic or cause secondary pancreatitis. Unfortunately, confirming a diagnosis of pancreatitis often remains a diagnostic dilemma unless a biopsy is obtained.

Amylase and lipase have historically been used to diagnose pancreatitis in the dog. The diagnostic value of their sensitivity and specificity remains highly debatable, however, and they are of little or no value in the diagnosis of feline pancreatitis. The following discussion relates to these analytes in dogs only. If amylase and lipase are used, tests should be performed simultaneously and the results should exhibit at least a twofold increase before they are considered clinically significant. These enzymes can be elevated in other conditions, such as renal and intestinal diseases, and corticosteroid therapy can result in lipase elevations. Interfering substances in the serum, such as lipemia, may also adversely affect their measurement.

Hyperamylasemia of 3 to 4 times the upper reference interval is highly suggestive of pancreatitis, and the probability of the animal having the disease increases with the magnitude of elevation. Amylase values of 7 to 10

Box 3. Exocrine pancreas and/or pancreatitis

Core tests
  Amylase
  Lipase
  BUN
  Calcium
  Cholesterol
  Triglycerides
  Glucose
  Albumin
  ALP
  ALT
Ancillary test
  Trypsin-like immunoreactivity (TLI)

times the upper limit of normal are possible with acute pancreatitis, but false-negative results are quite common. Increased amylase has a low specificity for pancreatitis unless it is severe. As with amylase, serum lipase activity elevations of at least 3 times the upper normal value are needed to diagnose acute pancreatitis, with more severe elevations being more confirmatory. Amylase and lipase activities should parallel one another when pancreatic pathologic findings are present. Renal disease can result in elevations of amylase and lipase of 2 to 3 times normal, however; thus, BUN testing and urinalysis may be needed to rule out renal pathologic changes.

Additional assays are usually needed to determine the presence of pancreatic disease. Alone, these assays are not specific for pancreatitis. When analyzed together and in conjunction with amylase and lipase, increased confidence in a diagnosis of pancreatitis is gained. Hypocalcemia is an occasional finding in patients with acute pancreatitis and results from an accompanying necrotizing steatitis with saponification of fat. Altered lipid metabolism and fat mobilization may lead to elevations in cholesterol and triglycerides. Hyperglycemia is a common feature, because insulin production is often decreased. Most animals with acute pancreatitis also demonstrate significant secondary liver abnormalities, such as elevations in ALP and ALT, that are associated with peritonitis, obstruction of the common bile duct, or fatty degeneration in the liver.

TLI seems to be a pancreatic-specific assay and is the test of choice in diagnosing EPI. With its high diagnostic specificity and sensitivity, decreased TLI concentrations are confirmatory for EPI. TLI is of slightly less utility in diagnosing pancreatitis, because elevations with necrotizing pancreatitis are an inconsistent finding. It seems that TLI may increase before amylase or lipase with acute pancreatitis, but additional research is needed to determine its worth in diagnosing this disease. Like amylase and lipase, decreased renal clearance can also result in mild elevations.

Gastrointestinal system

A list of core tests for the gastrointestinal system is provided in Box 4. There are no assays specifically indicated for the identification of intestinal disease, with the exception of the previously mentioned ancillary tests. Several nonspecific assays on the biochemical profile can provide valuable information when evaluated in the context of a clinical case and other analytes, however. Animals with protein-losing enteropathies exhibit panhypoproteinemia as evidenced by decreased albumin and globulin, whereas renal or liver disease typically results in decreased albumin only. Animals that are dehydrated because of loss of fluid from the gastrointestinal tract ordinarily have elevated albumin if levels were normal before the dehydrated state.

Electrolyte disturbances are also common in animals with gastrointestinal disease. Increases can occur with dehydration, but vomiting and diarrhea

---

Box 4. Gastrointestinal system

Core tests
   Total protein (albumin and globulin)
   Electrolytes: sodium, potassium, chloride
   TCO_2 and anion gap
   BUN and creatinine
Ancillary tests
   Vitamin B_{12} (cobalamin)
   Folate

---

can result in a loss of chloride and potassium. Decreased intake in anorectic animals may also result in hypochloremia and hypokalemia. Loss of hydrochloric acid from animals with high intestinal obstruction can result in a hypochloremic metabolic alkalosis with a high TCO_2. Conversely, loss of bicarbonate in a patient with intestinal disease can result in conservation of chloride by the kidney, a decrease in TCO_2, and an ensuing hyperchloremic metabolic acidosis. This particular pattern of abnormalities is also seen in patients with renal disease; thus, evaluation of electrolytes and acid base is important in animals with clinical evidence of disorders with either organ system. BUN and creatinine abnormalities may help to localize a disease, because animals with renal disease or even hypoadrenocorticism (Addison's disease) are sometimes presented with gastrointestinal signs as an initial complaint. Furthermore, elevated BUN with a normal creatinine level is suggestive of a gastrointestinal hemorrhage rather than renal disease.

The ancillary tests for vitamin B_{12} (cobalamin) and folate are fairly specific, because altered levels may occur with any primary intestinal disease that results in decreased absorption or bacterial overgrowth. A decreased level of vitamin B_{12} may arise from defective absorption in the ileum as a result of any disease that damages ileal mucosa. A preabsorptive defect, such as EPI or intestinal bacterial overgrowth, may also lead to reduced vitamin B_{12} levels. Regardless of the cause, decreased concentrations are not noted in the serum until body reserves are exhausted.

Folate concentration may be elevated or depressed with gastrointestinal disease. Small intestinal bacterial overgrowth can result in excessive microbial folate production and secondary digestive absorption. The underlying disease process allowing this overgrowth could be intestinal, such as reduced gastric acid secretion or depressed intestinal peristalsis. Extraintestinal disorders, such as EPI, can also result in bacterial overgrowth. Furthermore, folate absorption is optimized at a low pH; thus, a pathologic condition leading to an acidic intestinal environment could be associated with subsequently elevated serum folate levels. Disease conditions associated with decreased intestinal pH include excessive gastric acid production and impaired bicarbonate secretion secondary to EPI. As with vitamin B_{12}, decreased folate concentrations may occur with any disease that causes decreased intestinal absorption, such as damage of the proximal small intestinal mucosa [8].

Endocrine system

A list of core tests for the endocrine system is provided in Box 5. Endocrine disorders can be quite challenging to diagnose and treat, because many endocrine disorders mimic disease processes of other organ systems and some endocrine disorders resemble each other. Hyperadrenocorticism (Cushing's disease) and hypoadrenocorticism (Addison's disease) can hinder the kidney's ability to concentrate urine. Thus, isosthenuric urine is a laboratory finding common to adrenal and primary renal tubular pathologic findings. Diabetes mellitus and hyperadrenocorticism are characterized by hyperglycemia, although the underlying pathophysiologic findings are different. Additional routine diagnostic testing, such as urinalysis, and even specialized tests are often warranted to confirm an endocrinopathy. Urinalysis can help to rule out renal disease and may even lend additional diagnostic information, such as identifying glucosuria or ketonuria in a patient suspected of having diabetes mellitus.

Calcium and phosphorus are important for evaluation of parathyroid gland function. Patients with primary hyperparathyroidism and pseudohy-

---

Box 5. Endocrine system

Core tests
  Calcium
  Phosphorus
  Glucose
  ALP and AST
  Sodium and potassium
  BUN
  Triglycerides and cholesterol
  TCO_2 and anion gap
Ancillary tests
  Parathyroid hormone (PTH)
  Immunoreactive insulin/glucose (IRI/G) ratio
  Immunoreactive insulin (IRI)
  Corticotropin stimulation test
  Total thyroxine (tT_4), free thyroxine (fT_4), and thyrotropin (TSH)
  tT_4, fT_4, triiodothyronine (T_3) suppression test, and
     thyrotropin-releasing hormone (TRH) stimulation test

perparathyroidism associated with neoplasia demonstrate hypercalcemia with normal or decreased phosphorus. Serum PTH levels are elevated in primary hyperparathyroidism, whereas they are decreased with hypercalcemia of malignancy, because PTH-related protein (PTHrp) is not measured by the same assay. Simultaneous elevations in calcium and phosphorus are usually seen in renal secondary hyperparathyroidism. Calcium and, occasionally, phosphorus can also be altered by other endocrine disorders, however; approximately one third of dogs with Addison's disease are hypercalcemic. Patients with hypoparathyroidism, such as cats with excised parathyroid glands, develop significant hypocalcemia.

Glucose levels are easily affected by numerous disease states, including many that are not of endocrine origin. Thus, this analyte is not specific for a primary endocrine abnormality. With regard to assessment of the endocrine system, diseases of the endocrine pancreas usually affect glucose levels. Diabetes mellitus is characterized by hyperglycemia because of absolute insulin deficiency or insulin resistance. Administration of excessive insulin in diabetic patients can also result in a clinical finding of hyperglycemia. This phenomenon, known as the Somogyi effect, occurs when patients receive too much exogenous insulin, resulting in a sudden marked hypoglycemic state. Clinically, a rebound hyperglycemia is noted in response to the initiating hypoglycemia, but it may be incorrectly interpreted as the patient receiving too little insulin. When uncertainty exists, an IRI/G ratio can be used to help determine the cause of elevated glucose levels. Pancreatic β-cell neoplasia (insulinoma) is associated with excessive insulin secretion and subsequent hypoglycemia that is not followed by a rebound hyperglycemia. IRI assays can help to confirm a diagnosis of insulinoma.

Additional endocrine diseases associated with hyperglycemia that are not of pancreatic origin include hyperadrenocorticism and feline hyperthyroidism. Excessive glucocorticoids result in enhanced gluconeogenesis and antagonize insulin's actions. Hyperthyroidism seems to cause insulin resistance. Hypoglycemia may be noted with hypoadrenocorticism because of the decrease in glucocorticoids and ensuing absence of insulin antagonists, such that there is decreased gluconeogenesis and increased sensitivity of target cells.

ALP and ALT are liver enzymes that are often secondarily affected in patients with primary endocrine disorders, such as diabetes mellitus, dogs with hyperadrenocorticism, and cats with hyperthyroidism. Noting the classic electrolyte imbalances associated with hypoadrenocorticism, hyponatremia, and hyperkalemia often significantly aids in recognizing animals with Addison's disease. Other analytes, such as triglycerides and cholesterol, can be elevated in a number of endocrine disorders, including diabetes mellitus, hyperadrenocorticism, and hypothyroidism. TCO_2 is decreased and the anion gap is increased in animals with diabetic ketoacidosis and hypoadrenocorticism.

Ancillary tests may be needed to confirm an endocrine disorder. In addition to the aforementioned tests for assessing parathyroid and endocrine pancreas function, specialized tests exist for evaluating the adrenal and thyroid glands. Tests for assessing adrenal function include the plasma cortisol test, corticotropin stimulation test, low- and high-dose dexamethasone suppression tests, and urine cortisol/creatinine ratios. Serum thyroxine (T_4), TSH, and fT_4 help in the diagnosis of hypothyroidism and are often included in "thyroid panels." Serum tT_4 and fT_4 tests, the T_3 suppression test, and the TRH stimulation test are used to confirm hyperthyroidism. Reference values from the laboratory performing these tests should be used.

Musculoskeletal system

A list of core tests for the musculoskeletal system is provided in Box 6. The evaluation of the musculoskeletal system primarily involves enzymes that are elevated as a result of myositic leakage (eg, CPK, LDH, AST) or bone resorption (bone isoenzyme of ALP). In dogs, severe muscle disease may also result in elevated ALT. Although CPK is found in striated muscle and brain tissue, serum elevations are specific and sensitive for muscle damage because it cannot cross the blood-brain barrier. Because CPK is not elevated with liver disease, it may be useful in determining whether elevated AST, an enzyme common to striated muscle and hepatocytes, is a result of muscle or liver damage. The half-life of CPK is markedly shorter than that of AST; thus, CPK levels decline more rapidly once active muscle damage has subsided.

Creatinine is a waste product of muscle metabolism, and elevations in this analyte with a normal BUN level indicate muscle wasting rather than azotemia. Potassium is important to assess in cats, because decreases in this electrolyte are a defining feature of hypokalemic polymyopathy. If

---

Box 6. Musculoskeletal system

Core tests
  ALT
  CPK
  AST
  Creatinine and BUN
  Potassium
  ALP
Ancillary test
  Myoglobin in urine

additional diagnostics are warranted, evaluation of urine for myoglobinuria by means of the ammonium sulfate precipitation test to distinguish between hemoglobin and myoglobin could be pursued. ALP has been discussed extensively in previous sections and is included here because of its diagnostic utility in diagnosing bone disease. Elevations of ALP are attributed to bone pathologic changes if other biochemical abnormalities that would be more suggestive of another primary disease are not noted.

Cardiovascular system

A list of core tests for the cardiovascular system is provided in Box 7. Cardiovascular system disease is usually not diagnosed with biochemical profiling: diagnostic imaging and electrocardiography provide much better indications of cardiac function. Certain biochemical abnormalities often occur with cardiovascular disease, however, and can be used to assess the effects on other organ systems. Liver enzyme elevations of ALP and ALT are frequently seen in association with cardiovascular disease, particularly in dogs. The source of these elevations is associated with secondary effects of reduced blood flow and passive congestion in the liver. ALT may be elevated with increased systemic venous pressure or portosystemic shunts, thus providing an indirect means of evaluating the liver.

Minor elevations in AST and CPK result from striated muscle damage. The half-life of CPK is much shorter than that of AST; thus, this abnormality may be missed unless the damage is quite recent or ongoing. Ancillary testing may be pursued to localize these elevations to cardiac muscle. Although infrequently used in veterinary medicine, LDH_1 isoenzyme (α-hydroxybutyrate dehydrogenase) is often elevated in patients with cardiac muscle disease. Cardiac troponin I (cTnI) is a highly specific and sensitive marker for myocardial injury [9]. Serum elevations are associated with cellular injury and death [10], and recent research suggests that this may be a valuable diagnostic test for identifying cats with hypertrophic cardiac myopathy [11].

Box 7. Cardiovascular system

Core tests
  ALP and ALT
  AST
  CPK
Ancillary tests
  LDH_1 isoenzyme
  Cardiac troponin

Summary

Alterations in an individual analyte rarely provide an indication of the initiating circumstances that caused the abnormality. It is obvious from the previous discussion that multiple organs or organ systems can cause abnormal results in the same analyte. This fact underscores the importance of evaluating a biochemical profile in an integrated fashion, relating abnormalities of a particular analyte with the rest of the profile as well as with the signalment, history, and physical findings in the patient. Furthermore, assessment of abnormalities should be approached with some degree of skepticism because they may not be indicative of an actual disease.

References

[1] Mahaffey EA. Quality control, test validity, and reference values. In: Latimer KS, Mahaffey EA, Prasse KW, editors. Duncan and Prasse's veterinary medicine: clinical pathology. 4th edition. Ames: Iowa SP; 2003. p. 331–42.

[2] Weiser G. Sample collection, processing, and analysis of laboratory service options. In: Troy DB, editor. Veterinary hematology and clinical chemistry. Philadelphia: Lippincott Williams & Wilkins; 2004. p. 39–44.

[3] Gerstman BB, Cappucci DT. Evaluating the reliability of diagnostic test results. J Am Vet Med Assoc 1986;188(3):248–51.

[4] Alleman AR. Laboratory profiling in dogs and cats (part 1). Presented at the 75th Annual Western Veterinary Conference. Las Vegas, 2003.

[5] Biopure Corporation. Oxyglobin: questions and answers for veterinarians. Available at: http://www.biopure.com/products/vetQandA.cfm?CDID = 2&CPgID = 57. Accessed October 2, 2004.

[6] Stockham SL, Scott MA. Calcium, phosphorous, magnesium, and their regulatory hormones. In: Fundamentals of veterinary clinical pathology. Ames: Iowa SP; 2002. p. 401–32.

[7] Willard MD, Twedt DC. Gastrointestinal, pancreatic, and hepatic disorders. In: Small animal clinical diagnosis by laboratory methods. 4th edition. St. Louis: Elsevier; 2004. p. 208–46.

[8] Bounous DI. Digestive system. In: Latimer KS, Mahaffey EA, Prasse KW, editors. Duncan and Prasse's veterinary medicine: clinical pathology. 4th edition. Ames: Iowa SP; 2003. p. 215–30.

[9] Oyama MA, Solter PF, Prosek F, et al. Cardiac troponin-I levels in dogs and cats with cardiac disease. Presented at American College of Veterinary Internal Medicine Forum, Charlotte, NC, 2003.

[10] Diehl S, Lichtenberger M, Tilley L, et al. The value of cardiac troponin T concentrations in predicting outcome in dogs with congestive heart failure [abstract]. Presented at the 9th Annual International Veterinary Emergency and Critical Care Symposium, New Orleans, LA, 2003.

[11] Connolly DJ, Cannata J, Boswood A, et al. Cardiac troponin I in cats with hypertrophic cardiomyopathy. J Feline Med Surg 2003;5(4):209–16.

ELSEVIER
SAUNDERS

Vet Clin Small Anim
35 (2005) 557–569

VETERINARY
CLINICS
Small Animal Practice

Geriatric Pharmacology

Patricia M. Dowling, DVM, MSc

*Department of Veterinary Biomedical Sciences, Western College of Veterinary Medicine,
University of Saskatchewan, 52 Campus Drive, Saskatoon, Saskatchewan S7N 5B4, Canada*

The process of aging causes changes in pharmacokinetics (altered drug concentration at the site of action) and pharmacodynamics (altered drug action) [1]. Pharmacokinetics is what the body does to a drug; the processes of absorption, distribution to the various organs and tissues, metabolism of lipid-soluble drugs into water-soluble metabolites, and, finally, renal excretion. Pharmacodynamics is what the drug does to the body. It describes the drug action and responses of the patient. Pharmacokinetics and pharmacodynamics are interrelated in that pharmacokinetics determines the amount of drug that reaches the site of action and the intensity of a pharmacodynamic effect is associated with the drug concentration at the site of action. The definition of "geriatric" varies between species, and in small animals, it varies between breeds. Body composition and regional blood flow change with aging. Cardiac output decreases; thus, regional and organ blood flow also decreases [2]. Blood flow is preferably redistributed to the brain and heart; thus, there is an increase in the risk of drug toxicity in these organs. Gastrointestinal motility, gastric acid secretion, and absorptive capacity are reduced [1,3,4]. Hepatocyte number and function decrease along with hepatic and splanchnic blood flow [2]. As renal blood flow decreases, the glomerular filtration rate (GFR) and active secretory capacity of the nephron decrease, resulting in decreased renal clearance of drugs [2,3]. Lean body mass decreases, whereas fatty tissues increase. Increased body fat decreases total body water and cell mass [2,3,5]. The plasma concentrations of water-soluble (low volume of distribution [Vd]) drugs tend to increase, whereas the plasma concentrations of lipid-soluble (high Vd) drugs tend to decrease [6]. As the Vd increases for a drug, plasma elimination half-life increases, resulting in longer drug retention time in the body. Serum albumin decreases, whereas gamma globulins increase such that total plasma protein concentrations remain the same [1,2,5]. These age-related changes influence drug absorption, distribution, and elimination. Aging also

E-mail address: trishaw.dowling@usask.ca

doi:10.1016/j.cvsm.2004.12.012
vetsmall.theclinics.com

affects the response to many drugs because of changes in binding affinity to receptors, changes in the number or density of receptors on the target organ, and changes in homeostatic regulation [1]. Age-related changes are further affected by disease states common in elderly patients. In geriatric people, the frequency of adverse drug reactions is 3- to 10-fold higher than in the younger population [3,5,7]. Currently, there is limited information regarding geriatric pharmacology in dogs and cats, and most recommendations are extrapolated from findings in geriatric people [8]. Many geriatric patients have dysfunction of more than one major organ system. Altogether, these effects make it difficult to determine safe and effective drug dosages for geriatric veterinary patients, and the clinician must monitor elderly patients carefully. This review focuses on the disease states common in geriatric dogs and cats that significantly affect drug disposition: renal, hepatic, and cardiac disease.

Renal insufficiency and failure

The ultimate route for most drug elimination from the body is the kidney. With its small size and large blood flow, the kidney is exposed to higher drug concentrations than other tissues. Because of age-related changes in function, elderly human beings are routinely considered to be renal insufficient [6,9]. There is a close relationship between the incidence of adverse drug reactions in people and renal function [10]. It is estimated that 15% to 20% of geriatric dogs and cats are renal insufficient [11]; thus, it is likely that this is also true for geriatric dogs and cats. With the large variability in age-dependent changes in renal function, the only sure way to be certain about a geriatric animal's renal function is to measure it. An age-dependent decrease can be expected for all drugs that are eliminated by the kidney [3]. With reduced renal clearance, the parent drug or its metabolites may accumulate in the patient and cause toxicity. Loss of proteins and electrolytes in urine and the alterations in acid-base balance associated with renal failure affect the pharmacokinetics and pharmacodynamics of drugs. Enhanced drug activity or toxicity can occur because of synergy with uremic complications.

Renal clearance of drugs

Renal excretion is the major route of elimination from the body for most drugs. Drug disposition by the kidneys includes glomerular filtration, active tubular secretion, and tubular reabsorption, such that renal drug clearance is defined by the following equation [12]:

$$Cl_R = Cl_F + Cl_S - FR$$

where Cl_R is total renal clearance, Cl_F is clearance attributed to glomerular filtration, Cl_S is clearance attributed to active tubular secretion, and FR is fraction reabsorbed from the tubule back to circulation.

Clearance attributed to glomerular filtration occurs with small molecules (<300 molecular weight) of free drug (not bound to plasma proteins). Large molecules or protein-bound drugs do not get filtered at the glomerulus because of size and electrical hindrance. The kidneys receive approximately 25% of cardiac output, so the major driving force for glomerular filtration is the hydrostatic pressure within the glomerular capillaries. The GFR is estimated by measuring a substance or drug that is only eliminated by glomerular filtration, such as creatinine or inulin. In aging people from 40 to 80 years, GFR decreases by 1 mL/min each year as measured by creatinine clearance [1].

If total renal clearance is greater than clearance attributed to glomerular filtration, some tubular secretion is occurring. Active tubular secretion is a carrier-mediated transport system located in the proximal renal tubule. It requires energy input, because drug is moved against a concentration gradient. In patients with reduced functional renal tissue, remaining transport systems become easily saturated and drug accumulation occurs.

If total renal clearance is less than clearance attributed to glomerular filtration, tubular reabsorption of drug is occurring. Tubular reabsorption is an active process for endogenous compounds (eg, vitamins, electrolytes, glucose). It is a passive process for most drugs. It occurs along the entire nephron but primarily in the distal renal tubule. Factors that affect reabsorption include pKa of the drug, urine pH, lipid solubility, drug size, and urine flow. Drug reabsorption is highly dependent on ionization, which is determined by the drug's pKa and the pH of urine. According to the Henderson-Hasselbach equation, a drug that is a weak base is nonionized in alkaline urine and a weak acid is ionized in alkaline urine. The nonionized form of the drug is more lipid soluble and has greater reabsorption. The pKa of a drug is constant, but urinary pH is highly variable in animals and varies with the diet, drug intake, time of day, and systemic acidosis and/or alkalosis.

Bioavailability and absorption

Gastric emptying is delayed in uremic patients, which delays oral absorption of some drugs [13]. Renal failure also affects the absorptive capacity of the small intestine [1,14]. Gastrointestinal symptoms, such as vomiting and diarrhea, are common in uremic patients and may affect drug absorption. Drugs with pH-dependent bioavailability may be decreased by the concomitant administration of antacids or phosphate-binding drugs, which are commonly administered to patients with renal failure [15,16]. The fluoroquinolones, tetracyclines, ampicillin, and sulfonamides have reduced bioavailability when administered with antacids.

Drug distribution

The Vd of many drugs changes in geriatric patients with renal failure. Fluid retention is often a characteristic of renal failure, and the consequent change in body water alters the Vd of drugs that are predominantly distributed to extracellular water, such as penicillins, cephalosporins, aminoglycosides, and nonsteroidal anti-inflammatory drugs (NSAIDs). There is also a marked reduction in the degree of protein binding of many drugs, which is more than can be explained by the hypoalbuminemia that occurs in many glomerular diseases [17]. It is thought that there is a conformational change in the albumin molecule caused by "uremic toxins," which reduces the degree of drug binding [17,18]. Protein binding of acidic drugs is also altered by the accumulation of organic molecules that displace acidic drugs from their albumin-binding sites. Protein binding of basic drugs tends to be normal in patients with renal failure [18].

Hepatic metabolism in renal failure

Hepatic metabolism of some drugs is altered during renal insufficiency, and there is considerable species variation in this effect. Glycine conjugation, acetylation, and hydrolytic reactions are generally slowed in uremia [19]. Uremia does not seem to affect glucuronide synthesis, sulfate conjugation, or methylation pathways [19]. The metabolism of cephalothin, cortisol, hydralazine, insulin, procaine, procainamide, salicylate, and some sulfonamides is decreased in uremic people [20]. This results in drug accumulation if the overall drug elimination rate is decreased. Conversely, some drugs that are normally predominantly excreted by the kidney demonstrate a shift to hepatic metabolism and intestinal elimination. In dogs with experimentally induced renal failure, the clearance of the NSAID tolfenamic acid increased and plasma elimination half-life decreased, apparently from hepatic metabolism and elimination [21].

The formation of renally eliminated drug metabolites is also important in patients with renal failure, because some metabolites are pharmacologically active, such as enalaprilat, the active metabolite of enalapril [22,23]. In a canine experimental model, renal impairment reduced enalaprilat clearance from 40% to 55% of normal [22]. In the dog, enrofloxacin undergoes some hepatic metabolism to ciprofloxacin, which has greater antimicrobial activity than enrofloxacin against *Pseudomonas* spp [24]. The high incidence of adverse drug reactions in patients with renal failure is attributed, in part, to the accumulation of toxic metabolites. For example, the acetylation metabolites of sulfonamides are not antimicrobially active but retain the toxicity of the parent drugs [20].

Metabolic balance

The uremic patient is often in a state of altered acid-base balance, electrolyte derangement, and fluid depletion. Administration of sodium- or potassium-containing antimicrobials, such as sodium ampicillin or potassium penicillin, may result in serious sodium overload and potassium-induced neuronal disturbances. Administration of antacids, enemas, or laxatives may cause magnesium, aluminum, or phosphate intoxication. Acidosis, which occurs commonly in uremic patients, increases the free drug concentrations of some drugs, such as salicylate and phenobarbital, thereby increasing drug concentrations in the central nervous system [5]. Acidosis also increases ionic binding of the aminoglycosides, increasing accumulation in the renal tubular epithelium and enhancing nephrotoxicity [13]. Drug toxicity may also be enhanced by uremic complications. Uremia-induced functional changes in gastrointestinal and nervous system tissues allow adverse reactions to be more easily induced [5,19]. The blood-brain barrier is altered in uremia, allowing greater drug concentrations in the central nervous system [19]. The anabolic effect of tetracyclines and the catabolic effect of corticosteroids may worsen azotemia [13].

Hepatic insufficiency and failure

For many drugs, disposition and elimination that undergo hepatic metabolism are affected by hepatic blood flow, drug protein binding, and intrinsic hepatic clearance. Aging, diet, and hepatic and concurrent diseases greatly affect hepatic drug metabolism in geriatric small animals. In the elderly, there is a decrease in liver mass, a decrease in hepatic blood flow, and reduction in the intrinsic activity of drug-metabolizing enzymes [1]. The results of liver function tests typically remain normal in the absence of overt hepatic disease.

Hepatic clearance

Nonrenal clearance is assumed to be caused by hepatic metabolism and biliary excretion into the feces. Hepatic clearance (Cl_H) is determined by hepatic blood flow (Q_H) and intrinsic ability of the liver to extract the drug (hepatic extraction ratio [ER_H]) [12],

$$Cl_H = (Q_H)(ER_H)$$

Drugs with a high ER_H (approaching 1) have hepatic clearance equal to the hepatic blood flow. These drugs are called high-clearance drugs. Examples of drugs with a high ER_H are morphine, verapamil, lidocaine, propranolol, and isoproterenol. Clearance of drugs with a high ER_H is highly influenced by changes in hepatic blood flow. Lidocaine, an antiarrhythmic drug, has an average clearance of 21 mL/min/kg after intravenous administration in dogs. Hepatic plasma flow in dogs is 20 to 26 mL/min/kg. Lidocaine is not eliminated by any other route; therefore, the clearance of lidocaine is almost identical to hepatic blood flow. When given orally, these drugs are unable to achieve high concentrations in the circulation because of the high clearance; thus, they are known as high "first-pass effect" drugs.

Drugs that have a low ER_H (≤ 0.2) are not greatly affected by changes in hepatic blood flow. Their clearance is affected by changes in the hepatic microsomal enzyme systems and protein binding, however. A first-pass effect does not interfere with the systemic availability of these drugs. Drugs with a low ER_H include chloramphenicol, benzodiazepines, phenylbutazone, and phenobarbital.

The first-pass effect is reduced with aging, so the oral bioavailability drugs (eg, propranolol, lidocaine) may be increased in the geriatric animal [1,3]. Geriatric patients have a reduced rate of phase I metabolism reactions (oxidation, reduction, dealkylation, and hydroxylation), but phase II reactions (glucuronidation, acetylation, and sulfation) do not change significantly with age [1]. Because older patients are often on multiple medications, there is great potential for one drug to alter the metabolism of another. If geriatric patients on beta-blockers (which decrease cardiac output and hepatic blood flow) are given lidocaine (which normally undergoes dealkylation), they may develop lidocaine toxicity [5]. Enzyme induction seems to be unrelated to aging but is greatly affected by disease [3]. Reduced nutritional intake impairs drug metabolism and increases the risk of adverse drug effects [3,4].

Pharmacodynamic responses are caused by free drug concentrations, because protein-bound drugs are too large to cross biologic membranes. For drugs that are highly protein bound, decreases in serum proteins and interactions from other highly protein-bound drugs may cause adverse drug reactions. If the drug has a low ER_H, a decrease in protein binding initially causes an increase in the free drug fraction, causing an increase in the Vd of the drug and in clearance. With the increase in clearance, the total drug concentration decreases, but the free drug concentration remains the same and there is no change in pharmacodynamic response [5,25]. If the drug has a high ER_H, a decrease in protein binding causes an increase in the free drug fraction, with an increase in the Vd of the drug but no increase in clearance. The increase in Vd causes a decreased elimination rate and negates the decrease in total drug concentration by the conversion of bound drug to free drug and the movement of the free drug into tissues. The concentration of free drug increases, whereas the concentration of total drug remains the same. In this situation, the pharmacodynamic response is increased from the increased free drug with no change in total drug concentration [5].

Although it is difficult to determine the absolute changes in protein binding in an individual patient, is important to understand these effects to interpret the results of therapeutic drug monitoring correctly. For drugs with a high ER_H, a decrease in protein binding results in lower total drug concentrations but not lower free drug concentrations. "Therapeutic" concentrations of these drugs in geriatric patients are achieved at lower than normal therapeutic concentrations of these drugs in normal animals.

Cardiovascular disease

Cardiac disease in geriatric dogs and cats causes disturbances in sodium and water retention, and increased sympathetic nervous system output redistributes blood flow, leading to important changes in drug disposition and action. There is an age-dependent decline in chronotropic and inotropic responsiveness to α-adrenergic agents [5]. This is not from a loss of receptors but seems to be a decrease in responsiveness [5]. In congestive heart failure, the rate and absolute amount of furosemide absorbed are reduced [26]. Diuretic therapy can cause volume contraction, however, with subsequent reduced organ blood perfusion. The α-adrenergic blocking drugs and calcium channel blockers can produce significant negative inotropic effects, impairing ventricular function and advancing heart failure [5]. Tricyclic antidepressants (eg, clomipramine) and phenothiazines (eg, acepromazine) may potentiate ventricular arrhythmias [5]. In general, cardiac drug dosages should be reduced, and geriatric patients must be carefully monitored.

Dosage adjustments in geriatric patients

For most drugs, because equal doses are given at a constant dosage interval, the plasma concentration-time curve plateaus and a "steady state" is reached (Fig. 1). At steady state, the plasma drug concentrations fluctuate between a maximum concentration (C_{max} or peak) and a minimum concentration (C_{min} or trough). Once steady state is reached, C_{max} and C_{min} are constant and remain unchanged from dose to dose. The time to steady state depends solely on the elimination half-life of a drug. It takes six half-lives to reach 99% of steady-state concentrations. Dose and dosage

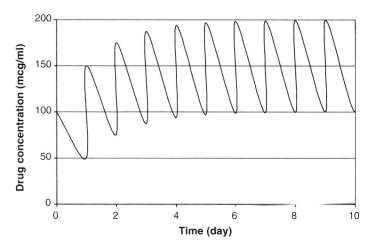

Fig. 1. With an elimination half-life and dosing interval of 1 day, steady-state drug concentrations are reached in 6 days (six half-lives) and the maximum concentration and minimum concentration remain unchanged from dose to dose.

frequency influence the values of C_{max} and C_{min} at steady state. If the drug is given at a dosage frequency that is shorter than the elimination half-life, drug accumulation occurs and the C_{max} at steady state is greater than the C_{max} after a single dose. Conversely, if the dosage frequency is less than the elimination half-life, drug accumulation does not occur to any significant degree. Dosage frequency and elimination half-life influence the amount of fluctuation between C_{max} and C_{min}.

The goal of dosage adjustment is to provide a drug concentration-time profile in the geriatric patient as similar as possible to that of a normal patient. The best approach to modifying drug therapy in geriatric patients is to carry out therapeutic drug monitoring and adjust the dosage for each patient. This is possible with some drugs, such as phenobarbital, digoxin, and the aminoglycoside antimicrobials, but it is impractical and cost-prohibitive for most drugs used in veterinary practice. The best approach for most drugs is to estimate a corrected dose from available renal function tests and then to monitor the patient closely for evidence of efficacy or toxicity. Most decisions on drug dosage adjustment can be based on creatinine clearance, because tubular secretion functions decrease at parallel rates [1]. Creatinine is an endogenous product of creatinine phosphate metabolism in muscle. It is removed by glomerular filtration, and serum concentrations are relatively constant in healthy people and animals. The elimination half-life of a drug that is eliminated in urine remains stable until creatinine clearance is reduced to 30% to 40% of normal, which is why drug dosage regimens are typically not adjusted until two thirds of renal function has been lost [27]. In human patients, creatinine clearance is quantified by determining urinary creatinine excretion over a 24-hour period. The measured creatinine clearance is then used in formulas to make drug dosage adjustments. Because of the difficulty of 24-hour urine collection, values for creatinine clearance are not usually available for veterinary patients. When creatinine clearance is not available, a single value of the patient's serum creatinine can be substituted into the formulas. The relationship between serum creatinine and creatinine clearance is not linear once serum creatinine is greater than 4 mg/dL (305 mmol/L) [27]. In addition, these formulas do not account for changes in the Vd, degree of protein binding, and nonrenal clearance mechanisms of the drug that may be caused by the renal dysfunction. Therefore, calculated dosage adjustments are preliminary estimations and need to be followed by adjustments based on observed clinical response.

With the dose-reduction method, the normal dosage regimen is adjusted by reducing the drug dose and maintaining the drug dosing interval [27] as follows:

Adjusted Dose = Normal Dose

$\times$ (Patient's Creatinine Clearance/Normal Creatinine Clearance)

or

Adjusted Dose = Normal Dose

$\times$ (Normal Serum Creatinine/Patient's Serum Creatinine)

With the interval-extension method, the drug dose is maintained and the drug dosing interval is extended [27] as follows:

Adjusted Interval = Normal Interval

$(1 \div [$Patient's Creatinine Clearance/Normal Creatinine Clearance$])$

or

Adjusted Interval = Normal Interval

$(1 \div [$Normal Serum Creatinine/Patient's Serum Creatinine$])$

Both methods attempt to keep the average plasma drug concentrations constant. The interval-extension method produces C_{max} and C_{min} values similar to those seen in healthy patients. It does produce substantial periods when drug concentrations may be subtherapeutic, however (Fig. 2). This is the preferred method with aminoglycosides, which have a long postantibiotic effect and where a low trough concentration is desirable to reduce the risk of nephrotoxicity, and the NSAIDs [13]. Depending on the relation of the elimination half-life to the dosage interval, significant drug accumulation may occur with the dose-reduction method, but at steady state, there are no periods when concentrations are subtherapeutic (Fig. 3). This is the preferred method for the penicillin and cephalosporin antimicrobials, where maintaining the plasma concentration at greater than the pathogen's minimum inhibitory concentration (MIC) correlates with efficacy and the drugs are relatively nontoxic even if accumulation occurs [13]. To decide

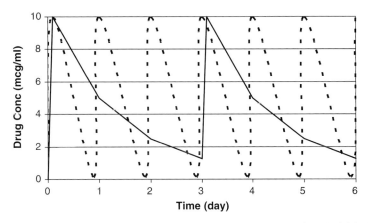

Fig. 2. Comparison of the interval-extension method in a geriatric patient (*solid line*) with a normal dosage regimen in a healthy patient (*dotted line*). Normal elimination half-life is 12 hours; in the geriatric patient, it increased to 24 hours.

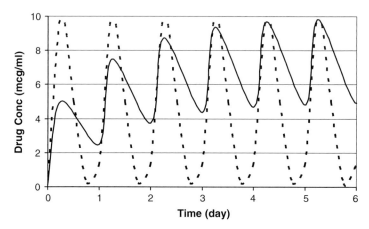

Fig. 3. Comparison of a dose-reduction regimen in a geriatric patient (*solid line*) with a normal dosage regimen in a healthy patient (*dotted line*). Normal elimination half-life is 6 hours; in the geriatric patient, it increased to 18 hours.

which method to use, the practitioner should determine if drug efficacy and toxicity are related to peak, trough, or average plasma concentrations and then select the method that balances efficacy against potential toxicity. The fixed-dose method is more convenient for clients, because the normal recommended dose is simply administered less frequently. If drugs are available only in fixed-dosage forms (eg, capsules, unbreakable tablets), it is easier to adjust the dosage interval.

Because the elimination half-life is prolonged in patients with renal disease and it always takes six half-lives to reach 99% of steady-state concentrations, there is a delay in reaching steady state in renal failure patients compared with animals with normal renal function. Therefore, a loading dose may need to be administered to achieve therapeutic drug concentrations rapidly [27]. If the dose-reduction method is used, this is achieved by giving the usual dose initially, followed by the reduced dose the next time. If the interval-extension method is used, this is accomplished by giving a double dose initially.

Summary

When faced with the geriatric dog or cat, the practitioner should consider the following:

1. Avoid using any drugs at all unless there are definite therapeutic indications. If the patient has some degree of renal insufficiency, try to select drugs that are hepatically metabolized and excreted in bile rather than eliminated by the kidneys (eg, doxycycline, tolfenamic acid). If hepatic insufficiency is present, select drugs that do not undergo metabolism before renal excretion (eg, penicillins, cephalosporins).

Table 1
General guidelines for dosage adjustment of drugs commonly used in geriatric veterinary patients

Antimicrobials	
Aminoglycosides	Contraindicated because of nephrotoxicity; Use IE method and TDM to individualize dosage regimen
Penicillins and cephalosporins	May accumulate in renal insufficiency but high therapeutic index; monitor electrolytes if sodium or potassium formulations are used; use DR method
Sulfonamides	Some risk of nephrotoxicity; increased risk of drug eruptions and bone marrow depression; decreased protein binding with uremia; use DR method
Tetracyclines	May accumulate in renal insufficiency (except doxycycline) and are nephrotoxic; worsen azotemia; use DR and IE methods
Fluoroquinolones	May accumulate in renal insufficiency but high therapeutic index; use IE method
Macrolides and lincosamides	No dosage adjustment required
Metronidazole	No dosage adjustment required
Nonsteroidal anti-inflammatory drugs	Decreased protein binding with uremia; most undergo hepatic metabolism; all are potentially nephrotoxic and/or hepatotoxic
Carprofen	Hepatic metabolism with elimination of metabolites in feces and urine; associated with idiosyncratic hepatotoxicity; use DR and IE methods
Deracoxib	Saturation of elimination mechanisms results in nonlinear elimination kinetics and unpredictable concentrations at doses greater than 8 mg/kg; high concentrations result in loss of cyclooxygenase-2 selectivity; hepatic metabolism with parent drug and metabolites eliminated in urine and feces but only metabolites eliminated in urine; use DR and IE methods
Etodolac	Hepatic metabolism and excretion in feces; associated with keratoconjunctivitis sicca; narrow therapeutic index; use DR and IE methods
Meloxicam	With chronic use, elimination half-life may increase; use DR and IE methods
Tepoxalin	Hepatic metabolism to an active metabolite that is eliminated in feces; no dosage adjustment required in renal insufficiency
Tolfenamic Acid	With renal insufficiency, shifts to hepatic elimination; no dosage adjustment required
Corticosteroids	Avoid when possible; increase number and sensitivity of α-adrenergic receptors; hepatic metabolism decreased in renal insufficiency and worsens azotemia; may exacerbate hypertension
Furosemide	Decreased oral absorption and diuretic response and increased elimination half-life; decreased protein binding with uremia; individualize patient therapy based on clinical response

(continued on next page)

Table 1 (*continued*)

Cardiac drugs	
α-Adrenergic blockers	Increased bioavailability, decreased hepatic metabolism, and prolonged elimination half-life; use IE and DR methods
Digoxin	Accumulates with renal insufficiency; decreased volume of distribution with loss of muscle mass; toxicity exacerbated by furosemide; use IE and DR methods and TDM to individualize therapy
Angiotensin-converting enzyme inhibitors	Hepatic metabolism to active metabolite may be reduced; decreased clearance with renal insufficiency; increased response to hypotensive effects
Pimobendan	Hepatic metabolism and elimination in feces
Anticonvulsants	
Phenobarbital	Decreased protein binding with uremia; decreased hepatic metabolism; potentially hepatotoxic; individualize therapy with TDM
Potassium bromide	Renal elimination; start with 50% of recommended dose in patients with renal insufficiency and use TDM to individualize therapy

Abbreviations: DR, dose-reduction method; IE, interval-extension method; TDM, therapeutic drug monitoring.

2. If therapeutic drug monitoring is available, tailor the drug dosage regimen to that specific patient (eg, phenobarbital, digoxin, aminoglycosides).
3. If therapeutic drug monitoring is unavailable, determine if there are clinically proven adjusted dosage regimens for specific drugs. The package insert on human pharmaceutics often gives guidelines for adjusting dosages in geriatric patients.
4. If the drug has not been sufficiently studied to have dosage adjustment recommendations, determine if there is sufficient information about its kinetics to estimate the proper drug dose in a geriatric patient. Some general guidelines for commonly used drugs in geriatric veterinary patients are provided in Table 1. In general, if the Vd changes in your patient, change the dose. If the elimination half-life changes, change the dosing interval.
5. Carefully monitor treated patients for signs of efficacy and toxicity.

References

[1] Ambrose PJ. Altered drug action with aging. Health Notes 2003;1(7):12–9.
[2] Mosier JE. Effect of aging on body systems of the dog. Vet Clin N Am Small Anim Pract 1989;19(1):1–12.
[3] Turnheim K. Drug dosage in the elderly. Is it rational? Drugs Aging 1998;13(5):357–79.
[4] Burkholder WJ. Age-related changes to nutritional requirements and digestive function in adult dogs and cats. J Am Vet Med Assoc 1999;215(5):625–9.

[5] Tumer N, Scarpace PJ, Lowenthal DT. Geriatric pharmacology: basic and clinical considerations. Annu Rev Pharmacol Toxicol 1992;32:271–302.

[6] Turnheim K. When drug therapy gets old: pharmacokinetics and pharmacodynamics in the elderly. Exp Gerontol 2003;38(8):843–53.

[7] Muhlberg W, Platt D. Age-dependent changes of the kidneys: pharmacological implications. Gerontology 1999;45(5):243–53.

[8] Aucoin DP. Drug therapy in the geriatric animal: the effect of aging on drug disposition. Vet Clin N Am Small Anim Pract 1989;19(1):41–7.

[9] Turnheim K. Pitfalls of pharmacokinetic dosage guidelines in renal insufficiency. Eur J Clin Pharmacol 1991;40(1):87–93.

[10] Dieppe P, Bartlett C, Davey P, et al. Balancing benefits and harms: the example of non-steroidal anti-inflammatory drugs. BMJ 2004;329(7456):31–4.

[11] Burkholder WJ. Dietary considerations for dogs and cats with renal disease. J Am Vet Med Assoc 2000;216(11):1730–4.

[12] Rowland M, Benet LZ, Graham GG. Clearance concepts in pharmacokinetics. J Pharmacokinet Biopharm 1973;1(2):123–36.

[13] St. Peter WL, Redic-Kill KA, Halstenson CE. Clinical pharmacokinetics of antibiotics in patients with impaired renal function. Clin Pharmacokinet 1992;22(3):169–210.

[14] Haney SL. Drug use in renal failure. Crit Care Nurs Clin N Am 2002;14(1):77–80.

[15] Rubin SI. Chronic renal failure and its management and nephrolithiasis. Vet Clin N Am Small Anim Pract 1997;27(6):1331–54.

[16] Nagode LA, Chew DJ, Podell M. Benefits of calcitriol therapy and serum phosphorus control in dogs and cats with chronic renal failure. Both are essential to prevent of suppress toxic hyperparathyroidism. Vet Clin N Am Small Anim Pract 1996;26(6):1293–330.

[17] Reidenberg MM, Drayer DE. Alteration of drug-protein binding in renal disease. Clin Pharmacokinet 1984;9(Suppl 1):18–26.

[18] Reidenberg MM, Drayer DE. Effects of renal disease upon drug disposition. Drug Metab Rev 1978;8(2):293–302.

[19] Reidenberg MM, Drayer DE. Drug therapy in renal failure. Annu Rev Pharmacol Toxicol 1980;20:45–54.

[20] Drayer DE. Active drug metabolites and renal failure. Am J Med 1977;62(4):486–9.

[21] Lefebvre HP, Laroute V, Alvinerie M. The effect of experimental renal failure on tolfenamic acid disposition in the dog. Biopharm Drug Dispos 1997;18(1):79–91.

[22] Toutain PL, Lefebvre HP, Laroute V. New insights on effect of kidney insufficiency on disposition of angiotensin-converting enzyme inhibitors: case of enalapril and benazepril in dogs. J Pharmacol Exp Ther 2000;292(3):1094–103.

[23] Lefebvre HP, et al. Effects of renal impairment on the disposition of orally administered enalapril, benazepril, and their active metabolites. J Vet Intern Med 1999;13(1):21–7.

[24] Kung K, Riond JL, Wanner M. Pharmacokinetics of enrofloxacin and its metabolite ciprofloxacin after intravenous and oral administration of enrofloxacin in dogs. J Vet Pharmacol Ther 1993;16(4):462–8.

[25] Toutain PL, Bousquet-Melou A. Free drug fraction vs free drug concentration: a matter of frequent confusion. J Vet Pharmacol Ther 2002;25(6):460–3.

[26] Sica DA. Pharmacotherapy in congestive heart failure: drug absorption in the management of congestive heart failure: loop diuretics. Congest Heart Fail 2003;9(5):287–92.

[27] Riviere J. Dosage adjustments in renal disease. In: Comparative pharmacokinetics: principles, techniques and applications. Ames (IA): Iowa State University Press; 1999. p. 283–95.

ELSEVIER
SAUNDERS

Vet Clin Small Anim
35 (2005) 571–580

VETERINARY
CLINICS
Small Animal Practice

Anesthesia for Geriatric Patients

Rachael E. Carpenter, DVM[a],*,
Glenn R. Pettifer, DVM, DVSc[b],
William J. Tranquilli, DVM, MS[a]

[a]Department of Veterinary Clinical Medicine, University of Illinois,
1008 West Hazelwood Drive, Urbana, IL 61802, USA
[b]Department of Veterinary Clinical Sciences, School of Veterinary Medicine,
Louisiana State University, Baton Rouge, LA 70803, USA

Veterinarians are seeing an increasing number of geriatric animals in their daily practice. Often, these patients need to be placed under general anesthesia for dental care, surgical procedures, diagnostic procedures, or treatment of chronic conditions. In 2002, the pet population in the United States was estimated at 100 million. Approximately 30% of those pets are expected to be geriatric [1]. Because there is wide species and breed variation in life expectancy, there is no one specific age that defines an animal as "geriatric"; however, it is generally accepted that a geriatric animal is one that has reached 75% of its expected life span [2]. Because there is little correlation between physiologic and chronologic age, each animal must still be evaluated as an individual. Many older animals remain remarkably fit, whereas others seem to age faster than expected. Age itself is not a disease, but age-related changes and diseases do affect anesthetic management.

Physiology of geriatric animals

Physiologically, elderly animals cannot be considered the same as younger adults. Aging causes a progressive and irreversible decrease in functional reserves of the major organ systems, leading to altered responses to stressors and anesthetic drugs. Such changes in organ system function are covert until the patient is stressed by an illness, hospital stay, or general anesthetic procedure.

---

* Corresponding author.
E-mail address: recrpntr@uiuc.edu (R.E. Carpenter).

Cardiovascular system

Geriatric animals have a decreased cardiac reserve compared with that of younger animals. In the older animal, this often translates into a decreased ability to respond appropriately to the changes brought about by anesthetic drugs. Geriatric animals have varying degrees of myocardial fiber atrophy, which can affect rate and rhythm if the conduction system is involved. The aged heart also has increasing myocardial fibrosis and valvular fibrocalcification. As ventricular compliance decreases in the aging heart, relatively small changes in intravascular volume or venous capacitance become increasingly important determinants of circulatory stability [3]. These changes mean that whereas the geriatric animal is volume dependent, it is also volume-intolerant, because the decreased ventricular compliance is associated with optimal hemodynamic functioning within a narrow range of end-diastolic volume and pressure. The maximal chronotropic response during physiologic stress decreases with age. Additionally, the response to exogenously administered autonomic drugs is decreased. Younger adults can increase cardiac output primarily by increasing heart rate. In geriatric animals, cardiac output is more dependent on increased stroke volume in association with an increase in end-diastolic volume. For this reason, volume depletion during the perioperative period is less well tolerated in geriatric animals than in younger animals [4].

Geriatric animals are increasingly likely to experience degenerative myocardial disease, usually in the form of chronic valvular disease. This degenerative change has the potential to increase the likelihood of myocardial hypoxia associated with the increased myocardial work and oxygen consumption of inefficient pump function [5].

Pulmonary system

Even mild or moderate respiratory depression associated with the administration of some anesthetics can produce significant hypoxia and hypercarbia in the geriatric animal. This arises as a result of a decreased functional reserve capacity in the aging lung. Aging is associated with a decrease in chest wall compliance because of the loss of intercostal and diaphragmatic muscle mass. Vital capacity, total lung capacity, and maximum breathing capacity also decrease. With a reduction or loss of lung elastin, pulmonary compliance is reduced [5]. Anatomic dead space and functional residual capacity increase with age, as do closing volume, air trapping, and ventilation-perfusion mismatch. All these changes tend to lower Pao_2 levels in older patients [6]. Pathologic events like pneumonia, pulmonary edema, or pulmonary fibrosis exacerbate these aging processes. Pulmonary aging serves to render a geriatric animal less tolerant of even transient hypoxia during the perianesthetic period.

Hepatic system

The overall mass of the liver decreases with increasing age, leading to a decrease in overall hepatic function, including drug clearance [3]. This decrease in hepatic function causes an increase in the plasma half-life of drugs dependent on hepatic excretion, metabolism, or conjugation. Other important considerations in the geriatric patient include the potential for hypoproteinemia, impaired clotting functions, and hypoglycemia from altered hepatic function [5].

Renal system

Normal aging can alter renal function in several ways. Renal blood flow is decreased, making geriatric patients more susceptible to renal failure when exposed to renal ischemia. There is a decrease in the total number of functional glomeruli, and the glomerular filtration rate decreases. As changes in the renal tubules occur, there is an increase in the resistance of the distal renal tubules to antidiuretic hormone. This results in an impaired ability to conserve sodium or concentrate urine, leading to a reduced ability to correct fluid, electrolyte, and acid-base disturbances [6]. Overall, this may make some geriatric animals much less tolerant of body water deficits or excessive fluid administration. Additionally, the plasma half-life of an anesthetic drug eliminated by renal excretion may be prolonged, necessitating a reduction in the dose when used in geriatric patients.

Aged patients are generally more susceptible to renal failure after general anesthesia. The effects of anesthesia and surgery can exacerbate preexisting renal pathologic conditions [5]. General anesthesia typically reduces renal blood flow and glomerular filtration, whereas surgery may result in blood loss, hypovolemia, and hypotension, which can further compromise renal perfusion.

Central nervous system

Cerebral perfusion and oxygen consumption decline with increasing age and may be related to an overall loss of brain mass that correlates with a loss of neurons rather than atrophy of the supportive glial cells. Cerebrospinal fluid volume increases to maintain normal intracranial pressure in the face of this reduction in brain mass [6]. Anatomic and functional redundancy compensates for the loss of cellular elements and neuronal interconnections; thus, function of the central nervous system (CNS) is generally maintained at levels close to those seen in young adults [3]. There are decreased amounts of neurotransmitters, such as dopamine, norepinephrine, tyrosine, and serotonin, in the aging brain, and these substances may demonstrate a reduced receptor affinity [6].

Although not completely understood, one of the overall results of these changes is that geriatric animals have a decreased requirement for anesthetic agents. It is well documented that minimum alveolar concentration (MAC) decreases linearly with age, and requirements for local anesthetics, opioids, barbiturates, benzodiazepines, and other intravenous drugs seem to be similarly reduced [3,6,7].

Preoperative assessment

Individual geriatric animals may require different anesthetic protocols. As with any animal that is to be anesthetized, a complete history should be taken, with particular attention to previous and current medical problems, current medications, vitamins, and supplements. A thorough physical examination and broad laboratory screening (ie, complete blood cell count [CBC], chemistry panel, urinalysis) are essential in the assessment of the functional status of different organ systems and in the identification of any preexisting problems. Careful auscultation of the heart should be performed in an attempt to identify any underlying cardiac disease or murmur. If a cardiac murmur or arrhythmia is detected, a cardiac workup (eg, chest radiographs, echocardiogram, electrocardiogram [ECG]) may be performed to determine the cause of the murmur. Whenever possible, any significant abnormalities detected by physical examination or preoperative blood work should be corrected before the induction of anesthesia.

Premedication

Preanesthetic sedation reduces stress in anxious patients and decreases the amount of anesthetics needed for induction and maintenance of anesthesia. The choice of premedication depends on the geriatric animal's physical condition, any concurrent disease processes, current medications, and the particular requirements for sedation and analgesia that are dictated by the intended procedure (suggested sedatives and preanesthetics are presented in Table 1).

Anticholinergics

Anticholinergics (eg, atropine, glycopyrrolate) should not be used indiscriminately in the geriatric patient. Patients with preexisting cardiac disease may not tolerate the increase in myocardial oxygen demand and work resulting from a marked increase in heart rate. Sinus tachycardia may precipitate acute myocardial failure [5]. In most cases, it is probably best to treat bradycardia as needed with judicious use of anticholinergic drugs on a case-by-case basis. Alternatively, α_2-agonist–mediated reductions in heart rate can be treated by titrating the reversal agent, atipamezole, to achieve the desired reversal of bradycardia. Although some clinicians recommend that α_2-agonists be given in combination with anticholinergics [8], others would suggest that this practice may result in a potentially undesirable

Table 1
Suggested drug doses (mg/kg) of anesthetic drugs in geriatric small animals

Drug	Dog	Cat
Anticholinergics		
Atropine	0.01–0.02 IM, IV	0.01–0.02 IM, IV
Glycopyrrolate	0.005–0.01 IM, IV	0.005–0.01 IM, IV
Sedatives and/or tranquilizers		
Acepromazine	0.01–0.05 IM, SC, IV	0.01–0.05 IM, SC, IV
Diazepam	0.2–0.4 IV	0.2–0.4 IV
Medetomidine	0.002–0.004 IM	0.006–0.008 IM
Midazolam	0.1–0.3 IM, SC, IV	0.1–0.3 IM, SC, IV
Opioids		
Buprenorphine	0.005–0.01 IM, SC, IV	0.005–0.01 IM, SC, IV, PO
Butorphanol	0.2–0.4 IM, SC, IV	0.2–0.4 IM, SC, IV
Hydromorphone	0.1–0.2 IM, SC, IV	0.1–0.2 IM, SC, IV
Morphine	0.05–1 IM, SC	0.002–0.1 IM, SC
Oxymorphone	0.1–0.2 IM, SC, IV	0.05–0.1 IM, SC, IV
Induction[a]		
Etomidate	0.5–1.5 IV	0.5–1.5 IV
Ketamine and/or valium	3–5/0.2–0.4 IV	3–5/0.2–0.4 IV
Propofol	4–6 IV	4–6 IV
Thiopental	2–6 IV	2–6 IV

Abbreviations: IM, intramuscular; IV, intravenous, PO, by mouth; SC, subcutaneous.
[a] All recommended doses should be titrated slowly to effect.

increase in myocardial work and possible arrhythmias [9]. Because of the potential for development of serious side effects, α_2-agonists should be reserved for use in cardiovascularly healthy geriatric animals.

Opioids

Opioids often provide adequate sedation in geriatric animals, with the added benefit of providing analgesia. μ-Agonists (OP_3-agonists; morphine, hydromorphone, and oxymorphone) provide the greatest sedation but may also cause the greatest cardiovascular and respiratory depression. Morphine (and other μ/OP_3-agonists) has the potential to induce vagally mediated bradycardia, which may be prevented with an anticholinergic if needed [10]. Lowering the heart rate can reduce myocardial oxygen demand and consumption and may actually be desirable in some aged patients. Partial agonists (eg, buprenorphine) and agonist-antagonists (eg, butorphanol) provide only mild to moderate analgesia and sedation but also cause minimal cardiovascular and respiratory depression. These agents may be quite useful in the geriatric animal, where concern for cardiopulmonary instability is present but mild sedation and analgesia are desired for the procedure.

Tranquilizers and sedatives

Even though geriatric animals may be calmer than their younger counterparts, it may still be quite valuable to include a tranquilizer in the anesthetic protocol to reduce the stress associated with hospitalization, treatment, anesthesia, and surgery. The benzodiazepines (eg, diazepam, midazolam) are reversible and produce little to no cardiovascular or respiratory depression, making them appropriate for many geriatric animals. Although benzodiazepine-induced sedation can be unreliable in younger animals, this is less of a concern in geriatric animals. If needed, benzodiazepines can be combined with other premedicants, such as opioids, to achieve the desired level of sedation. In addition, benzodiazepines like diazepam or midazolam can be combined with ketamine for the induction of anesthesia in selected geriatric animals.

In healthy geriatric animals, low doses of acepromazine may be a suitable choice for premedication. Acepromazine produces general CNS depression and sedation without analgesia. Nevertheless, it has a peripheral vaso-dilating effect that can cause significant hypotension, which contributes to the development of hypothermia in geriatric animals. When acepromazine is combined with the opioid analgesics, remarkably low doses of the tranquilizer can be used to maximize sedation and minimize the unwanted side effects.

The α_2-agonists may be considered for sedation and premedication in healthy geriatric animals because they are reversible and thus are not dependent on hepatic or renal clearance for recovery. A recent study showed that safe effective sedation could be performed in geriatric cancer patients undergoing daily radiation therapy using a combination of low-dose medetomidine, butorphanol, and glycopyrrolate [11]. Although these animals were all older (average of 8.9 years for dogs and 10.8 years for cats) and had a variety of age-related diseases, they were all identified as being in good cardiopulmonary health before drug administration. The α_2-agonists can cause serious side effects, such as bradycardia, atrioventricular conduction block, increased peripheral vascular resistance, and hypertension, making appropriate patient selection a must, especially when considering use in a geriatric population.

Anesthetic induction

Anesthetic induction may be accomplished using injectable anesthetics or by mask delivery of inhalant anesthetics if necessary. Because many injectable anesthetics demonstrate altered pharmacokinetics and pharma-codynamics, decreased plasma protein binding, and decreased hepatic and renal metabolism and excretion in geriatric animals, the use of these drugs should be undertaken cautiously.

Barbiturates

Barbiturates are highly protein bound and depend on redistribution and hepatic metabolism for termination of activity. As such, they should be used

cautiously in geriatric animals. Decreased protein binding and hypoproteinemia may lead to enhanced drug effects in geriatric animals [3,10]. To
minimize the potential for a relative overdose, the lowest possible dose that
produces the desired effect should be used. Barbiturates can cause significant
cardiovascular and respiratory depression, and their use should be reserved
for the healthy geriatric animal.

Dissociative anesthetic agents

The N-methyl-D-aspartate (NMDA) antagonist ketamine may be used for
the induction of anesthesia in geriatric animals. Ketamine may improve
cardiovascular function through stimulation of the sympathetic nervous
system [12,13]; however, this may not always be desirable in the geriatric
animal. NMDA antagonists may increase heart rate, causing a marked
increase in myocardial oxygen demand and consumption that may not be
well tolerated by animals with preexisting cardiovascular disease. Because
ketamine causes muscle stiffness and rigidity, it is typically combined with
a benzodiazepine to ameliorate this undesirable side effect. The effects of
ketamine may be prolonged in patients with failing hepatic and renal
systems, necessitating the administration of decreased doses in these animals.

Etomidate

Etomidate is a sedative-hypnotic agent with a rapid onset of action and
rapid recovery. At doses normally used to produce general anesthesia,
etomidate maintains cardiovascular stability, making it a good choice for the
induction of anesthesia in animals with clinically significant cardiac disease
[10]. Debilitated or sedated patients normally have a smooth anesthetic
induction when etomidate is titrated intravenously to effect. Excited animals
may exhibit undesirable side effects, such as retching, myoclonus, and apnea,
during induction.

Inhalant induction

Inhaled anesthetics may be used for the induction of anesthesia in
otherwise sedated or debilitated patients. There are many caveats to the use
of inhaled anesthetics for induction. These include the associated severe
physiologic stress of protracted induction in the animals and unwanted
environmental pollution and exposure of personnel to waste anesthetic gases.
An excessive depth of anesthesia can be attained rapidly during the induction
of anesthesia with inhalant anesthetics, and animals must be closely monitored and assessed to prevent overdose.

Propofol

Propofol is a good choice for use in most geriatric patients because it is
rapidly cleared from the body by many different routes. Recovery is

generally rapid in dogs, even after repeated doses, and metabolism is not dependent on the function of a single organ system. Propofol can induce significant respiratory and cardiovascular depression and should be titrated to achieve the desired effect. Premedication decreases the amount of propofol needed and helps to minimize side effects. Propofol has been shown to cause increased Heinz body production in cats when used for daily induction and maintenance (for an average of 6 days) and should thus be used with caution in this species if daily anesthesia is needed [14].

Anesthetic maintenance

Inhalant anesthetics are the agents of choice for anesthetic maintenance in geriatric animals, particularly for procedures lasting longer than 10 to 15 minutes. Halothane, isoflurane, and sevoflurane may be used with success in geriatric animals as long as close attention is paid to the monitoring of anesthetic depth and cardiopulmonary function during the anesthetic period.

Halothane

Halothane has been the cornerstone of anesthetic practice in veterinary medicine for many years, and many geriatric animals have been successfully anesthetized using halothane. With the newer inhalants available, however, it is generally held that the use of halothane should be reserved for healthy animals and avoided in higher risk animals. Halothane causes significant dose-related cardiovascular depression that may not be well tolerated in older patients. Heart rate, contractility, and cardiac output are significantly decreased in a dose-dependent manner [10]. Halothane can also cause profound hypotension because of vasodilation and direct depression of the vasomotor center. Halothane is also known to sensitize the myocardium to catecholamines; thus, it should be avoided in patients with the potential for dysrhythmias. Hepatitis has been reported in human patients after exposure to halothane; thus, chronic liver dysfunction should probably be considered a relative contraindication to its use.

Isoflurane

Compared with halothane, isoflurane better maintains cardiac output in anesthetized animals [10]. In addition, it does not sensitize the heart to catecholamines to the same degree as halothane. Because isoflurane has the potential to cause significant hypotension due to a direct effect on vasomotor tone, the lowest concentration necessary to achieve the desired level of anesthesia should be administered. Overall, there are fewer con-traindications to the use of isoflurane in geriatric animals than to the use of halothane.

Sevoflurane

Sevoflurane is a newer inhaled anesthetic that produces extremely rapid induction and recovery. Sevoflurane is less pungent than isoflurane, making it a better choice during the induction of anesthesia with an inhaled anesthetic. Faster induction and recovery, coupled with the increased acceptance of sevoflurane's odor, reduces the stress of inhalant induction and minimizes delay in achieving airway control with endotracheal intubation. Generally speaking, this makes sevoflurane preferable to isoflurane when the induction of anesthesia is performed with an inhaled anesthetic [15].

Monitoring and support

Geriatric animals are less tolerant of a busy hospital environment and are likely to become more stressed than younger animals when taken out of their normal daily routine. Every effort to make their hospitalization stress-free should be made.

Geriatric animals may have some degree of arthritis or muscle wasting, making it harder for them to lie down comfortably on a cage or run floor. If possible, their cages should be well bedded with soft materials (eg, padded beds, orthopedic foam) to ensure their comfort while hospitalized. Additionally, they may be less flexible than younger animals, and care should be taken when their legs are secured during surgery so that they are not pulled too tight, potentially causing soreness in the postoperative period.

Because geriatric animals have decreased thermoregulatory capacity, every effort should be made during the perianesthetic period to keep them warm with warmed fluids, circulating water blankets, and forced air warmers. Hypothermia increases the incidence of arrhythmias, leads to a catabolic state and delayed healing, adversely affects immune function, leads to hypoxia and metabolic acidosis, and prolongs the effects of anesthetic agents [16]. When the body attempts to rewarm itself after surgery by shivering, there is a 200% to 300% increase in oxygen consumption that may lead to increased myocardial work and ischemia or systemic hypoxia in the postoperative period. This may be especially relevant in the geriatric animal with significant loss in functional cardiopulmonary reserve. It is easier to maintain a core body temperature in animals while they are anesthetized and vasodilated than to try to rewarm them externally as the effects of anesthetic drugs are wearing off and they become more vasoconstricted during the recovery period.

As discussed previously, geriatric animals are less tolerant of volume overload than juvenile or middle-aged animals. Aggressive fluid therapy may result in excessive intravascular and extravascular volume, leading to congestive heart failure and pulmonary edema in geriatric animals that are unable to excrete a salt and water load efficiently [6]. The goal for fluid therapy in aged animals should be the correction of any specific deficits and the maintenance of adequate tissue perfusion and oxygen delivery.

Summary

Choosing the best anesthetic agents for each geriatric animal does not in itself ensure a successful outcome. Aggressive, careful, vigilant monitoring during the anesthetic and recovery periods is required to detect and correct alterations in homeostasis that may develop during the perianesthetic period. With appropriate preoperative screening, informed choice and judicious dosing of anesthetics, and careful monitoring and supportive care, the risk of anesthesia in geriatric animals can be greatly reduced.

References

[1] Wise JK, Heathcott BL, Gonzalez ML. Results of the AVMA survey on companion animal ownership in US pet-owning households. J Am Vet Med Assoc 2002;221:1572–3.

[2] Goldston RT. Introduction and overview of geriatrics. In: Goldston RT, Hoskins JD, editors. Geriatrics and gerontology of the dog and cat. Philadelphia: WB Saunders; 1995. p. 1–10.

[3] Muravchick S. Anesthesia for the elderly. In: Miller RD, editor. Anesthesia. 5th edition. Philadelphia: Churchill Livingstone; 2000. p. 2140–56.

[4] Thurmon JC, Tranquilli WJ, Benson GJ. Anesthesia for special patients: neonatal and geriatric patients. In: Thurmon JC, Tranquilli WJ, Benson GJ, editors. Lumb and Jones' veterinary anesthesia. 3rd edition. Baltimore: Williams & Wilkins; 1996. p. 844–8.

[5] Paddleford RR. Anesthesia. In: Goldston RT, Hoskins JD, editors. Geriatrics and gerontology of the dog and cat. Philadelphia: WB Saunders; 1995. p. 363–77.

[6] Pettifer GR, Grubb TC. Anesthesia for selected patients and procedures: neonatal and geriatric patients. In: Thurmon JC, Tranquilli WJ, Grimm KA, editors. Lumb and Jones' veterinary anesthesia. 4th edition. Baltimore: Williams & Wilkins; in press.

[7] Eger EI. Anesthetic uptake and action. Baltimore: Williams & Wilkins; 1974. p. 1–25.

[8] Grimm KA, Thurmon JC, Olson WA, et al. The pharmacodynamics of thiopental, medetomidine, butorphanol and atropine in beagle dogs. J Vet Pharmacol Ther 1998;2: 133–7.

[9] Ko JC, Fox SM, Mandsager RE. Effects of preemptive atropine administration on incidence of medetomidine-induced bradycardia in dogs. J Am Vet Med Assoc 2001;218:52–8.

[10] Stoelting RK. Pharmacology and physiology in anesthetic practice. 3rd edition. Philadelphia: Lippincott, Williams & Wilkins; 1999. p. 36–157.

[11] Grimm JB, deLorimier LP, Grimm KA. Medetomidine-butorphanol-glycopyrrolate sedation for radiation therapy: an eight-year study [abstract]. In: Proceedings of the Veterinary Midwest Anesthesia and Analgesia Conference. Columbus: The Ohio State University; 2004. p. 18.

[12] Kohrs R, Durieux ME. Ketamine: teaching an old drug new tricks. Anesth Analg 1998;87: 1186–93.

[13] Wright M. Pharmacologic effects of ketamine and its use in veterinary medicine. J Am Vet Med Assoc 1996;209:967–8.

[14] Andress JL, Day TK, Day D. Effects of consecutive day anesthesia on feline red blood cells. Vet Surg 1995;24:277–82.

[15] Johnson RA, Striler E, Sawyer DC, et al. Comparison of isoflurane with sevoflurane for anesthesia induction and recovery in adult dogs. Am J Vet Res 1998;59:478–81.

[16] Kaplan RF. Hypothermia/hyperthermia. In: Gravenstein N, editor. Manual of complications during anesthesia. New York: JB Lippincott; 1991. p. 121–50.

ELSEVIER
SAUNDERS

Vet Clin Small Anim
35 (2005) 581–596

VETERINARY
CLINICS
Small Animal Practice

Early Detection of Renal Damage and Disease in Dogs and Cats

Gregory F. Grauer, DVM, MS

*Department of Clinical Sciences, College of Veterinary Medicine, 111B Mosier Hall,
Kansas State University, Manhattan, KS 66506, USA*

Renal damage and disease can be caused by acute or chronic insults to the kidney. The terms *renal disease* and *renal damage* are used to denote the presence of renal lesions; however, the terms imply nothing about renal function or the cause, distribution, or severity of the renal lesions. Acute renal damage (ARD) often results from ischemic or toxic insults and usually affects the tubular portion of the nephron. In contrast, chronic renal disease (CRD) can be caused by diseases and/or disorders that affect any portion of the nephron, including its blood supply and supporting interstitium. Early detection of ARD facilitates appropriate intervention that can arrest or at least attenuate tubular cell damage and the development of established acute renal failure (ARF). Similarly, early detection of CRD, before the onset of renal azotemia and chronic renal failure (CRF), should facilitate appropriate intervention that stabilizes renal function or at least slows its progressive decline.

Acute renal damage and acute renal failure

In many cases, ARD leading to ARF inadvertently develops in the hospital setting in conjunction with diagnostic or therapeutic procedures. For example, ARD may result from decreased renal perfusion associated with anesthesia and surgery or with the use of vasodilators and nonsteroidal anti-inflammatory drugs (NSAIDs). Similarly, acute tubular damage frequently occurs in patients treated with potential nephrotoxicants, such as gentamicin, amphotericin, and cisplatin. Ischemic and nephrotoxic insults usually involve the most metabolically active portions of the nephron (ie, the proximal convoluted tubule and the thick ascending limb of Henle). This

---

E-mail address: ggrauer@ksu.edu

tubular damage may lead to ARF, which is not always reversible; animals that do recover adequate renal function often require prolonged and expensive intensive care. Several recent retrospective studies have documented the poor prognosis associated with ARF in dogs and cats. In a study of hospital-acquired ARF, the survival rate was only 40% [1]. In another retrospective study of 99 dogs with all types ARF, 22% died, 34% were euthanized, 24% survived but progressed to CRF, and only 19% regained normal or adequate renal function [2]. Similarly, in a retrospective study of 25 cats with all types of ARF, 20% died, 36% were euthanized, 20% survived but progressed to CRF, and only 24% regained normal or adequate renal function [3]. These studies underscore the importance of early detection of ARD and prevention of ARF. Several risk factors have been identified that predispose dogs to gentamicin-induced ARF (Box 1) [4]; however, it is likely that many of these risk factors also predispose dogs and cats to other types of toxicant-induced as well as ischemic-induced ARD. A combination of decreased renal perfusion or use of nephrotoxic therapeutic agents superimposed on more chronic preexisting renal disease is often responsible for ARD and ARF in the clinical setting. Age has been identified as a risk factor, because many geriatric dogs and cats have preexisting renal lesions and subclinical loss of renal function.

Box 1. Potential risk factors for development of acute renal damage and acute renal failure in dogs and cats

Preexisting renal disease
Advanced age
Fever
Sepsis
Trauma
Diabetes mellitus
Hypoalbuminemia
Liver disease
Multiple organ involvement
Dehydration[a]
Decreased cardiac output[a]
Hypotension[a]
Hyperviscosity syndromes[a]
Dietary protein level[a]
Acidosis[a]
Electrolyte imbalances[a]
Concurrent use of potentially nephrotoxic drugs[a]

---

[a] Risk factors that are potentially correctable (see text).

ARF has three distinct phases, which are categorized as (1) initiation, (2) maintenance, and (3) recovery. During the initiation phase, therapeutic measures that reduce the renal insult can prevent development of established ARF. Tubular lesions and established nephron dysfunction characterize the maintenance phase. Therapeutic intervention during the maintenance phase, although potentially life saving, usually does little to diminish existing renal lesions or improve dysfunction. The recovery phase is the period when renal lesions resolve and function improves, although not all ARF is reversible. Identification of patients at risk for developing ARF allows the clinician to increase the monitoring of these patients during procedures and therapies that may insult the kidney. This increased monitoring aids in the detection of acute tubular damage in the initiation phase of ARF when appropriate intervention has the potential to prevent development of established lesions.

Risk factors for acute renal damage

Dehydration and volume depletion are perhaps the most common and most important risk factors for development of ARF (see Box 1). Studies in people indicate that volume depletion increases a patient's risk of developing ARF by a factor of 10 [5]. Hypovolemia not only decreases renal perfusion, which can enhance ischemic damage, but decreases the volume of distribution of nephrotoxic drugs and results in decreased tubular fluid flow rates and enhanced tubular absorption of toxicants. In addition to hypovolemia, renal hypoperfusion may be caused by decreased cardiac output, decreased plasma oncotic pressure, increased blood viscosity, systemic hypotension, and decreased renal prostaglandin synthesis (eg, use of NSAIDs). Any of these conditions can increase the risk of ARF in the hospital setting.

Preexisting renal disease and advanced age, which are often associated with some degree of decreased renal function, can increase the potential for nephrotoxicity and ischemic damage by several mechanisms. The pharmacokinetics of potentially nephrotoxic drugs can be altered in the face of decreased renal function. Gentamicin clearance is decreased in dogs with subclinical renal dysfunction [6], and the same is probably true for other nephrotoxicants that are excreted via the kidneys. Animals with renal insufficiency also have reduced urine-concentrating ability and, therefore, decreased ability to compensate for prerenal influences. Renal disease may also compromise the local production of prostaglandins that help to maintain renal vasodilatation and blood flow [7].

Decreased serum concentrations of several electrolytes can increase the risk of renal damage and ARF. Hyponatremia exacerbates or potentiates intravenous contrast media–induced ARF in dogs [8]. Additional studies in dogs have demonstrated that dietary potassium restriction exacerbates gentamicin nephrotoxicity [9], possibly because potassium-depleted cells are more susceptible to necrosis. It is important to note that gentamicin administration in dogs is associated with increased urinary excretion of potassium [9]. This increased urinary excretion of potassium could result in potassium depletion and increased nephrotoxicity in clinical patients. Therefore, serum electrolyte concentrations should be closely monitored in patients receiving potentially nephrotoxic drugs, especially if these patients are anorexic or vomiting or have diarrhea.

Administration of potentially nephrotoxic drugs or a drug that may enhance nephrotoxicity obviously increases the risk of ARF. Concurrent use of furosemide and gentamicin in dogs is associated with increased risk and severity of ARF (Fig. 1) [10]. Furosemide probably potentiates gentamicin-induced nephrotoxicity by causing dehydration, reducing the volume of distribution of gentamicin, and increasing the renal tubular absorption of gentamicin. Fluid repletion minimizes but does not avoid the potentiating effect of furosemide on gentamicin nephrotoxicity in the dog, because furosemide facilitates cellular uptake of gentamicin independent of hemodynamic changes. Use of NSAIDs can also increase the risk of ARF (Fig. 2) [11]. Renal prostaglandin production may be compromised in patients receiving NSAIDs, which can result in decreased renal blood flow, especially if superimposed on dehydration or decreased cardiac output. Anesthesia, hypotension, hyponatremia, sepsis, nephrotic syndrome, and hepatic disease are additional conditions in which prostaglandin-induced renal vasodilatation helps to maintain renal blood flow and the susceptibility to NSAIDs is increased [12].

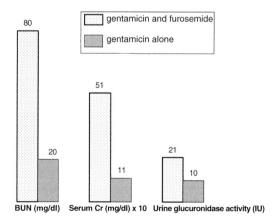

Fig. 1. The detrimental effects of combination treatment with gentamicin and furosemide compared with gentamicin treatment alone. After 8 days of treatment, azotemia and enzymuria are significantly greater in dogs treated with gentamicin and furosemide. (*From* Adelman RD, Spangler WL, Beasom F, et al. Furosemide enhancement of experimental gentamicin nephrotoxicity: comparison of functional and morphological changes with activities of urinary enzymes. J Infect Dis 1979;140:342–52; with permission.)

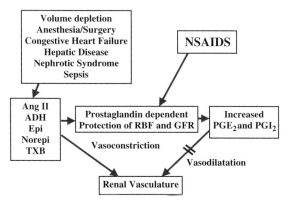

Fig. 2. The potential effects that nonsteroidal anti-inflammatory drugs can have on renal blood flow.

Recent evidence in dogs suggests that the quantity of protein fed before a nephrotoxic insult can significantly affect subsequent renal damage and dysfunction. Feeding high dietary protein before and during gentamicin administration reduces nephrotoxicity, enhances gentamicin clearance, and results in a larger volume of distribution compared with feeding medium or low dietary protein [13]. The beneficial effects of high dietary protein are likely associated with increased glomerular filtration and, therefore, improved toxicant excretion. High dietary protein also results in increased urinary excretion of protein, which may compete for nephrotoxicant reabsorption by tubular epithelial cells. Similar to potential causes of decreased electrolyte stores, anorexia, vomiting, and diarrhea have the potential to decrease dietary protein intake and thus increase the risk of nephrotoxicant-induced ARD.

Risk factors are additive, and any complication occurring in high-risk patients increases the potential for ARD and ARF. Patients with shock, acidosis, sepsis, and major organ system failure are at increased risk, and these are the patients that are likely to require aggressive treatment, including prolonged anesthesia, surgery, or chemotherapeutics, which are potentially damaging to the kidneys. For example, ARF is relatively common in dogs with pyometra and *Escherichia coli* endotoxin-induced urine-concentrating defects, especially if fluid therapy is inadequate during anesthesia for ovariohysterectomy or during the recovery period. Trauma, extensive burns, vasculitis, pancreatitis, fever, diabetes mellitus, and multiple myeloma are additional conditions associated with a high incidence of ARF.

Early recognition of acute renal damage

Because therapeutic intervention is most successful when initiated during the induction phase of ARF, early recognition of renal damage and/or dysfunction is important. Physical examination of the patient at risk for ARF should include evaluation of pulse quality and hydration status. Monitoring body weight, packed cell volume, and plasma total solids in comparison to baseline values may indicate subtle changes in hydration status. Blood pressure measurement identifies hypotensive and hypertensive patients, both of which may be at increased risk for renal injury. In patients with palpable kidneys, renal swelling or pain, although subjective, may be associated with acute ischemic or toxic insult.

Numerous urine parameters can herald the development of ARF. Urine output should be monitored in all high-risk patients that undergo anesthesia; once a patient is anesthetized, placement of an indwelling urinary catheter and measurement of urine production is relatively easy. Closed catheter systems hooked up to empty sterile fluid bags should be used to quantitate urine production. Normal urine output is approximately 1 to 2 mL/h/kg of body weight. Decreased renal perfusion during anesthesia can result in oliguria (<0.25 mL/hr/kg) or anuria, which signals the need for prompt treatment. Nonoliguric ARF is being recognized with increasing frequency, and increases in urine production may thus also signal the onset of renal damage. Examples of nonoliguric ARF include that induced by gentamicin and cisplatin. Increased urine turbidity or changes in urine sediment (increasing numbers of white blood cells [WBCs], red blood cells [RBCs], renal epithelial cells, or cellular or granular casts) are other indications of ARD, along with increased excretion of sodium and chloride. Finally, the acute onset of tubular glucosuria (normoglycemic glucosuria) or proteinuria may also be indicative of ARD. The interpretation of these parameters is enhanced by knowledge of baseline values.

Detection of enzymes in the urine, such as gamma-glutamyl trans-peptidase (GGT) and N-acetyl-beta-D-glucosaminidase (NAG), has proven to be a sensitive indicator of early renal tubular damage (Fig. 3) [13,14]. These enzymes are too large to be filtered by the glomerulus normally; therefore, enzymuria indicates cell leakage, usually associated with tubular epithelial damage or necrosis. Urinary GGT originates from the proximal tubule brush border, and NAG is present in proximal tubule lysosomes. In a study of gentamicin-treated dogs, increased urinary GGT and NAG activity was one of the earliest markers of renal damage and/or dysfunction (see Fig. 3) [13,14]. Interpretation of enzymuria is aided by baseline values obtained before a potential renal insult; two- to threefold increases over baseline suggest significant tubular damage. Urine enzyme/creatinine ratios have been shown to be accurate in dogs before the onset of azotemia, obviating the need for timed urine collections [15]. False-positive enzymuria can potentially occur with severe glomerular damage, resulting in increased glomerular filtration of serum enzymes. False-negative results can occur after severe tubular damage depletes tubular enzyme stores.

In the specific case of aminoglycoside administration, measurement of serum trough concentrations of the antibiotic can help to prevent

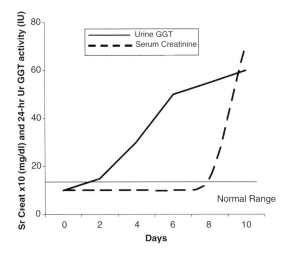

Fig. 3. In dogs treated with gentamicin, detection of enzymuria precedes the development of azotemia by approximately 6 days. (*From* Greco DS, Turnwald GH, Adams R, et al. Urinary gamma-glutamyl transpeptidase activity in dogs with gentamicin-induced nephrotoxicity. Am J Vet Res 1985;46:2332–5; with permission.)

nephrotoxicity. Renal tubular damage increases with elevated serum trough concentrations (>2 µg/dL for gentamicin and >5 µg/dL for amikacin) [16]. Administering the same total daily dose once or twice daily versus three times daily seems to maintain antimicrobial efficacy while reducing serum trough concentrations and the potential for nephrotoxicity [17]. Serum aminoglycoside concentrations can be measured by most reference laboratories.

Knowledge of the predisposing risk factors allows the clinician to assess the risk-benefit ratio in individual cases in which an elective anesthetic procedure is considered or the use of potentially nephrotoxic drugs is indicated. In some cases, predisposing risk factors can be corrected before any potential renal insults occur. In other cases, such as geriatric patients with suspected preexisting renal disease, more intensive monitoring of the patient may allow detection of ARD and/or ARF in its early phase before the onset of established failure.

Chronic renal disease and chronic renal failure

CRD leading to CRF is a major cause of morbidity and mortality in dogs and cats. The prevalence of CRD increases with age, and the underlying lesions are often irreversible as well as progressive. Whether the underlying disease process primarily affects glomeruli, tubules, interstitial tissue, or the blood supply to the nephron, irreversible damage to any of these components renders the entire nephron nonfunctional. Healing of irreversibly damaged nephrons occurs by means of replacement fibrosis. Renal histopathologic preparations usually show some combination of a loss of tubules with replacement fibrosis and mineralization, glomerulosclerosis and glomerular atrophy, and foci of mononuclear cells (small lymphocytes, plasma cells, and macrophages) within the interstitium. These histopathologic changes are not process-specific; therefore, the underlying cause of the renal disease is usually unknown. Because of the large functional renal reserve and the compensatory hypertrophy of remaining viable nephrons, clinical signs and laboratory data compatible with CRF are not present in most cases until greater than 80% to 85% of all nephrons are nonfunctional. At this point, improvement of renal function is often not possible, and management of the CRF patient is aimed at reducing "renal workload," reducing the clinical signs associated with the decreased renal function, and reducing the progressive nature of the disease process. Early detection of canine and feline chronic kidney disease (CKD), before the onset of azotemia and CRF, should improve our ability to manage these patients (Fig. 4).

Early detection of chronic renal disease

Most acquired (versus hereditary or familial) canine and feline CRD and CRF occur in middle-aged to older patients. An annual health examination that includes a complete blood cell count, serum biochemistry profile, and urinalysis is one of the best ways to detect declining renal function (Box 2). Special attention should be paid to decreases in appetite, body weight, packed cell volume, and urine specific gravity. Conversely, increases in serum urea nitrogen, creatinine, and phosphorus or urinary excretion of protein or albumin may signal the onset of renal disease. Plotting the inverse of the serum creatinine concentration versus time can demonstrate a decrease in renal excretory function; the steeper the slope, the more progressive is the functional decline. Developing a data flow chart is an excellent way to keep

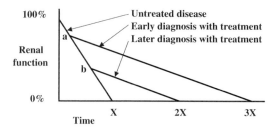

Fig. 4. The potential benefit of early diagnosis and treatment of chronic renal disease. Treatments initiated at points a and b were equally effective in slowing the progressive decline of renal function; however, treatment initiated at point a resulted in longer patient survival compared with treatment initiated at point b.

Box 2. Clinicopathologic findings that may be associated with early chronic renal disease in dogs and cats

Annual health examinations
  Decreases in
    Appetite
    Body weight
    Packed cell volume
    Urine specific gravity
  Increases in
    Water consumption/urine production
    Serum urea nitrogen concentration
    Serum creatinine concentration
    Serum phosphorus concentration
    Urine protein excretion/MA
    Bacteriuria/urinary tract infections

---

track of changes in body weight and clinicopathologic values. Longitudinal assessment of serum creatinine, for example, can indicate declining renal function even if values stay within the normal range [18]. A serum creatinine concentration of 1.2 mg/dL may be overlooked on a single biochemistry profile; however, if previous results showed a serum creatinine concentration of 0.6 mg/dL, a 50% or greater loss of renal excretory function may have occurred. It is important to keep in mind that prerenal factors like hydration status can influence serum creatinine concentrations; concurrent assessment of urine specific gravity can aid in the interpretation of serum creatinine and urea nitrogen values. Dogs and cats may also become more susceptible to bacterial urinary tract infections as their ability to concentrate urine decreases and the antibacterial properties of their urine decrease. If any of these parameters suggests the possibility of renal disease, an ultrasound examination should be used to evaluate kidney tissue architecture. Pyelonephritis, renoliths, and renal cortical fibrosis can be demonstrated by ultrasound. Percutaneous or ultrasound-guided renal biopsy can also be used to confirm or define renal cortical disease further.

Importance of proteinuria as a diagnostic marker of early chronic renal disease

Persistent proteinuria with an inactive urine sediment has long been the clinicopathologic hallmark of CKD in dogs and, more recently, in cats. Beyond this diagnostic marker utility, the potential for proteinuria to be associated with the progression of renal disease has been recently recognized in dogs and cats (Fig. 5). The implication that proteinuria may be a mediator of renal disease progression has stimulated a discussion about what level of protein in the urine is normal. The development of species-specific albumin enzyme-linked immunoassay (ELISA) technology that enables detection of low concentrations of canine and feline albuminuria has helped to drive this re-evaluation process. Perhaps somewhat similar to our changing definition and treatment guidelines for systemic hypertension, the need to recognize and treat proteinuria, which was considered normal not long ago, is increasing.

Albuminuria and microalbuminuria

Albuminuria accounts for most of the urine protein in most CRD states. Microalbuminuria (MA) is defined as concentrations of albumin in the urine that are greater than normal but below the limit of detection using conventional semiquantitative urine protein-screening methodology. Urine albumin concentrations can be adjusted for differences in urine concentration by dividing by urine creatinine concentrations. For example, a urine albumin/creatinine ratio greater than 0.03 is considered abnormal in people [19]. Alternatively, urine can be diluted to a standard concentration, such as a urine specific gravity of 1.010, before assay (eg, the Heska E.R.D.-HealthScreen urine test, Heska, Fort Collins, CO). In one study of dogs, normalizing urine albumin concentrations to a 1.010 specific gravity yielded results similar to the urine albumin/creatinine ratio [20]. Using urine that has been diluted to a specific gravity of 1.010, MA is usually defined as a urine albumin concentration greater than 1.0 mg/dL but less

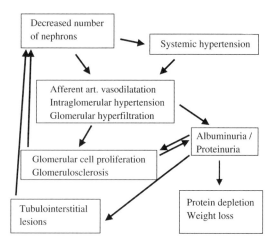

Fig. 5. Proposed pathogenesis of progressive chronic renal disease. Note the potential contribution of proteinuria to glomerular and tubulointerstitial disease.

than 30 mg/dL. Albuminuria above this limit is referred to as overt albuminuria and can often be detected using the urine protein/creatinine ratio (UP/C).

The prevalence of MA in dogs has been evaluated in several studies. In 86 dogs whose owners were not seeking veterinary care, the prevalence of MA was 19% [21]. The prevalence was higher (36%) in 159 dogs whose owners were seeking veterinary care for routine health screening, elective procedures, and evaluation of health problems at a veterinary teaching hospital [21]. In dogs evaluated at another veterinary teaching hospital for health problems, the prevalence of MA was 30%, although MA was more rigidly defined (2–20 mg/dL) [22]. In 3041 dogs owned by the staff from more than 350 veterinary clinics, the prevalence of MA was 25% [23]. Although the health status of these 3041 dogs was not reported, a statistically significant correlation was found between increasing age and MA in this study. The increasing prevalence of glomerular lesions and CRD in dogs as they age tends to corroborate the age-related prevalence of MA [24,25].

The prevalence of MA in apparently healthy cats seems to be approximately 15%, and similar to the situation in dogs, it is correlated with increasing age (Heska, Fort Collins, CO, unpublished data, 2003) [26]. Interestingly, when cats with medical conditions were evaluated, the overall prevalence increased to greater than 40% and the correlation with age was less apparent (Heska, Fort Collins, CO, unpublished data, 2003).

Causes of microalbuminuria

MA reflects the presence of intraglomerular hypertension or generalized vascular damage and endothelial cell dysfunction in human beings [27]. It is interesting to note that the presence of MA has been shown to be an accurate predictor of subsequent renal disease in people with systemic hypertension and diabetes mellitus, and it has also been observed in people with systemic diseases that are associated with glomerulopathy [28–32]. Importantly, early detection of albuminuria and institution of appropriate treatment have slowed the progression of kidney disease in people [33].

Based on recent studies, MA seems to be a good indicator of early renal disease in dogs, particularly those diseases that involve the glomerulus [20,34,35]. Albuminuria was evaluated in 36 male dogs with X-linked hereditary nephropathy, a rapidly progressive glomerular disease that is secondary to a defect in type IV collagen, a structural component of the glomerular basement membrane [20]. In these dogs, ultrastructural lesions in the glomerular basement membrane become apparent by 8 weeks of age. In a longitudinal study, persistent MA was detected in dogs with X-linked hereditary nephropathy between 8 and 23 weeks of age, 0 to 16 weeks before the onset of overt proteinuria, which occurred at 14 to 30 weeks of age.

In 12 healthy dogs that were experimentally infected with *Dirofilaria immitis* L3 larvae and evaluated over time, all the dogs developed MA, with 82% of all samples collected over the 14- to 23-month postinfection period of study being positive for MA [34]. The onset of MA corresponded to the onset of antigenemia. The magnitude of MA increased over time, and MA preceded the development of overt proteinuria, as measured by UP/C. At the end of the study, all the dogs had histologic evidence of glomerular disease by light or electron microscopy [34].

Finally, in 20 Soft-Coated Wheaten Terriers that were genetically at risk for the development of protein-losing enteropathy and nephropathy, the prevalence of MA was 76% [35]. The magnitude of MA increased over time, and 43% of the dogs with MA eventually developed abnormal UP/Cs. Significantly persistent MA developed in these dogs at approximately the same time that mesangial hypercellularity and segmental glomerular sclerosis were observed histologically. The results of these three studies demonstrate the utility of MA as a marker of early CRD.

Similar to what is observed in people, MA is also observed in dogs and cats with systemic diseases that can alter glomerular permeability to plasma proteins (see previous discussion on the prevalence of MA). Inasmuch as the Soft-Coated Wheaten Terriers discussed previously were predisposed to inflammatory bowel disease, the MA observed in some of the dogs that did not progress to overt proteinuria may have been primarily associated with intestinal inflammation rather than progressive CRD. Other conditions have been reported in dogs with MA, including infectious, inflammatory, neoplastic, metabolic, and cardiovascular disease [22,36]. Results of an ongoing study of MA in dogs with lymphosarcoma and osteosarcoma demonstrated that urine albumin concentrations were significantly increased in dogs with these tumors, even though UP/Cs may not be increased above the reference range [37]. Urine albumin concentrations did not, however, consistently decrease with decreased tumor burden. The prevalence of MA in dogs admitted to intensive care unit (ICU) is higher than in other reported patient populations and seems to vary with different classifications of disease [22,36]. As reported in people with acute inflammatory conditions, transient MA occurred in some of these dogs. Conversely, a large percentage of dogs that were euthanized or died had MA, suggesting that, as in people, the presence of MA may be a negative prognostic indicator.

Dogs and cats with persistent MA (ie, MA present on three urinalyses ≥2 weeks apart) are at greatest risk for CRD or systemic diseases that can adversely affect the kidneys. Similarly, MA that is not only persistent but increases over time should be of more concern than MA that is stable. The appropriate response to albuminuria and/or proteinuria should first be continued monitoring. In cases of persistent albuminuria and/or proteinuria or increasing albuminuria and/or proteinuria, further investigation is warranted and may include blood pressure measurement, imaging, serology, and biopsy. This investigation should be designed to rule out underlying and/or concurrent systemic diseases and to define the CRD further. Perhaps the best treatment for albuminuria and/or proteinuria is the identification and correction of underlying or concurrent disease processes. Dietary therapy (early renal failure diets) and angiotensin-converting enzyme inhibition have been recommended for treatment of persistent or increasing "idiopathic" albuminuria and/or proteinuria; however, in the case of MA, these treatments have not been evaluated in a prospective controlled fashion.

Implications of proteinuria and/or albuminuria

In addition to the classic complications of heavy proteinuria (hypoalbuminemia, edema, ascites, hypercholesterolemia, hypertension, and hypercoagulability), there is increasing evidence in laboratory animals and human beings that proteinuria can cause glomerular and tubulointerstitial damage and result in progressive nephron loss (see Fig. 5). Proteinuria can occur secondary to immune-mediated or structural glomerular damage or as a consequence of intraglomerular hypertension and/or hyperfiltration secondary to the compensatory hypertrophy that occurs in remaining viable nephrons in the face of any type of CRD. Plasma proteins that have crossed the glomerular capillary wall can accumulate within the glomerular tuft and stimulate mesangial cell proliferation and increased production of mesangial matrix [38]. In addition, excessive amounts of protein in the glomerular filtrate can be toxic to tubular epithelial cells and can lead to interstitial inflammation, fibrosis, and cell death by means of several mechanisms [39–41]. These mechanisms include tubular obstruction, lysosomal rupture, complement-mediated damage, and peroxidative damage as well as increased production of cytokines and growth factors.

Evidence linking proteinuria to the progression of renal disease in dogs and cats is also beginning to accumulate. In dogs with the remnant kidney model of renal failure, there is an association between proteinuria and individual nephron hyperfiltration [42]. In 45 dogs with naturally occurring CRF, the relative risk of uremic crisis and mortality was approximately three times higher in dogs with a UP/C of 1.0 or greater (n = 25) compared with dogs with a UP/C less than 1.0 (n = 20) [43]. The risk of adverse outcomes was approximately 1.5 times greater for every unit increase in UP/C [43]. In addition, the decline in renal function, as measured by serum creatinine, was greater in dogs with higher UP/Cs [43]. Similar findings have been observed in cats with the remnant kidney model of CRF, where proteinuria was associated with nephron hypertrophy, intraglomerular hypertension, and glomerular hyperfiltration [44]. In cats with naturally occurring CRF, relatively mild proteinuria (UP/C >0.43) was a negative predictor of survival [45]. Interestingly, low-level proteinuria within the conventional normal reference range also seems to be a predictor of survival in healthy nonazotemic cats [46]. In one study, the median UP/C for cats that died was 0.3, compared with a UP/C of 0.16 for cats that were alive at the end of the study or lost to follow-up [46]. Finally, in dogs with naturally occurring protein-losing nephropathies (x-linked hereditary nephritis in male Samoyeds and idiopathic immune complex glomerulonephritis) treated with angiotensin-converting enzyme inhibitors having renoprotective effects that decrease or delay progression of disease, a reduction in proteinuria was also observed [47,48].

In summary, proteinuria is a common disorder in the dog and cat that can indicate the presence of CRD before the onset of azotemia. Tests for MA can detect abnormal albuminuria at its earliest stage and seem to be valuable adjunctive tests for early detection of CRD. In addition to being a diagnostic marker of renal disease, albuminuria and/or proteinuria may also contribute to the progressive nature of canine and feline renal disease.

References

[1] Behrend EN, Grauer GF, Mani I, et al. Hospital-acquired acute renal failure in dogs: 29 cases (1983–1992). J Am Vet Med Assoc 1996;208:537–41.

[2] Vaden SL, Levine J, Breitschwerdt EB. A retrospective case-control of acute renal failure in 99 dogs. J Vet Intern Med 1997;11:58–64.

[3] Worwag S, Langston C. Retrospective, acute renal failure in cats: 25 cases (1997–2002) [abstract]. J Vet Intern Med 2004;18:416.

[4] Brown SA, Barsanti JA, Crowell WA. Gentamicin-associated acute renal failure in the dog. J Am Vet Med Assoc 1985;186:686–90.

[5] Brezis M, Rosen S, Epstein FH. Acute renal failure. In: Brenner BM, Rector FC, editors. The kidney. 4th edition. Philadelphia: WB Saunders; 1991. p. 993–1061.

[6] Frazier DL, Aucoin DP, Riviere JE. Gentamicin pharmacokinetics and nephrotoxicity in naturally acquired and experimentally induced disease in dogs. J Am Vet Med Assoc 1988; 192:57–63.

[7] Clive DM, Stoff JS. Renal syndromes associated with nonsteroidal anti-inflammatory drugs. N Engl J Med 1984;310:563–71.

[8] Margulies KB, McKinley LJ, Cavero PG, et al. Induction and prevention of radiocontrast-induced nephropathy in dogs with heart failure. Kidney Int 1990;38:1101–8.

[9] Brinker KR, Bulger RE, Dolgan DC, et al. Effect of potassium depletion on gentamicin nephrotoxicity. J Lab Clin Med 1981;98:292–301.

[10] Adelman RD, Spangler WL, Beasom F, et al. Furosemide enhancement of experimental gentamicin nephrotoxicity: comparison of functional and morphological changes with activities of urinary enzymes. J Infect Dis 1979;140:342–52.

[11] Kore AM. Toxicology of nonsteroidal anti-inflammatory drugs. Vet Clin North Am Small Anim Pract 1990;20:419–30.

[12] Wilkes BM, Mailloux LU. Acute renal failure: pathogenesis and prevention. Am J Med 1986;80:1129–36.

[13] Grauer GF, Greco DS, Behrend EN, et al. Effects of dietary protein conditioning on gentamicin-induced nephrotoxicosis in healthy male dogs. Am J Vet Res 1994;55:90–7.

[14] Greco DS, Turnwald GH, Adams R, et al. Urinary gamma-glutamyl transpeptidase activity in dogs with gentamicin-induced nephrotoxicity. Am J Vet Res 1985;46:2332–5.

[15] Grauer GF, Greco DS, Behrend EN, et al. Estimation of quantitative enzymuria in dogs with gentamicin-induced nephrotoxicosis using urine enzyme/creatinine ratios from spot urine samples. J Vet Intern Med 1995;9:324–7.
[16] Brown SA, Engelhardt JA. Drug-related nephropathies, part I: mechanisms, diagnosis and management. Compend Contin Educ Pract Vet 1987;9:148–60.
[17] Frazier DL, Riviere JC. Gentamicin dosing strategies for dogs with subclinical renal dysfunction. Antimicrob Agents Chemother 1987;31:1929–34.
[18] Lees GE, Bahr A, Russell KE, et al. Comparison of serum cystatin C and creatinine concentrations as indices of declining glomerular filtration rate in dogs with progressive renal disease [abstract]. J Vet Intern Med 2002;16(3):378.
[19] Jones CA, Francis ME, Eberhardt MS, et al. Microalbuminuria in the US population: third national health and nutrition examination survey. Am J Kidney Dis 2002;39(3):445–59.
[20] Lees GE, Jensen WA, Simpson DF, et al. Persistent albuminuria precedes onset of overt proteinuria in male dogs with X-linked hereditary nephropathy [abstract]. J Vet Intern Med 2002;16:353.
[21] Jensen WA, Grauer GF, Andrews J, et al. Prevalence of microalbuminuria in dogs [abstract]. J Vet Intern Med 2001;15:300.
[22] Pressler BM, Vaden SL, Jensen WA. Prevalence of microalbuminuria in dogs evaluated at a referral veterinary hospital [abstract]. J Vet Intern Med 2001;15:300.
[23] Radecki S, Donnelly R, Jensen WA, et al. Effect of age and breed on the prevalence of microalbuminuria in dogs [abstract]. J Vet Intern Med 2003;17:406.
[24] Muller-Peddinghaus R, Trautwein G. Spontaneous glomerulonephritis in dogs 1. Classification and immunopathology. Vet Pathol 1977;14:1–13.
[25] Rouse BT, Lewis RJ. Canine glomerulonephritis: prevalence in dogs submitted at random for euthanasia. Can J Comp Med 1975;39:365–70.
[26] Grauer GF, Moore LE, Smith AR, et al. Comparison of conventional urine protein test strips and a quantitative ELISA for the detection of canine and feline albuminuria [abstract]. J Vet Intern Med 2004;18:418–9.
[27] Kruger M, Gordjani N, Burghard R. Post exercise albuminuria in children with different duration of type-1 diabetes mellitus. Pediatr Nephrol 1996;10:594–7.
[28] Hebert LA, Spetie DN, Keane WF. The urgent call of albuminuria/proteinuria: heeding its significance in early detection of kidney disease. Postgrad Med 2001;110:79–96.
[29] Gerstein HC, Mann JF, Yi Q, et al. Albuminuria and risk of cardiovascular events, death, and heart failure in diabetic and nondiabetic individuals. JAMA 2001;286:421–6.
[30] Osterby R, Hartmann A, Nyengaard JR, et al. Development of renal structural lesions in type-1 diabetic patients with microalbuminuria. Observations by light microscopy in 8-year follow-up biopsies. Virchows Arch 2002;440:94–101.
[31] Bakris GL. Microalbuminuria: what is it? Why is it important? What should be done about it? J Clin Hypertens 2001;3:99–102.
[32] Pinto-Sietsma SJ, Janssen WM, Hillege HL, et al. Urinary albumin excretion is associated with renal functional abnormalities in a nondiabetic population. J Am Soc Nephrol 2000;10:1882–8.
[33] Keane WF, Eknoyan G. Proteinuria, albuminuria, risk, assessment, detection, elimination (PARADE): a position paper of the National Kidney Foundation. Am J Kidney Dis 1999;33:1004–10.
[34] Grauer GF, Oberhauser EB, Basaraba RJ, et al. Development of microalbuminuria in dogs with heartworm disease [abstract]. J Vet Intern Med 2002;16:352.
[35] Vaden SL, Jensen WA, Longhofer SL, et al. Longitudinal study of microalbuminuria in soft-coated wheaten terriers [abstract]. J Vet Intern Med 2001;15:300.
[36] Whittemore JC, Jensen WA, Prause L, et al. Comparison of microalbuminuria, urine protein dipstick, and urine protein creatinine ratio results in clinically ill dogs [abstract]. J Vet Intern Med 2003;17:437.

[37] Pressler BM, Proulx DA, Williams LE, et al. Urine albumin concentration is increased in dogs with lymphoma or osteosarcoma [abstract]. J Vet Intern Med 2003;17:404.

[38] Jerums G, Panagiotopoulos S, Tsalamandris C, et al. Why is proteinuria such an important risk factor for progression in clinical trials? Kidney Int 1997;52(Suppl):S87–92.

[39] Tang S, Sheerin NS, Zhou W, et al. Apical proteins stimulate complement synthesis by cultured human proximal tubular epithelial cells. J Am Soc Nephrol 1999;10:69–76.

[40] Abrass CK. Clinical spectrum and complications of the nephrotic syndrome. J Invest Med 1997;45:143–53.

[41] Eddy A. Role of cellular infiltrates in response to proteinuria. Am J Kidney Dis 2001; 37(Suppl):S25–9.

[42] Brown SA, Finco DR, Crowell WA, et al. Single-nephron adaptation to partial renal ablation in the dog. Am J Physiol 1990;258:F495–503.

[43] Jacob F, Polzin D, Osborne J, et al. Association of initial proteinuria with morbidity and morality in dogs with spontaneous chronic renal failure [abstract]. J Vet Intern Med 2004;18: 417.

[44] Brown SA, Brown CA. Single-nephron adaptations to partial renal ablation in cats. Am J Physiol 1995;269:R1002–8.

[45] Syme HM, Elliott J. Relation of survival time and urinary protein excretion in cats with renal failure and/or hypertension [abstract]. J Vet Intern Med 2003;17:405.

[46] Walker D, Syme HM, Markwell P, et al. Predictors of survival in healthy, non-azotemic cats [abstract]. J Vet Intern Med 2004;18:417.

[47] Grauer GF, Greco DS, Getzy DM, et al. Effects of enalapril vs placebo as a treatment for canine idiopathic glomerulonephritis. J Vet Intern Med 2000;14:526–33.

[48] Grodecki KM, Gains MJ, Baumal R, et al. Treatment of X-linked hereditary nephritis in Samoyed dogs with angiotensin converting enzyme (ACE) inhibitor. J Comp Pathol 1997; 117:209–25.

ELSEVIER
SAUNDERS

Vet Clin Small Anim
35 (2005) 597–615

VETERINARY
CLINICS
Small Animal Practice

Geriatric Heart Diseases in Dogs

Robert L. Hamlin, DVM, PhD

*Department of Veterinary Biosciences, The Ohio State University College of Veterinary
Medicine, 1920 Coffey Road, Columbus, OH 43210, USA*

In human beings, ageing is characterized by at least three changes in cardiovascular physiology [1,2]. The β_1-adrenergic effects, heart rate, and myocardial contractility do not increase in response to adrenergic stimulation, and β_2-adrenergic vasodilatation is also blunted in ageing patients. This is not attributable to a reduction in the ability to increase catecholamines or to a reduction in β-receptor density in target tissues. The abnormal adrenergic responses stem from some point in calcium cycling between the sarcoplasmic reticulum and cytosol or between the cytosol and calcium receptors (eg, troponin-C). It is thought that beta-blockers and exercise retard or reverse this process of abnormal adrenergic response of ageing [3]. An increase in vascular stiffness results from the deposition of abnormal collagen in the vascular media and intima. The myocardium also becomes stiffer, impairing diastolic filling, because of hypertrophy, the presence of abnormal collagen, and the impaired rate of resequestration of calcium from troponin-C to the sarcoplasmic reticulum. Ventricular filling seems to be impaired principally after the rapid-filling phase. Angiotensin-converting enzyme (ACE) inhibitors are thought to minimize the hypertrophic process in blood vessels and the myocardium and to retard the process of abnormal collagen deposition. It is important to note that much of the beneficial effect of ACE inhibitors stems from their ability to block bradykininase, thus increasing the beneficial effects of bradykinin. Because nonsteroidal anti-inflammatory drugs (NSAIDs) block the brady-kininase inhibition of ACE inhibitors, the use of NSAIDs with ACE inhibitors is contentious [4]. Mitochondria in hearts of aged patients seem to be unable to produce increased amounts of ATP to fuel contraction or relaxation in response to stress. The β-adrenergic blocking agents may improve exercise capacity dramatically. Which of these issues is applicable to the ageing pet is unknown.

E-mail address: hamlin.1@osu.edu

0195-5616/05/$ - see front matter © 2005 Elsevier Inc. All rights reserved.
doi:10.1016/j.cvsm.2005.01.003   *vetsmall.theclinics.com*

Slightly more than 10% of dogs and an equal percentage of cats seen by a veterinarian have some form of heart disease, with more than 75% of the dogs having mitral regurgitation [4–6]. With an ageing population, close to 90% of the dogs with heart disease have mitral regurgitation, although we are recognizing that more and more ageing dogs have systemic arterial hypertension and pulmonary hypertension. The reason why the percentage afflicted with mitral regurgitation increases with age is that it is a developmental (possibly degenerative) disease; most dogs born with congenital heart disease died when they were young and did not reach old age or had the defect corrected surgically (eg, patent ductus arteriosus), and the defect is thus of no concern in old age. Mitral regurgitation (Fig. 1) is extremely important in the ageing population because it must be treated; if it is not, the cause of the symptoms for which the dog was presented must be known so that other causes may be sought. The second most common heart disease of old age, principally in larger dogs and English Cocker Spaniels, is probably dilated cardiomyopathy (Fig. 2A, B) [7]. The convenient feature of mitral regurgitation and dilated cardiomyopathy is that, with rare exceptions (eg, cardiomyopathy caused by L-carnitine deficiency), they are treated the same. We do not treat the "name of the disease"; rather, we treat to achieve general and specific goals (Box 1). Because we have the same goals for treating mitral regurgitation and dilated cardiomyopathy, they are treated the same.[1]

Myocardial fibrosis (see Fig. 2C) resulting from arteriosclerosis of small coronary arteries (see Fig. 2D) also occurs in aged dogs, often concomitantly with mitral regurgitation [5,6]. The importance of myocardial fibrosis depends on how extensive it is and whether or not peri-infarcted areas serve as a substrate for arrhythmia (see Fig. 2E). When extensive, the amount of contractile myocardium is reduced, resulting in reduced systolic function, and the substitution of fibrotic scars for contractile units makes the myocardium stiff and decreases ventricular filling. Finally, although not a primary heart disease but occurring commonly with heart disease and complicating the heart disease, pulmonary fibrosis with chronic obstructive lung disease occurs in dogs. This may result in pulmonary arterial hypertension and cor pulmonale heart disease secondary to lung disease.

Elevation of systemic arterial pressure (arterial hypertension) in dogs has become of greater interest in the ageing population. We are not certain precisely how important it is, because we do not know for certain what the normal limits of pressure are for dogs (particularly among different breeds and age groups) and the methods of measuring pressure are difficult (sometimes impossible) and contentious. Nonetheless, it is axiomatic, if we may extrapolate from human medicine, that systemic arterial hypertension

---

[1] It probably matters little whether a dog is ill as a result of one or the other.

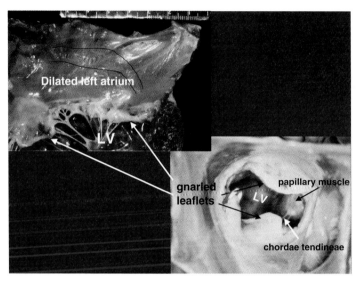

Fig. 1. Endocardiosis: thickened and gnarled leaflets of the mitral valve. Notice the left atrial tear, which healed naturally, between the black lines in the dilated left atrium and the leaflets of the mitral valve manifesting the endocardiosis. Note that these diseased leaflets allow you to view the left ventricle through the mitral orifice.

is important itself, and when combined with mitral regurgitation, it can become lethal.

Mitral regurgitation

For most dogs, with the exception being Cavalier King Charles Spaniels [8–12],[2] the prevalence of mitral regurgitation increases almost linearly with age, beginning at 5 or 6 years of age. Approximately 10% of dogs 6 years old have mitral regurgitation, but it may be present in as many as 60% of dogs that are 12 years old. It is more prevalent in male dogs and in small-breed dogs, particularly in breeds that are chondrodysplastic (eg, Cocker Spaniels, Dachshunds). This indicates a genetic (familial) basis for the disease. Ageing dogs with mitral regurgitation commonly have a plethora of other abnormalities, and it is not known whether they are merely concomitant because of ageing or if they may produce one another. For example, some believe [13,14] that periodontal disease with continual seeding of the bloodstream with bacteria results in endocardiosis, or at least aggravation of endocardiosis, producing mitral regurgitation. Presuming

---

[2] With Cavalier King Charles Spaniels, mitral regurgitation may begin at 2 to 3 years of age, and it usually progresses in severity much faster than in other breeds.

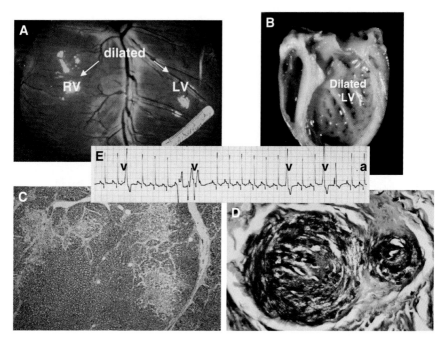

Fig. 2. (*A*) "Basketball-shaped" heart as a result of generalized cardiomegaly. (*B*) Heart section showing left ventricular dilatation. (*C*) Myocardial fibrosis (gray matter) "riddling" the myocardium. (*D*) Myointimal thickening of the small coronary artery with virtual obstruction of the lumen. (*E*) Ventricular (v) and atrial (a) premature depolarizations resulting from myocardial stretch or irritation around fibrotic regions.

that periodontal disease is a contributor to the development of mitral regurgitation, it is extremely important that good oral health be maintained.[3]

When the leaflets of the mitral valve become thickened and gnarled because of abnormal deposition of glycosaminoglycans (see Fig. 1), they fail to close the mitral orifice during ventricular contraction and blood leaks from the left ventricle into the left atrium (Fig. 3). The amount that leaks (ie, the seriousness of the disease) depends on the difference in pressure between the left ventricle and the left atrium, the size of the regurgitant orifice, and the duration that pressure in the left ventricle exceeds that in the left atrium. The volume of blood ejected by the left ventricle is the sum of blood normally traveling into the aorta and blood traveling regurgitantly

[3] I, for one, recommend that dogs with murmurs of mitral regurgitation receive a broad-spectrum antibiotic during dental or the procedures that might seed the bloodstream with bacteria. The thought is that the bacteria would never cause problems in hearts with a normal structure, but with structural defects, bacteria may adhere to the defect and accelerate the pathologic process. This has yet to be proven.

Box 1. General and specific goals of therapy

General goals of therapy (eg, how to achieve them)
1. Prolong life (eg, ACE inhibitors, spironolactone, carvedilol)
2. Decrease symptoms (eg, furosemide, theophylline)
3. Retard or reverse disease process (eg, ACE inhibitors, spironolactone, carvedilol)
4. Avoid and/or reduce troublesome events (ie, monitor therapeutic responses, understand potential for drug interactions)
5. Reduce need for resources

Specific goals for treating mitral regurgitation and dilated cardiomyopathy
1. Minimize vascular and myocardial remodeling
2. Adjust heart rate and rhythm
3. Reduce edema
4. "Upregulate" high-pressure baroreceptors
5. Improve cardiac output
6. Improve oxygenation

---

into the left atrium. The ratio of the amount regurgitating to the amount traveling into the aorta is termed the *regurgitant fraction*. The regurgitant fraction may not be large, but enough mitral regurgitation may occur so as to enlarge the left atrium sufficiently to compress the left mainstem bronchus (Fig. 4), and the dog may exhibit a hacking cough in the absence of pulmonary edema or reduced systemic arterial pressure. When the regurgitant fraction reaches or exceeds 100% (ie, as much of the left ventricular stroke volume regurgitates into the left atrium as travels antegrade into the aorta) congestion of pulmonary vessels and pulmonary edema often develop and cardiac output may be inadequate to sustain normal function.

Symptoms resulting from mitral regurgitation may include cough, dyspnea, exercise incapacity, and syncope [4–6]. Classes of mitral regurgitation are shown in Box 2, and functional classification is shown in Box 3. The classes represent a continuum in which the disease state never reverses. For example, an aged dog is always in at least class A; once that dog develops endocardiosis but is asymptomatic, it can never return to class A or become less than class B. This method of classification helps the veterinarian to talk with clients about their pet's health and to understand the need for a level of surveillance or therapy.

An animal may be in a functional class and progress to a higher functional class or may actually reverse in response to therapy. For example, a dog may be severely exercise intolerant and be in functional class III but

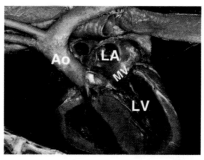

Normal   **Regurgitation**

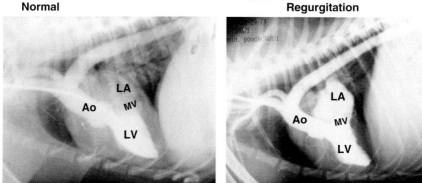

Fig. 3. Left lateral section of the thorax (*top*) and angiocardiograms (*bottom*) with indicator injected into the left ventricle. Note opacification of the left atrium with mitral regurgitation. LA, left atrium; LV, left ventricle; MV, mitral orifice; Ao, aorta.

may return to functional class II with an ACE inhibitor and diuretic. Thus, it is reasonable to rate a dog with geriatric mitral regurgitation as A, B, C, or D, followed by I, II, III, or IV; however, class D and functional class IV are quite similar, with the difference being that a dog may be reduced (albeit rarely) from functional class IV to functional class III but can never be reduced from class D to class C. This method of classifying heart disease may prove useful for determining a therapeutic strategy, for prognosis, and, again, for proposing a level of surveillance.[4]

Although unproven in dogs, people with heart failure have a worse prognosis if they have concurrent elevation of serum creatinine[5] and microalbuminuria, indicating renal disease, hypoalbuminemia, or hyponatremia. The same is probably true with dogs; therefore, frequent measure-

---

[4] My opinion is that any dog considered old should be auscultated carefully to search for a murmur every 6 months to a year and that yearly thoracic radiographs might also be indicated to serve as a standard against which to compare subsequent radiographs and search for cardiomegaly and pulmonary disease (eg, neoplasia, pulmonary fibrosis).

[5] Even if the creatinine remains within "normal"limits but is elevated from a previous time, the elevation carries increased risk for worsening of heart failure.

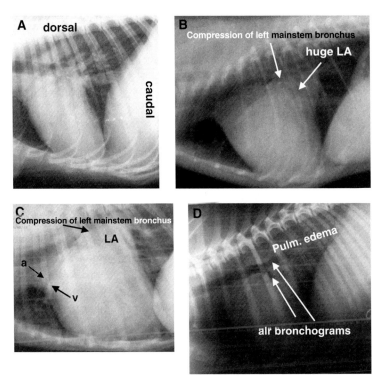

Fig. 4. Lateral thoracic radiographs from dogs. (*A*) Normal dog. (*B*) Gigantic left atrium compressing left mainstem bronchus. (*C*) Same as in *B* but also pulmonary venous (v) engorgement. Note that the venous engorgement is larger than pulmonary artery (a) in the same lobe of lung. (*D*) Pulmonary edema in caudal-dorsal lung lobes. LA, left atrium.

ments of serum creatinine, sodium, and albumin as well as a search for microalbuminuria are indicated; every effort should be made to sustain renal function as normally as possible[6] and to sustain serum sodium and albumin within normal limits.

Pharmacologic classification of heart disease

It is tempting to try to prevent an ageing dog, a younger Cavalier King Charles Spaniel, or a dog with periodontal disease (by definition, in class A) on a therapeutic regimen from evolving to class B or to prevent a dog in class B from progressing to class C or D or to functional class II, III, or IV

---

[6] My personal belief is that this is a further indication for administration of ACE inhibitors (which are proven to stabilize glomerular function in all instances of kidney disease) so as to limit diuretics to what is absolutely necessary to control pulmonary congestion and to make certain that the patient does not become dehydrated for other reasons.

Box 2. Classes (continuum) of heart disease

A. Prone and/or at risk to develop heart disease (eg, Cavalier King Charles Spaniel, old age, possibly periodontal disease)
B. Anatomic or physiologic cardiovascular abnormality (eg, endocardiosis, left-sided cardiomegaly)
C. Symptoms at one time or another related to heart disease (eg, cough, shortness of breath, syncope, exercise intolerance)
D. Severe symptoms and/or limitations, high risk of dying

---

from functional class I. There is serious and active debate as to whether cessation or slowing of progression can be accomplished, at least with ACE inhibitors [11,12], the drug class purported to retard the progression. This debate stems from the absence of knowledge of the origin of these diseases and what determines their evolution because of the heterogeneity of the population of afflicted dogs and because large multicenter studies have not been conducted. Nonetheless, the following is an attempt to address the issue of precisely when, in the course of ageing dogs with mitral regurgitation or at risk for developing mitral regurgitation, each drug should be given, how to identify success or failure, and when enough of each drug has been given. The classification is based on observations of signs and symptoms through the physical examination, radiography, electrocardiography, echocardiography, and blood chemistry. Whatever decisions are to be made about therapy, or whether or not a diagnostic test should be ordered, there should be a reasonable expectation that the test or drug is likely to change the outcome of the case or provide the client with information that he or she desires (eg, prognosis).[7] If we use data on file with the US Food and Drug Administration (FDA) proving safety and efficacy for a drug to treat heart disease, we would use only enalapril,[8] because that is the only drug with proven safety and efficacy. Digitalis and furosemide are approved, but there is no evidence for efficacy and little for safety.[9] Table 1 summarizes a scheme to determine objective criteria on precisely when to give each drug.

Approach to the patient

The patient should be approached with the intent of improving comfort, doing something to slow or reverse the trend of disease, and allowing

---

[7] The client should not be expected to pay for the drug or the test just because it is available, because others do it, or because of intellectual curiosity on the part of the veterinarian.
[8] Furosemide, digitalis, benazepril, ramipril, and pimobendan are approved in Canada, Europe, and Japan.
[9] I personally believe that furosemide and digitalis are efficacious.

Box 3. Functional classification of heart disease

I. Heart disease but no physical limitations (asymptomatic)
II. Symptoms present with only the most severe activity
III. Symptoms with slight activity
IV. Symptoms at rest

---

reasonable prognostication, which are things the client may expect. Although it may be intellectually rewarding to uncover a cause, we can rarely, if ever,[10] remove the causative agent in degenerative cardiovascular diseases of old age, and arriving at a diagnosis or placing a name on a pathologic entity does not necessarily mean that we can alter the outcome. We identify specific pathologic features (eg, dilatation, hypertrophy, tachycardia, regurgitation) that we hope to modify to prevent worsening morbidity or mortality. For example, aged dogs with mitral regurgitation or dilated cardiomyopathy may have left ventricular and left atrial dilatation, a rapid ventricular response (ie, high ventricular rate), and pulmonary edema, which lead to worsening morbidity and to mortality; our job is to identify and mitigate the causes of worsening, and it matters little what specific causes resulted in those symptoms.[11] What does matter, however, is that we know enough about the disease process so that we can (hopefully) intervene to make the patient more comfortable and live longer. Table 1 contains a list of pathologic features (and drugs used to modify them) that we must identify in our approach to the patient.

Because most cardiovascular diseases of ageing dogs affect the left side of the heart and result in dyspnea or exercise intolerance, we must identify, and hopefully ameliorate, the causes of dyspnea and exercise incapacity.

Auscultation

Although history, anamnesis, and inspection should initiate any approach to a patient, for the sake of this discussion, we presume that the dog is aged, has a systolic murmur heard with maximal intensity at the left fifth or sixth intercostal space near the costochondral juncture, and that the murmur becomes softer during inspiration and louder during expiration. Although it has been reported in Cavalier King Charles Spaniels [10,15] that

---

[10] A notable exception is the seemingly miraculous cure accomplished by giving L-carnitine to a dog with dilated cardiomyopathy resulting from carnitine deficiency.

[11] With ability to modify mitral regurgitation by surgery, it may be more important to identify its presence; however, most experiences with attempts to modify the regurgitation surgically are extremely expensive and/or failures.

Table 1
Objective criteria on when to use each drug for treating mitral regurgitation

Criterion	Drug	Goal
Left atrial enlargement	Angiotensin-converting enzyme inhibitor	↓ regurgitation and ↑ cardiac output by ↓ afterload, ↓ remodeling, protects against tachyphylaxis to nitroglycerin
Left ventricular enlargement	a. Digitalis b. Spironolactone c. Carvedilol	a. Heart rate, ↓ regurgitant fraction, ↑ baroreceptors, ↑ diaphragm b. ↓ remodeling c. ↓ heart rate, arrhythmia, oxidant stress
Pulmonary venous engorgement and/or wheezing	theophylline	↓ bronchoconstriction
Ventricular ectopia	sotalol	↓ heart rate, ↓ irritability
Atrial fibrillation	diltiazem	↓ ventricular response
Pulmonary edema	furosemide	↑ urine by affecting loop of Henle, ↓ ventricular preload by venodilatation
Refractory pulmonary edema	a. Thiazide b. Nitroglycerin	a. ↑ urine by affecting distal convolute tubule b. Venodilate and shift blood from lungs to peripheral veins

Abbreviations: ↓, decrease; ↑, increase.

the louder the murmur, the more serious the disease (ie, the greater the morbidity and mortality), the same is not true in people with mitral regurgitation, that is not my opinion in most dogs with mitral regurgitation, and there are theoretic arguments against that conclusion. In particular, the intensity of a murmur depends on (1) the velocity of blood regurgitating (eg, how vigorously the left ventricle contracts), (2) the area of the regurgitant jet, (3) the direction that the regurgitant jet takes into the left atrium, (4) the acoustic conducting properties of the thorax (eg, lung volume, subcutaneous fat), and (5) the phase of respiration (louder murmur during expiration than during inspiration). The primary impact of auscultating a left apical systolic murmur in an ageing dog is that it indicates mitral regurgitation. It is not an indication for treatment, but it is an indication to examine the dog more extensively, principally by radiography, to determine if a requirement for therapy exists.

Because heart disease almost always worsens, and worsening is manifested by cardiomegaly, increased heart rate, atrial or ventricular arrhythmia, myocardial fibrosis, or arteriosclerosis (morphologic and electrophysiologic changes termed *remodeling*), it may be appropriate to initiate anti-remodeling therapy early in the disease course. Thus, spironolactone, ACE inhibitors, and the β-adrenergic blocker carvedilol may be indicated not at the first sign of murmur but at the first sign of cardiomegaly.

Bronchial breath sounds

Bronchial breath sounds are abnormally intense inspiratory, much louder than expected, and higher pitched expiratory vesicular breath sounds caused by air tumbling through larger airways. Vesicular breath sounds are, in fact, murmurs produced not by high-velocity blood flow but by high-velocity air flow. When the pulmonary parenchyma is wet, heavy (as in congestion), or dense, the vesicular breath sounds "made" by air flowing through large airways are transmitted with greater than usual intensity through the dense lungs to the surface of the thorax. A murmur of mitral regurgitation and bronchial breath sounds in an ageing dog are indications for the use of diuretics to reduce the pulmonary edema.

Crackles

Crackles are so-called "adventitious" (ie, not caused by air flowing into or out of the lungs) breath sounds. They are produced by airways "scrunching" closed during end-expiration and "popping" open during midinspiration. Crackles occur when the lung is wet and heavy, such as occurs with pneumonia or pulmonary edema, or when the pulmonary parenchyma is shrunken and gnarled, such as occurs with pulmonary fibrosis. Edematous or pneumonic crackles are most often soft and high pitched, whereas crackles of fibrosis are usually extremely loud and "ugly" sounding. If the crackles result from edema, this is a clear indication for use of a diuretic. Because crackles indicate airways closing, a form of chronic obstructive lung disease, it is appropriate to initiate bronchodilator therapy with theophylline or terbutaline. In addition, theophylline strengthens ventilation muscles and may return tidal volume toward normal. Animals with crackles are commonly cyanotic. Cyanosis results from too much unoxygenated hemoglobin enters the arterial blood. This occurs because airways, which have collapsed and thus produce crackles, do not contain enough oxygen to oxygenate the pulmonary capillary blood.

Dyspnea and tachypnea

Dyspnea or labored breathing reflects increased effort of ventilation or an increased rate of ventilation; tachypnea is an increase in the rate of respiration. Tachypnea is detected best when the pet is quiet or sleeping. Most dogs or cats (as well as people) breathe fewer than 18 times a minute. The size of the animal does not influence the respiratory rate; a sleeping

Chihuahua breathes at the same rate as a sleeping Great Dane. When the motion of the lung is limited for any reason (eg, edema, pneumonia, fibrosis, space-occupying mass), the animal can achieve normal ventilation more easily by decreasing the tidal volume than by increasing the breathing rate. A minute ventilation of 2400 mL/min is achieved by a healthy dog at a respiratory rate of 18 breaths per minute with a tidal volume of 150 mL/breath, whereas a dog with a stiff lung may achieve the same 2400-mL/min ventilation at a respiratory rate of 36 breaths per minute and a tidal volume of 75 mL. The reduced tidal volume minimizes the risk of fatiguing muscles of ventilation when the lung is stiff because of congestion or edema. Because tachypnea in the presence of mitral regurgitation usually indicates pulmonary congestion and edema, as mentioned previously, it indicates the need for diuretics. If diuretics are inadequate, it may be useful to initiate therapy with a venodilator, such as nitroglycerin. Nitroglycerin, intravenously administered furosemide, and ACE inhibitors are venodilators. Venodilatation results in the "stealing" of blood from the lungs and subsequent reduction of pulmonary congestion and edema.

Percussion

A veterinarian skilled in the practice of percussion can detect a relatively dense lung or pleural effusion, because when he or she "thumps" (percusses) on a region of the thorax below which there is an increase in density (lung or pleural fluid), the note of percussion is relatively dull when compared with the note of percussion over an air-filled structure. Thus, in the hands of an unusually skilled diagnostician,[12] percussion may be used as a complement or, at times, even as a substitute to auscultation and radiography.

Radiography

Well-positioned lateral and dorsoventral thoracic radiographs (Figs. 5 and 6) of an ageing dog produce an enormous amount of potentially valuable information on which diagnostic, prognostic, and therapeutic decisions can be based. It is reasonable to obtain thoracic radiographs from any patient with a murmur of mitral regurgitation. The murmur tells us that the disease is present, but the radiographs tell us if specific treatment is necessary. Specific observations from radiographs allow for semiquantitation of the severity of heart disease and imply specific goals of therapy (see Fig. 4; Fig. 7). For example, the degree of left atrial enlargement in an aged dog predicts how limiting the disease process may be to longevity and quality of life (Fig. 8);

---

[12] It is "magical" to watch an examiner who is skilled in percussion identify a state of disease; however, few examiners practice percussion today.

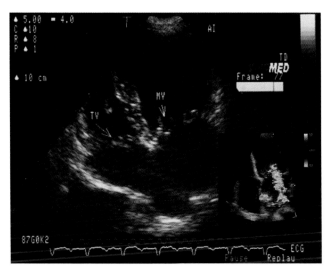

Fig. 5. Echocardiogram from a dog with mitral regurgitation. Mitral valve (MV) leaflet, with arrow pointing from left ventricle toward left atrium. Inset shows color-Doppler image with blood regurgitating through the mitral orifice into the left atrium. (Courtesy of Bruce Keene, DVM, PhD, North Carolina State University, Raleigh, NC.)

thus, it indicates a need to reverse the disease process (which can be done only rarely) or to retard (eg, with ACE inhibitors, spironolactone, carvedilol) the pathogenetic process (ie, remodeling) to which the enlargement is attributed. With the rare exception of mitral stenosis, the more severe the disease is, the larger is the left ventricle. This must be a reality, because the left atrium may

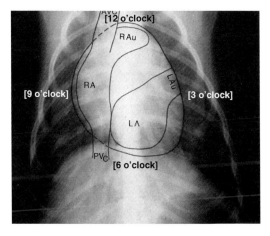

Fig. 6. Dorsoventral radiograph of thorax with contribution of left auricle from 1 to 3 o'clock. AVC, anterior vena cava; LA, left atrium; LAu, left auricle; PV$_C$, posterior vena cava; RA, right atrium; RAu, right auricle.

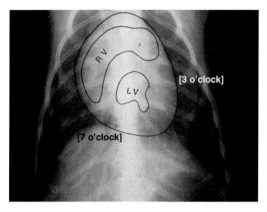

Fig. 7. Dorsoventral radiograph of the thorax demonstrating contribution of the ventricle from 3 to 7 o'clock. LV, left ventricle; RV, right ventricle.

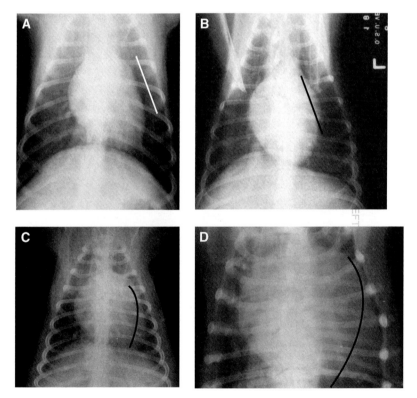

Fig. 8. Dorsoventral thoracic radiographs from a normal dog (*A*), a dog with left atrial enlargement and a "bowing-out" cardiac silhouette from 1 to 3 o'clock (*B*), a dog with left atrial and early left ventricular enlargement (*C*), and a dog with generalized cardiomegaly (*D*).

only become enlarged if the pressure within it is elevated. Because left atrial pressure (along with pleural pressure and left ventricular myocardial stiffness) is a prime determinant of left ventricular volume, left atrial dilatation precedes left ventricular dilatation. Left ventricular distention is particularly bad, because stretching myocardial fibers injures them and may result in arrhythmia, causing them to generate increased tension to attain the same pressure, and causes them to demand more oxygen. The increased tension and myocardial oxygen demand may result in myocardial oxygen deprivation, which leads to further reductions in systolic and diastolic function. Thus, left ventricular distention indicates the need for a positive inotrope (eg, digitalis, pimobendan), an anti-remodeling agent (eg, spirono-lactone, ACE inhibitor), and a compound (eg, carvedilol) that is antiarrhythmic and a scavenger of free radicals of oxygen. Pulmonary congestion, pulmonary edema, pleural effusion, pulmonary neoplasia, and pulmonary fibrosis may also be observed on thoracic radiographs. In fact, as may be implied from Table 1, it may be possible to select drugs based on observations made from thoracic radiographs. For this reason, it seems reasonable to obtain thoracic radiographs yearly if a murmur of mitral regurgitation is present and certainly any time that the patient manifests a significant change in symptoms or signs. When interrogated by a client as to why a radiograph is being taken, the answer should be, "because the radiograph provides information about the need for additional therapy."

Electrocardiography

A complete multilead electrocardiogram (ECG) or a single lead II (Fig. 9), aVF, or V3 ECG may be useful in the approach to an aged pet. Although the ECG has many false-negative results in identifying chamber enlargement (ie, limited sensitivity), when an ECG criterion for enlargement is present, chamber enlargement usually is present (ie, high specificity). The ECG has no equal for studying heart rate and rhythm, however. When the heart rate exceeds 150 beats per minute, it is extremely difficult to count; it may be quantified without error from an ECG. When premature depolarizations indicating electrophysiologic abnormalities occur, however, the ECG is the most reliable method for detecting their presence and the focus (or foci) of origin (ie, supraventricular, ventricular). Myocardial disease may be identified by a broadening of the descent of the R waves (Fig. 10), whereas premature depolarizations and atrial fibrillation, common sequelae to left atrial enlargement of any cause, may be identified and the ventricular rate quantified. One of the most important goals in treating ageing dogs with atrial fibrillation caused by mitral regurgitation or dilated cardiomyopathy is to slow the ventricular rate. Thus, the ECG may be the only means of determining that the heart rate is, for example, 240 beats per minute; that the rhythm is, in fact, atrial fibrillation and not ventricular tachycardia; and that the ventricular rate slows in response to a digitalis

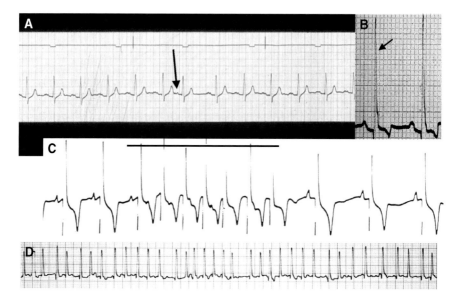

Fig. 9. Lead II electrocardiograms from dogs with mitral regurgitation showing broad notched P waves of left atrial enlargement and atrial premature depolarization (*arrow*) (*A*), a tall R wave (*arrow*) indicating left ventricular enlargement (*B*), a bout of atrial tachycardia (*line on top*) (*C*), and atrial fibrillation (no P waves and rapid and irregular appearances of QRS complexes (*D*).

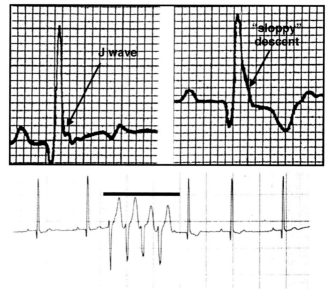

Fig. 10. (*Top*) Lead II electrocardiograms from a normal dog (*left*) and a dog with an aged myocardium showing "sloppy" descent of an R wave (*arrow*). Do not confuse the sloppy descent with the normal J wave at the bottom of the R wave.

glycoside (digoxin), a calcium channel blocker (diltiazem), or a β-adrenergic blocker (carvedilol).

Echocardiography

Echocardiography (see Fig. 5) has added a new dimension to the understanding of the pathophysiology of heart disease and to the diagnosis and quantification of complex cardiovascular disease [15–17]. The contribution of echocardiography to therapy is less impressive, and the actual contribution of echocardiography in changing the outcome of cases of ageing pets with heart disease is seldom discussed, probably because it, too, is less impressive. In the hands of a skillful operator, the echocardiogram has no equal for confirming the diagnosis of pericardial disease, cardiac neoplasms, pulmonary hypertension, or restrictive cardiomyopathies (which constitute less than 5% of geriatric heart disease); however, the specific knowledge gained by echocardiography, compared with that acquired by means of the physical examination and radiography, does not often translate into benefits for the patient.

Blood chemistry

As mentioned previously, analysis of blood chemicals may be extremely important for the diagnosis, prognosis, and therapy of heart disease in animals of any age. Azotemia (elevation of creatinine) in the presence of heart disease indicates a worse prognosis. It may indicate that cardiac output and renal blood flow are severely compromised because of the failing circulation. In addition, it may indicate that therapy with diuretics is too aggressive or needs to be so aggressive to relieve congestion and edema that prerenal azotemia is produced. Reductions in serum sodium or albumin carry extremely guarded prognoses—a reduction in sodium, because it indicates the need for such aggressive diuresis, and a reduction in protein, because it indicates hepatic involvement resulting in failure to produce albumin or gastrointestinal pathologic change (edema) limiting absorption of products required for production of protein. Hypokalemia also carries a more guarded prognosis. It, too, indicates that the heart disease is so bad that aggressive diuresis is necessary; in addition, hypokalemia increases the risk of digitalis toxicity, decreases efficacy of lidocaine and other antiarrhythmics, and may sensitize the animal to the development of the ventricular arrhythmias.

If we may extrapolate knowledge gained from experience in treating aged people with heart disease, some interesting questions arise with respect to treating aged dogs with heart disease [3,18–20]. Are there monumental difficulties in extrapolating from human beings to dogs because of the important role that the coronary artery disease plays in people and the insignificant role that it probably plays in dogs? ACE inhibitors reduce morbidity and mortality significantly in people with heart disease, but β-adrenergic blockers decrease mortality even more. At what time in dealing with aged dogs with heart disease should they be given these agents...if at all? What doses should be used and at what frequency? Which geriatric heart diseases might benefit most, or at all, from therapy? What is the importance of an aerobic exercise program? In people, it has been proven to reduce morbidity and mortality.

Many ageing pets with heart disease constitute an ethical dilemma. This is particularly pertinent to the veterinarian, because euthanasia is legal and acceptable. We must deal with more than the issue of whether we can sustain the pet's life. We must ask, what are the financial and psychologic burdens to the owner? Are we sustaining the pet's life because we can; does our ego prohibit us from recommending euthanasia (ie, we are too good to let the pet die)? Is it worth prolonging a pet's life for 2 days, 2 weeks, or 2 months, after which time the owner still must make a decision about euthanasia or continued treatment? The veterinarian has a responsibility to the owner, but I believe even more so to the pet. I believe it is our responsibility to recommend euthanasia when we believe the quality of the pet's life has reached a particular threshold. I believe it is appropriate to plant the seed of euthanasia in the minds of the owners or at least to give the owner your opinion about when enough is enough (eg, dyspnea at rest, anorexia, indifference to the owner). Clearly, the decision is made by the owner, but many owners do not know how to make the decision, and I believe it is unethical for a veterinarian to withhold a recommendation for euthanasia until the owner asks when a pet may be miserable, and the veterinarian is the person most qualified to steer the process.

There is a potential to slow the progression of heart disease in dogs with mitral regurgitation by surgical interventions [17,21–23], but these remain in the experimental stage, have high operative mortality, are rather expensive, and are not performed at many centers.

In conclusion, it is clear that (1) a discussion of the diagnosis and therapy of heart disease in an aged pet does not differ significantly from that in a pet of any age, (2) mitral regurgitation constitutes by far the most important geriatric heart disease, and (3) the selection of drugs to treat heart disease of ageing pets is based on identification of specific pathologic features (eg, atrial fibrillation, left atrial enlargement) for which each aspect of treatment (eg, diuretics, ACE inhibitors, spironolactone) is specific.

References

[1] Lakatta EG. Circulatory function in younger and older humans in health. In: Hazzard WR, Blass JP, Ettinger WH, et al, editors. Principles of geriatric medicine and gerontology. 4th edition. New York: McGraw Hill; 1999. p. 645–60.
[2] Rich M. The cardiovascular system. Heart failure. In: Hazzard WR, Blass JP, Ettinger WH, et al, editors. Principles of geriatric medicine and gerontology. 4th edition. New York: McGraw Hill; 1999. p. 679–700.

[3] Bean JF, Vora A, Frontera WR. Benefits of exercise for community-dwelling older adults. Arch Phys Med Rehabil 2004;85(7 Suppl 3):S31–42.

[4] Buchanan JW. Valvular disease (endocardiosis in dogs). Adv Vet Sci Comp Med 1979;21: 75–99.

[5] Detweiler DK, Patterson DF. The prevalence and types of cardiovascular diseased in dogs. Ann NY Acad Sci 1965;127:481–93.

[6] Detweiler DK, Luginbuhl H, Buchanan JW, et al. The natural history of acquired cardiac disability in the dog. Ann NY Acad Sci 1968;147:318–29.

[7] Tidholm A, Haggstrom J, Borgarelli M, et al. Canine idiopathic dilated cardiomyopathy. Part I: aetiology, clinical characteristics, epidemiology and pathology. Vet J 2001;162: 92–107.

[8] Haggstrom J, Duelund Pedersen H, Kvart C. New insights into degenerative mitral valve disease in dogs. Vet Clin N Am Small Anim Pract 1998;28:1057–62.

[9] Haggstrom J, Hansson K, Kvart C, et al. Chronic valvular disease in the Cavalier King Charles spaniel in Sweden. Vet Rec 1992;131:549–53.

[10] Haggstrom J, Kvart C, Hansson K. Heart sounds and murmurs: changes related to severity of chronic valvular disease in the Cavalier King Charles spaniel. J Vet Intern Med 1995;9: 75–85.

[11] Kvart C, Haggstrom J, Pedersen HD. ACE inhibitors in dogs with subclinical chronic mitral insufficiency [in German]. Tijdschr Diergeneeskd 2003;128:76–7.

[12] Kvart C, Haggstrom J, Pedersen HD, et al. Efficacy of enalapril for prevention of congestive heart failure in dogs with myxomatous valve disease and asymptomatic mitral regurgitation. J Vet Intern Med 2002;16:80–8.

[13] DeBowes LJ, Mosier D, Logan E, et al. Association of periodontal disease and histologic lesions in multiple organs from 45 dogs. J Vet Dent 1996;13:57–60.

[14] DeBowes LJ. The effects of dental disease on systemic disease. Vet Clin Pract 2004;34: 1209–26.

[15] Pedersen HD, Haggstrom J, Falk T, et al. Auscultation in mild mitral regurgitation in dogs: observer variation, effects of physical maneuvers, and agreement with color Doppler echocardiography and phonocardiography. J Vet Intern Med 1999;13:56–64.

[16] Choi H, Lee K, Lee H, et al. Quantification of mitral regurgitation using proximal isovelocity surface area method in dogs. J Vet Sci 2004;5:163–71.

[17] Sadanaga KK, MacDonald MJ, Buchanan JW. Echocardiography and surgery in a dog with left atrial rupture and hemopericardium. J Vet Intern Med 1990;4:216–21.

[18] Ahmed A, Dell'Italia LJ. Use of beta-blockers in older adults with chronic heart failure. Am J Med Sci 2004;328:100–11.

[19] Hanon O. Heart failure, a disease of the elderly [in French]. Presse Med 2004;33:1079–82.

[20] Le Couteur DG, Hilmer SN, Glasgow N, et al. Prescribing in older people. Aust Fam Physician 2004;33:777–81.

[21] Buchanan JW, Sammarco CD. Circumferential suture of the mitral annulus for correction of mitral regurgitation in dogs. Vet Surg 1998;27:182–93.

[22] Griffiths LG, Orton EC, Boon JA. Evaluation of techniques and outcomes of mitral valve repair in dogs. J Am Vet Med Assoc 2004;224:1941–5.

[23] Kollar A, Kekesi V, Soos P, et al. Left ventricular external subannular plication: an indirect off-pump mitral annuloplasty method in a canine model. J Thorac Cardiovasc Surg 2003; 126:977–82.

ELSEVIER
SAUNDERS

Vet Clin Small Anim
35 (2005) 617–634

VETERINARY
CLINICS
Small Animal Practice

Liver Disease in the Geriatric Patient

Johnny D. Hoskins, DVM, PhD*

DocuTech Services Inc., Choudrant, LA 71227, USA

Hepatic diseases of the dog

Chronic inflammatory hepatopathies

Infections, drugs, or copper accumulation can cause chronic hepatitis, or it can possibly occur in an immune-mediated form. The pathologic process involved in chronic hepatitis often begins with necrosis, followed by infiltration of the liver with lymphocytes, plasma cells, or macrophages, which may lead to hepatic fibrosis and cirrhosis. Viral infection, such as infectious canine hepatitis and canine acidophil hepatitis, and bacterial infection, such as canine leptospirosis, can cause acute and chronic hepatitis. Although these diseases tend to cause hepatic necrosis in their early stages, they may result in the same type of chronic injury seen with other chronic hepatopathies.

Almost any drug has the capacity to produce an idiosyncratic reaction in any given individual; some drugs are more likely to be associated with chronic hepatic inflammation in dogs, especially older animals. Administration of primidone, phenobarbital, clomipramine, oxibendazole-diethyl-carbamazine, or nonsteroidal anti-inflammatory drugs (NSAIDs) has been associated with periportal hepatitis and hepatic vacuolar change.

A familial predisposition to develop chronic hepatitis has been suggested in certain dog breeds. Breeds at increased risk for chronic hepatitis include the Bedlington Terrier, West Highland White Terrier, Doberman Pinscher, American and English Cocker Spaniel, Skye Terrier, Labrador Retriever, Standard Poodle, and others (Box 1).

Abnormal hepatic retention of dietary copper and copper hepatopathy occurs in Bedlington Terrier dogs [1]. An autosomal recessive mode of inheritance is involved; only individuals homozygous for the recessive gene develop the excess copper accumulation in hepatic lysosomes. Hepatic

* PO Box 389, Choudrant, LA 71227, USA.
   E-mail address: jdhoskins@mindspring.com

Box 1. Dog breeds with increased chronic hepatic disease associated with copper accumulation

Airedale Terrier
Bedlington Terrier[a]
Boxer
Bulldog
Bull terrier
American and English Cocker Spaniel
Collie
Dachshund
Dalmatian
Doberman Pinscher[a]
Wire-Haired Fox Terrier
German Shepherd Dog
Golden Retriever
Keeshond
Kerry Blue Terrier
Labrador Retriever
Norwich Terrier
Old English Sheepdog
Pekingese
Standard Poodle
Samoyed
Schnauzer
Skye Terrier[a]
West Highland White Terrier[a]

---

[a] Hereditary mechanism for increased hepatic copper.
Data from Rolfe DS, Twedt DC. Copper-associated hepatopathies in dogs. Vet Clin North Am Small Anim Pract 1995;25:399.

---

copper concentrations exceeding 2000 µg/g of dry tissue are consistently associated with morphologic and functional evidence of the progressive hepatopathy that progresses to chronic hepatitis and cirrhosis over time [1,2]. Diagnosis of copper-associated hepatopathy in Bedlington Terrier dogs can be made by examination of hepatic tissue for excessive copper storage or by performing genetic tests on DNA samples collected from suspected dogs. The frequency of the recessive gene in Bedlington Terrier dogs is estimated to be as high as 50% in the United States, with a similar frequency in England. This means that more than 25% of Bedlington Terrier dogs are "affected," and another 50% are "carriers."

The DNA samples can be collected using a soft cheek brush that is provided by a commercial genetic laboratory. By gently brushing the inside of the dog's cheek, cells containing DNA are removed. The collected DNA samples then are analyzed to determine the genetic status of the suspect dog. Useful for dogs of any age, the DNA sample collection and analysis activities can be completed before puppies are purchased at 6 to 10 weeks. The results of the DNA testing also may be formally registered with the Orthopedic Foundation for Animals. For further information about the Orthopedic Foundation for Animal's Registry for Copper Toxicosis in Bedlington Terriers, contact the Orthopedic Foundation for Animals (2300 East Nifong Boulevard, Columbia, MO 65201–3856; available at: http://www.offa.org/dnageninfo.html).

Primary hepatobiliary disease associated with an increased accumulation of hepatic copper, albeit smaller amounts of tissue copper than in Bedlington Terriers, has been described in Doberman Pinscher, Skye Terrier, West Highland White Terrier, and American and English Cocker Spaniel dogs [3–5]. The chronic hepatitis associated with an increased liver copper content in Doberman Pinscher dogs occurs primarily in middle-aged female dogs. A familial copper-associated liver disease occurs in West Highland White Terrier dogs [5]. Hepatic copper concentrations in affected dogs have ranged as high as 3500 ppm, which is considerably lower than the maximal values recorded for Bedlington Terriers. Liver disease has also been observed with unexpected frequency in American and English Cocker Spaniel dogs [3]. The liver disease seems to be progressive, and dogs dying because of hepatic cirrhosis have had hepatic copper concentrations three to five times normal.

Primary copper hepatopathy as the inciting cause of liver disease should be considered in those breeds known to have an increased incidence of copper retention (see Box 1). The diagnosis is confirmed by liver biopsy, revealing copper-containing granules in excess of what might be considered normal for the degree of cholestasis and fibrosis seen [6].

Dogs with chronic hepatitis of any cause usually have a slowly progressive onset of disease characterized by depression, weight loss, anorexia, and polyuria (PU) and/or polydipsia (PD). Laboratory evaluation of dogs with chronic hepatitis can vary depending on the stage of disease. Initially, affected dogs have marked increases in serum alanine aminotransferase (ALT) and aspartate aminotransferase (AST) activities, with little evidence of cholestasis or liver dysfunction. As the disease progresses, cholestasis develops, with increases in serum alkaline phosphatase (ALP) activity and total bilirubin concentration. Liver function progressively decreases, first seen in serum bile acid concentrations and later obvious in serum albumin, urea nitrogen, glucose, and coagulation factor concentrations.

Abdominal radiographs are unremarkable, except when a small liver or ascites accompanies advanced stages of the liver disease. Ultrasonography of the liver may be normal in the early stages of chronic hepatitis, or nonspecific changes in echogenicity may be detected. Potential ultrasonographic findings with hepatic cirrhosis include a small liver, irregular liver lobe margins, focal lesions representing regenerative nodules, increased parenchymal echogenicity associated with fibrous tissue, and ascites. Splenomegaly may also be detected.

The histopathologic findings from liver biopsies include piecemeal necrosis, bridging necrosis (presence of inflammatory cells bridging the limiting plate between lobules), and active cirrhosis. Specimens should also be stained to detect copper, although the presence of excess copper in a liver with severe cholestasis and cirrhosis could be secondary copper hepatopathy. If sufficient liver tissue is obtained, copper concentrations within the liver should be determined.

If a probable cause of hepatic injury can be determined, specific treatment is directed at removing the primary cause, such as replacing anticonvulsant primidone or phenobarbital therapy with potassium bromide therapy, treating for canine leptospirosis with antimicrobial agents, or chelating hepatic copper with penicillamine. In most cases, specific treatment is not available. Some of the drugs used in the treatment of chronic hepatitis are presented in Table 1 [7].

Therapy for copper-associated hepatopathy includes reduction in dietary copper and chelation therapy. Currently, drugs used for copper chelation are penicillamine and trientine dihydrochloride. Penicillamine is effective at reducing hepatic copper concentrations, although the rate of hepatic "decoppering" is slow [8]. Trientine is as effective as penicillamine at reducing hepatic copper concentrations and is currently being used when penicillamine-associated vomiting occurs. Bedlington Terriers, West Highland White Terriers, and, possibly, Doberman Pinschers may benefit from copper chelation or oral zinc therapy as part of their therapeutic plan.

Other therapies that can be considered in dogs with chronic hepatitis include corticosteroids and antifibrotic drugs. Corticosteroids have immu-

Table 1
Drugs used in the management of chronic hepatitis in older dogs

Drug	Dosage	Indication
D-penicillamine	10–15 mg/kg q 12 hours	Copper chelation, antifibrotic
Trientine	15–30 mg/kg q 12 hours	Copper chelation
Zinc acetate	1.5–4 mg/kg elemental zinc q 24 hours	Decrease copper absorption
Prednisone	0.5–2.0 mg/kg q 24–48 hours	Immunosuppressive, anti-inflammatory, antifibrotic
Azathioprine	1.0 mg/kg q 24–48 hours	Immunosuppressive
S-adenosyl-L-methionine (SAMe)	18 mg/kg q 12–24 hours	Increase hepatic glutathione, antioxidant
Ursodeoxycholic acid	10–15 mg/kg q 24 hours	Stimulates bile flow, cytoprotective, immunomodulatory effects
Vitamin E	10 IU/kg q 24 hours	Antioxidant
Milk thistle (silymarin)	4–8 mg/kg q 24 hours	Antioxidant

Abbreviation: q, every.

nosuppressive, anti-inflammatory, and antifibrotic effects. Other antifibrotic agents, such as colchicine, can be used to prevent or treat hepatic fibrosis and cirrhosis. Free radicals may contribute to oxidative hepatocellular injury if not counteracted by cytoprotective mechanisms. Antioxidants, such as S-adenosylmethionine and vitamin E, are important in scavenging free radicals and preventing oxidative injury. Ursodeoxycholic acid is believed to be beneficial by expanding the bile acid pool and displacing potentially hepatotoxic hydrophilic bile acids that may accumulate in cholestasis. It also stimulates bile flow, stabilizes hepatocyte membranes, and has cyto-protective and immunomodulatory effects on the liver.

Chronic hepatopathies frequently cause alterations in plasma proteins (hypoalbuminemia) and vascular hydrostatic pressures, resulting in ascites or edema. Chronic hepatopathies increase resistance to blood flow in the liver (portal hypertension), which can lead to acquired portosystemic shunts, increased lymph formation, increased plasma volume, and ascites and/or edema. Liver-induced ascites can be diagnosed by physical examination and laboratory evaluation of peritoneal fluid, blood, and urine. Ascitic fluid of liver disease is usually a transudate or modified transudate, which is further substantiated by the presence of hypoalbuminemia. Peripheral edema may occur in end-stage liver disease. Mechanisms similar to those that trigger ascites may cause peripheral edema (ie, distal legs, ventral abdomen and thorax, ventral neck region).

To re-establish the osmotic gradient in ascitic animals with hypoalbuminemia, administer intravenous colloids, such as hetastarch or dextrans at a dose of 10 to 20 mL/kg given over 1 to 2 hours and repeated as needed after several infusions. Diuretics and a low-sodium diet are used in the management of ascites and/or edema [9,10]. Spironolactone is used to reduce ascites and/or edema without causing hypokalemia. If these measures are ineffective, furosemide may be substituted, although serum electrolyte concentrations should be evaluated frequently.

Hepatic fibrosis and cirrhosis

The liver can respond to severe damage and necrosis by regeneration, mineralization, or fibrosis, depending on the severity of the challenge and the degree of damage to the supporting connective tissue structure. Loss of hepatocytes and connective tissue integrity caused by any disease can lead to hepatic fibrosis; thus, identification of hepatic fibrosis is not specific for any particular liver disease. When hepatic fibrosis is severe and leads to formation of small or large regenerative nodules limited by fibrous tissue, the term *cirrhosis* is used. Hepatic cirrhosis is considered an end-stage liver disease. Because hepatic cirrhosis is advanced, most affected dogs have significant clinical and laboratory evidence of hepatic dysfunction. As cirrhosis progresses, portal hypertension develops, and many dogs with hepatic cirrhosis have ascites and acquired portosystemic shunts [9]. Most chronic hepatopathies progress slowly, and fibrosis occurs in concert with the progression of necrosis and inflammation. Radiographic evaluation may reveal a small liver, and ultrasonography shows an increase in hepatic echogenicity and, possibly, the presence of acquired portosystemic shunts. Liver biopsy is required for definitive diagnosis of hepatic fibrosis and cirrhosis [11].

Treatment for hepatic fibrosis is aimed at treating the underlying disease process and managing the complications of liver disease. Inhibition of collagen formation and lysis of excess hepatic fibrous tissue would be additional goals of therapy for hepatic cirrhosis. When used for treatment of hepatic fibrosis in affected dogs, colchicine has produced improvement in clinical signs for several months [12]. Corticosteroids and azathioprine have antifibrotic properties. Other drugs for the treatment of hepatic fibrosis include penicillamine, which inhibits collagen polymerization secondary to its copper-chelating effects, and oral zinc, which decreases intestinal copper absorption and also has antifibrotic and hepatoprotective properties.

Chronic infiltrative hepatopathies

Alterations in hepatic structure and function may occur when hepatocytes are infiltrated with lipid, glycogen, amyloid, or other substances. Although hepatic lipidosis is a common histopathologic finding in dogs with diabetes mellitus, it seldom becomes a clinical problem associated with liver dysfunction. Other less common infiltrative disorders include amyloid deposition and hemochromatosis [11]. Exogenous glucocorticoids and naturally occurring hyperadrenocorticism often lead to steroid hepatopathy in older dogs. Impairment of liver function can occur with severe steroid hepatopathy, but most dogs do not develop signs referable to hepatic dysfunction [13].

Laboratory evaluation of dogs with steroid hepatopathy usually reveals a marked increase in serum ALP and glutamyltransferase (GGT) activity, occasionally up to a 60-fold increase over normal values [14]. Values for hepatocellular enzyme activities (ALT and AST) are usually increased but not to the magnitude of serum ALP and GGT. Serum total bilirubin concentrations are usually normal, which supports the idea that serum ALP activity increase is secondary to steroid induction and cholestasis. If liver function tests are performed, there may be mild increases in fasting and postprandial serum bile acid concentrations [11]. Liver biopsy is seldom performed, but expected changes of increased hepatic vacuolization are seen on histopathologic evaluation.

Hepatocutaneous syndrome

Hepatocutaneous syndrome, also known as superficial necrolytic dermatitis or metabolic dermatosis, is an uncommon dermatosis seen in dogs and has been described rarely in the cat. Superficial necrolytic dermatitis in dogs has been associated with hepatopathies in most cases [15]. The most common hepatopathy is an idiopathic hepatocellular collapse. Other findings may include cirrhosis, hepatopathy secondary to ingestion of mycotoxins, and hepatopathy possibly associated with primidone or phenobarbital administration. Nonhepatic associations have included glucagon-producing pancreatic adenocarcinoma, hyperglucagonemia and glucagon-secreting liver metastases, and gastric carcinoma. Affected dogs may become diabetic, although the cause of the diabetes mellitus is not known. Idiopathic pancreatic atrophy has been noted.

Superficial necrolytic dermatitis is generally seen in middle-aged to older dogs, with the average age being 10 years. Male dogs are more commonly affected. The history of skin lesions may span weeks to several months and may wax and wane. Skin lesions are usually noted to affect the feet first, including interdigital erythema, crusting, erosions, hyperkeratosis, and fissuring of footpads. Toenail loss has been noted. Skin lesions may become pruritic and painful. Symmetric erythema, alopecia, crusts, and erosions and/or ulcers may be noted around the mouth, muzzle, eyes, hock and elbow pressure points, vulva, and scrotum. Bulla-like lesions may be noted. Bullae seem to represent necrotic epidermal tissue and are not usually filled with appreciable amounts of purulent material. The skin lesions are prone to secondary staphylococcal and *Malassezia* infections, secondary candidiasis, and dermatophytosis. The importance of the underlying disease in the predisposition to these infections is demonstrated in the observation that therapy for the underlying disease may result in the spontaneous resolution of the secondary infections.

Skin lesions have a characteristic histopathologic appearance of marked diffuse parakeratosis. There is marked ballooning degeneration of the upper layers of the stratum spinosum (intracellular and extracellular edema of the upper layers of the epidermis). Edematous spaces are filled with neutrophils, necrotic epithelial cells, and eosinophilic debris. Marked epidermal hyperplasia is present, and there is mild neutrophilic perivascular inflammation in the superficial dermis. These changes have been termed the red (parakeratosis), white (edema), and blue (hyperplasia) signs suggestive of superficial necrolytic dermatitis.

Most dogs with superficial necrolytic dermatitis have preexisting liver disease. Clinical signs related to the liver disease vary from no signs to weight loss, depression, lethargy, PU and/or PD, jaundice, and anorexia. There is often a mild to moderate nonregenerative anemia to a mildly regenerative anemia. The serum chemistry profile usually shows increases in serum liver enzymes in 95% of cases, which are characterized by increases in serum ALP and ALT. Hypoproteinemia and fasting hyperglycemia are common, but only a small percentage of dogs are overtly diabetic at time of initial diagnosis. If a dog is euglycemic at presentation, a fasting hyperglycemia generally develops at some point in the future. If diabetes mellitus is encountered, it is usually late in the course of superficial necrolytic dermatitis. It is uncommon to see dogs proceed to the development of diabetic ketoacidosis. Increased serum glucagon concentrations have been noted in approximately 30% to 40% of affected dogs, and hypoaminoacidemia has been present in 85% to 90% of cases. Serum bile acids are abnormal in most cases.

Ultrasonography of the liver generally shows a characteristic "Swiss cheese" pattern that some think is pathognomonic for superficial necrolytic dermatitis. In dogs with idiopathic hepatocellular collapse as the cause for their liver disease, the liver is usually grossly nodular. Histopathologically, there is moderate to severe hepatocellular collapse and vacuolar degeneration accompanied by nodular regeneration. This severe hepatic vacuolar alteration suggests a metabolic or hormonal disease, but the initiating cause has not been established. In some dogs, the liver is classically cirrhotic.

Clinical signs associated with glucagonomas include depression, anorexia, diarrhea, vomiting, weight loss, and a normocytic and normochromic anemia. Increased serum liver enzymes may be seen in 40% to 50% of cases; hyperglycemia is common with overt diabetes mellitus in approximately 30% of cases. Hyperglucagonemia, hypoalbuminemia, and hypoaminoacidemia are common. Abnormal serum bile acids usually are not found. A pancreatic mass is usually noted in a small percentage of cases based on abdominal ultrasonography.

The diagnosis of the skin disease is based on histopathologic examination. Skin lesions should not be surgically prepared for biopsy, and biopsies should come from the margins and lesional areas. Skin lesions should routinely have cytologic preparations of skin scrapings, impression smears, and/or tape preparations to document secondary *Malassezia*, staphylococcal, and *Candida* infections. Samples for dermatophyte cultures are taken. Support for a diagnosis of an underlying hepatopathy is based on the results of the complete blood cell count (CBC), serum chemistry profile, urinalysis, serum bile acids analysis, radiography, ultrasonography, and liver biopsy. Support for a diagnosis of glucagonoma is based on the CBC, serum chemistry profile, urinalysis, serum bile acids analysis, radiography, ultrasonography, CT scan, arteriography, measurement of plasma glucagon (usually 5–10 times above the normal range), and exploratory surgery. In liver- or glucagonoma-related cases, consideration should be given to measuring amino acids, zinc, and fatty acids.

The treatment for superficial necrolytic dermatitis should include the following for consideration:

1. A diet high in good-quality protein (eg, supplement with Hill's A/D [Hill's Pet Nutrition, Topeka, Kansas] or a similar diet) may be needed.
2. Enteral or parenteral feeding procedures may be needed.
3. Manage diabetes mellitus, if present, and the response to insulin may be erratic.

4. Symptomatic treatment for secondary infections (systemic antibiotics and germicidal shampoo; if secondary bacterial pyoderma is present, use benzoyl peroxide or, if benzoyl peroxide is irritating, chlorhexidine shampoo; if secondary *Malassezia* infection is present, consider miconazole or ketoconazole shampoo) may be needed. Exudative lesions may be treated with a germicidal and/or astringent soak (one part chlorhexidine to three parts Domeboro solution [Bayer, Morristown, New Jersey]).

5. Amino acid supplementation:

   A. Egg yolk supplementation (three to six yolks daily) has been noted to be of some benefit, perhaps because of the amino acid profile provided. Others have used protein supplements favored by human body builders.

   B. Intravenous amino acid therapy has been noted to benefit dogs with hepatopathy-related superficial necrolytic dermatitis. Aminosyn 10% Crystalline Amino Acid Solution (Abbott Laboratories, Abbott Park, Illinois) is used for this purpose. Each 100 mL contains a total of 10 g of amino acids. Use 500 mL per dog administered slowly over approximately 8 to 12 hours in a large central vein, such as the external jugular vein. Consideration should be given to measuring serum bile acids before this amino acid infusion in that it is possible to contribute to hepatic encephalopathy with this therapy. If significant improvement is noted, no further amino acid infusions are given. Prolonged remissions have been noted after only a single infusion. If minimal to no response is noted, the infusions are repeated every 7 to 10 days for four treatments. If an individual dog does not respond by this time, it is generally not likely to respond. The amino acid infusion is repeated with each exacerbation of the skin lesions. Dogs may go several months between amino acid infusions, but some dogs require monthly infusions to maintain remission. As the disease progresses, the need for amino acid infusions is likely to increase.

6. Essential fatty acid supplementation may be needed, using primarily ω-3 fatty acids at twice the bottle dosage of a high-potency ω-3 fatty acid supplement.

7. Zinc supplementation using zinc methionine at a dose of 2 mg/kg/d is instituted in all individuals.

8. Niacinamide therapy may also be used at a dose of 250 to 500 mg per dog administered two to three times daily.

9. For focal inflammatory lesions, such as pododermatitis, that have been controlled as well as possible, consider the use of topical glucocorticoids, such as initially generic triamcinolone acetonide administered twice

daily. Gradually reduce the frequency of use, and, if possible, switch to hydrocortisone for long-term maintenance therapy.
10. Systemic steroids (prednisone starting at a dose of 1 mg/kg/d) may be beneficial some dogs. Effects are usually transient, and symptoms eventually become refractory to these therapeutic dosages.
11. Ketoconazole has been used with some benefit at a dose of 5 to 10 mg/kg administered twice daily because of its effects on secondary *Malassezia* infections or perhaps for its anti-inflammatory and antipruritic effects.

The treatment for glucagonoma-related superficial necrolytic dermatitis includes supportive care, treating the diabetes mellitus if present, surgical debulking and/or removal of the primary pancreatic tumor, octreotide (a long-acting analogue of somatostatin that temporarily inhibits glucagon secretion), intravenous amino acid therapy as for the liver-related superficial necrolytic dermatitis, and zinc and fatty acid supplementation as for the liver-related superficial necrolytic dermatitis.

The prognosis for dogs with idiopathic hepatocellular collapse is generally poor. Even with the amino acid therapies and other supportive care, the longest lengths of survival have been not more than 2.5 years. The prognosis for glucagonoma-related superficial necrolytic dermatitis is generally grave. Most of these dogs already have metastatic disease at the time of diagnosis or develop metastatic disease.

Vascular diseases

The most common vascular disease of the liver in older dogs is congenital or acquired portosystemic shunts. Congenital portosystemic shunting is the same condition as noted in young dogs. Acquired portosystemic shunting occurs secondarily to portal hypertension, advanced liver disease, and hepatic fibrosis or cirrhosis. As portal pressures increase, small vessels routing the portal circulation to the systemic circulation increase in size and volume capacity, thus providing a "pop-off valve" for the increased portal pressures. Treatment of portosystemic shunts is aimed primarily at treatment of the associated hepatoencephalopathy (HE). Attenuation of congenital portosystemic shunts is warranted, whereas that of acquired portosystemic shunts is contraindicated because this immediately results in extremely increased portal pressures, shock, and death.

Other vascular disorders of the liver include acquired arteriovenous (AV) fistulas and portal vein thrombosis. In dogs, acquired AV fistulas are usually the result of trauma [16]. The clinical signs associated with hepatic AV fistulas in dogs include ascites and HE. Diagnosis is based on contrast imaging studies, and surgical resection of the affected liver lobe usually results in resolution of clinical signs. Portal vein thrombosis resulting in altered laboratory parameters indicative of cholestasis, hepatocellular injury, and impaired liver function occurs in dogs [17]. Thrombosis may be diagnosed based on mesenteric venography, but treatment is usually not attempted.

Hepatoencephalopathy

HE refers to the neurologic derangements that occur secondary to liver dysfunction [18,19]. Neurologic signs may be seen at any time, often being more prominent after ingestion of a high-protein meal or blood loss into the gastrointestinal tract. Initial signs of HE include depression, lethargy, and mild behavior changes ranging from increased docility to aggression. Aimless pacing or circling, apparent blindness, and head pressing may ensue, followed by stupor, seizure activity, or coma. The diagnosis of HE is based on identification of liver dysfunction and response to treatment. Fasting serum ammonia and serum bile acid concentrations are usually markedly increased in HE.

Medical management is directed toward minimizing the signs of HE and includes manipulation of dietary proteins and intestinal flora and avoidance of medications or substances capable of inducing encephalopathic signs. A restricted protein diet (2.0–2.5 mg/kg) composed of proteins rich in branched-chain amino acids with comparatively smaller amounts of aromatic amino acids is recommended. Foods containing milk protein (dried milk or cottage cheese) are best. The bulk of the caloric intake should consist of simple carbohydrates, such as boiled white rice. Meals should be frequent and in small amounts to maximize digestion and absorption so that minimal residue is passed into the colon, where intestinal anaerobic bacteria degrade nitrogenous compounds to ammonia. Commercial diets formulated for liver or renal dysfunction and a diet formulated for intestinal disease are used with success in most animals with encephalopathic signs.

Manipulation of intestinal flora with antimicrobial agents and lactulose also produces marked clinical improvement. For animals presenting in encephalopathic crisis, intravenous isotonic electrolyte solutions supplemented with 2.5% or 5.0% dextrose solution and potassium chloride; cleansing enemas with warmed 0.9% saline solution; or enemas with added neomycin (15–20 mL of 1% solution three to four times daily), lactulose (5–10 mL diluted at a ratio of 1:3 with water three to four times daily), or povidone-iodine solution (10% solution, rinse after 10 minutes with warm water) are recommended. For long-term medical management of encephalopathic signs, lactulose is given orally at a dose of 0.25 to 1.0 mL per 4.5 kg of body weight, with the dose adjusted to the frequency and consistency of the stools passed each day. Two to three soft or pudding-consistency stools indicate an optimal dose. Too great a dose may result in flatulence, severe diarrhea, dehydration, and acidemia. To manipulate the intestinal flora further, neomycin (22 mg/kg administered orally two to three times daily), metronidazole (7.5 mg/kg administered orally two to three times daily), ampicillin (5 mg/kg administered orally two to three times daily), or amoxicillin (2.5 mg/kg administered orally two times a day) may be used intermittently for several weeks.

Neoplasia

Neoplasias involving the liver are primary hepatic tumors, metastatic carcinomas and sarcomas, and hemolymphatic tumors. In dogs, metastatic neoplasia is most common and can originate from the pancreas, spleen, mammary glands, adrenal glands, bones, lungs, thyroid glands, and gastro-intestinal tract. Primary hepatic tumors may be epithelial or mesodermal in origin and benign or malignant. Benign tumors of the hepatocytes are called hepatocellular adenoma or hepatoma, and its malignant counterpart is called hepatocellular carcinoma. Hepatocellular carcinoma is the most common primary hepatic tumor in dogs [20]. The cause of these spontaneous primary hepatic tumors in dogs is not known.

Primary hepatic tumors are most common in dogs that are 10 years of age or older. Dogs with hepatic tumors usually show vague nonspecific signs of hepatic dysfunction that often do not appear until the more advanced stages of hepatic disease. The most consistent signs are anorexia, lethargy, weight loss, PD, PU, vomiting, and abdominal distention. Other less frequent findings include icterus, diarrhea, and excessive bleeding. Signs of central nervous dysfunction, such as depression, dementia, or seizures, can be attributed to HE, hypoglycemia, or central nervous system metastasis.

On physical examination, a cranial abdominal mass or marked hepatomegaly is commonly detected in dogs with primary hepatic tumors. Ascites or hemoperitoneum may contribute to abdominal distention. Tumor rupture and hemorrhage are most likely with hepatocellular adenoma, hepatocellular carcinoma, and hepatic hemangiosarcoma. Generally, labo-ratory evaluation shows mild to moderate increases in liver enzyme activities, with some dogs displaying abnormal liver function based on serum bile acid concentrations [20]. Hypoglycemia occurs in some dogs with hepatocellular carcinoma and other hepatic neoplasms. Abdominal radiographic findings include symmetric or asymmetric hepatomegaly or ascites. A right cranial abdominal mass causing caudal and left gastric displacement most often occurs. Thoracic radiographs should be obtained to determine pulmonary metastasis.

Potential ultrasonographic findings include focal, multifocal, or diffuse changes in hepatic echotexture. Primary or secondary hepatic neoplasia and nodular hyperplasia often appear as focal or multifocal hypoechoic or mixed echogenic lesions. The diagnosis of primary or metastatic hepatic tumor cannot be made on the basis of ultrasonographic findings alone. Definitive diagnosis of hepatic neoplasia requires liver biopsy and histopathologic examination. The procedure of choice for a single large hepatic mass is laparotomy, because the excision of the mass can be performed concurrently. Ultrasound-guided biopsy is useful for diagnosing focal or diffuse involvement, but the small size of the biopsy sample can make the differentiation of nodular dysplasia versus primary hepatic tumor difficult. A surgical wedge biopsy is often necessary.

Surgical removal of the affected liver lobe is the treatment of choice for primary hepatic tumors that involve a single lobe, such as hepatocellular adenoma or carcinoma. Removal of a single mass lesion of hepatocellular carcinoma typically provides 1 year of quality life after surgery. Therefore, early detection before metastasis to other liver lobes provides the best chance for surgical control. A complete evaluation of the abdominal cavity for evidence of metastasis should be performed, and a biopsy specimen of hepatic lymph nodes should always be obtained. When all liver lobes are affected, the prognosis is poor. At the current time, chemotherapy is not an effective treatment for control of hepatocellular carcinoma.

Hepatic diseases of the cat

Inflammatory liver disease

Inflammatory liver diseases of older cats are probably best referred to as feline cholangitis and/or cholangiohepatitis syndrome (CCHS) [21]. This syndrome can then be described as being suppurative CCHS or non-suppurative CCHS. Affected cats with suppurative CCHS usually are male. A sudden-onset history of vomiting and diarrhea is common. Affected cats are icteric, febrile, lethargic, and dehydrated on initial presentation. Less then 50% of cats have hepatomegaly. The most common organisms associated with suppurative CCHS are *Escherichia coli*, *Staphylococcus*, α-hemolytic *Streptococcus*, *Bacillus*, *Actinomyces*, *Bacteroides*, *Enterococcus*, *Enterobacter*, and *Clostridium* species.

Most cats with suppurative CCHS show a moderate increase in serum ALT, AST, ALP, and GGT activities. Some cats have left-shifted leukograms with an accompanying leukocytosis. On ultrasonography, severe ascending cholangitis associated with thickening of the extrahepatic biliary system and inflammation within the lumen of the intrahepatic bile ducts may be observed. Ultrasonography also may show coexisting extrahepatic bile duct obstruction (enlarged gallbladder, distended and tortuous common bile duct, and obvious intrahepatic bile ducts), cholecystitis (thickened laminar appearance to the gallbladder wall and adjacent fluid accumulation), and pancreatitis (prominent and easily visualized enlarged pancreas with adjacent hyperechoic fat). Cytologic evaluation of liver aspirates or imprints may reveal suppurative inflammation.

Most cats with nonsuppurative CCHS have been ill for several months [21]. Clinical signs are subtle and may include only episodic vomiting, diarrhea, and anorexia. Most cats have hepatomegaly, are icteric, and may have ascites. Concurrent disorders frequently include inflammatory bowel disease, low-grade lymphocytic pancreatitis, and cholecystitis. Cats with lymphoplasmacytic inflammation tend to have greater magnitudes of increased serum ALT, AST, ALP, and GGT activities than cats with just lymphocytic inflammation. Cats with lymphocytic inflammation may develop a lymphocytosis (total lymphocyte counts greater than 14,000 per μL) without other evidence of malignant lymphoproliferative disease. Similar to cats with suppurative CCHS, abdominal radiographs rarely show important diagnostic information. In most cats with nonsuppurative CCHS, a multifocal hyperechoic pattern is recognized ultrasonographically, which represents peribiliary inflammation and fibrosis. In some cats, ultrasonography may fail to show any abnormalities. Cytologic preparations from liver aspirates may lack evidence of inflammation or may disclose only a few inflammatory cells. A wedge biopsy of the liver for histopathologic evaluation is preferable for a definitive diagnosis because it more reliably demonstrates whole acinar units and portal triads [21].

Treatment of suppurative CCHS incorporates appropriate antimicrobial therapy based on identification of infectious organisms (Box 2). If bacteria

---

Box 2. Medical management used in treatment of feline inflammatory liver disease

1. Fluid therapy according to the cat's needs
2. Prednisone (2–4 mg/kg administered orally once a day or divided twice daily with titration to the lowest effective dose over the next several months)
3. Metronidazole (5.0–7.5 mg/kg administered orally two to three times daily), ampicillin (20 mg/kg administered orally three to four times daily), or enrofloxacin (5 mg/kg administered orally two times daily)
4. Oral potassium gluconate at a dose of at least 2 to 3 mEq/d (no matter what the serum potassium value is)
5. Oral vitamin E (100–200 IU/d) or S-adenosylmethionine (18 mg/kg/d)
6. Oral pancreatic enzyme supplementation
7. Supplementation with L-carnitine at a dose of 250 mg per cat daily, water-soluble vitamins (two times the normal maintenance dose), and vitamin K_1 (0.5–1.5 mg/kg administered subcutaneously or intramuscularly for three doses at 12-hour intervals and then once a week for 1 or 2 additional weeks) may be provided
8. Periodic oral lactulose as needed to control abnormal mental behavior
9. Diet that the cat eats well

are cytologically observed, a Gram's stain facilitates selection of antimicrobial agents. Cats with extrahepatic bile duct obstruction should have their biliary occlusion decompressed if possible. If biliary tract decompression cannot be accomplished, the biliary pathway may be rerouted by means of a cholecystoenterostomy. Biliary diversion is a vital early therapeutic intervention in the prevention or control of sepsis in obstructive suppurative cholangitis. Aerobic and anaerobic bacterial cultures should be collected from bile, tissue adjacent to any focal lesion, the gallbladder wall, and liver tissue.

Any icteric cat suspected of having suppurative or nonsuppurative CCHS should be evaluated for coexistent extrahepatic bile duct obstruction, pancreatitis, and inflammatory bowel disease as well as coexistent hepatic lipidosis. If lipid vacuolation is detected, nutritional support with a commercially prepared feline diet should be included in the treatment plan.

Immunosuppressive therapy for cats with nonsuppurative CCHS includes a combination of prednisone (initial dose of 2–4 mg/kg administered orally once a day or divided twice daily), with titration to the lowest effective dose over the next several months, and metronidazole (7.5 mg/kg administered orally two to three times daily) [21]. Supplementation with L-carnitine at a dose of 250 mg per cat per day, water-soluble vitamins (two times the normal maintenance dose), and vitamin K_1 (0.5–1.5 mg/kg) administered subcutaneously or intramuscularly for three doses at 12-hour intervals and then once a week for 1 or 2 additional weeks may be provided. Oral S-adenosylmethionine (18 mg/kg/d) or vitamin E (100–200 IU/d) can also be added as a supplement to ensure its adequacy as a free radical scavenger. Ursodeoxycholic acid (10–15 mg/kg/d administered orally) is given to all cats with CCHS once extrahepatic bile duct obstruction is corrected and cholecystitis has resolved. Monthly serum liver enzyme activities and total bilirubin concentrations may be used to monitor treatment response as well as how well the cat is doing at home.

Pyogranulomatous hepatitis (feline infectious peritonitis)

Feline infectious peritonitis virus (FIPV) can induce a multisystemic disease process that may affect the liver by inducing pyogranulomatous hepatitis. Effusive and noneffusive forms of FIPV may affect the liver. Common clinical signs seen with pyogranulomatous hepatitis are anorexia, weight loss, fever, depression, icterus, and abdominal distention secondary to fluid accumulation. Laboratory evaluation of cats with FIPV-induced liver disease may reveal leukocytosis, nonregenerative anemia, and hyperglobulinemia. In addition, increased serum ALT, AST, and ALP activities as well as an increased total bilirubin concentration may be present. Ultrasonography may confirm the presence of abdominal effusion and define nodular involvement of the liver secondary to the pyogranulomatous inflammation. Alternatively, fine-needle aspiration cytology of the liver may reveal pyogranulomatous inflammation. Liver biopsy is the most reliable method to confirm FIPV of the liver. There is no specific treatment for FIPV-induced liver disease in cats. Supportive measures can be used, along with good nutrition and nursing care.

Secondary hepatic lipidosis

Secondary hepatic lipidosis is characterized by progressive infiltration of hepatocytes with fat and concomitant hepatic dysfunction. The usual clinical findings include a period of anorexia in a previously obese cat, obvious weight loss, muscle wasting, icterus, and vomiting [22]. Icterus is usually seen in the later stages of disease, and some cats have palpable hepatomegaly. Laboratory evaluation shows evidence of cholestatic liver disease. Ultrasonography shows a fine and diffuse increase in echogenicity [23]. Cytologic evaluation of fine-needle aspirates shows hepatocytes with marked vacuolar change [24]. Histopathologic evaluation of a liver biopsy specimen demonstrates marked macro- or microvesicular vacuolar change in most hepatocytes and evidence of bile stasis. Treatment is directed at restoring nutritional status and managing the underlying cause of the systemic illness. Enteral nutritional support by means of nasoesophageal, pharyngostomy, esophagostomy, or gastrostomy tube feeding is recommended.

Neoplasia

Primary neoplasia of the liver is uncommon in older cats. Primary nonhematopoietic tumors of the liver include bile duct adenoma and/or adenocarcinoma, hepatocellular carcinoma, and hemangiosarcoma [25]. Metastatic lymphosarcoma occurs commonly in cats, and other metastatic neoplasias seen in older cats include myeloproliferative diseases and mast cell tumors [26]. Clinical signs may include anorexia, lethargy, hepatomegaly, and icterus. If biliary obstruction is complete, clinical signs of extrahepatic bile duct obstruction can also be observed. Fine-needle aspiration for cytologic evaluation can be helpful with diffuse metastatic neoplasia, such as lymphosarcoma, mast cell tumor, or myeloproliferative disorders [24]. Treatment for primary neoplasia is primarily surgical. Treatment of metastatic neoplasia is directed at the primary tumor.

Summary

Normal functioning of the liver does not seem to change significantly in dogs and cats as a result of age. Despite this, older dogs and cats are at greater risk for the development of liver disease. The diagnosis of liver disease is initiated by the veterinarian's suspicion that liver disease might be present, followed by the case history and a physical examination. The initial workup for the older dog or cat with suspected liver disease should begin with a CBC, serum chemistry profile, and urinalysis. This may be followed by a liver function test, radiographic or ultrasonographic imaging studies, hepatic fine-needle aspiration, and, ultimately, liver biopsy.

References

[1] Hultgren B, Stevens J, Hardy R. Inherited, chronic, progressive hepatic degeneration in Bedlington terriers with increased liver copper concentrations: clinical and pathologic observations and comparison with other copper-associated liver diseases. Am J Vet Res 1986;47:365.

[2] Twedt D, Hunsaker H, Allen K. Use of 2,3,2-tetramine as a hepatic copper chelating agent for treatment of copper hepatotoxicosis in Bedlington Terriers. J Am Vet Med Assoc 1988; 192:52.

[3] Crawford MA, Schall WD, Jensen RK, et al. Chronic active hepatitis in 26 doberman pinschers. J Am Vet Med Assoc 1985;187:1343.

[4] Thornburg LP, Rottinghaus G. What is the significance of hepatic copper values in dogs with cirrhosis? Vet Med 1985;50.

[5] Thornburg L, Rottinghaus G, Gage H. Chronic liver disease associated with high hepatic copper concentration in a dog. J Am Vet Med Assoc 1986;188:1190.

[6] Thornburg L, Rottinghaus G, Koch J, et al. High liver copper levels in two Doberman Pinschers with subacute hepatitis. J Am Anim Hosp Assoc 1984;20:1003.

[7] Flatland B. Botanicals, vitamins, and minerals and the liver: therapeutic applications and potential toxicities. Compend Contin Educ Pract Vet 2003;25:514.

[8] Brewer G, Dick R, Schall W, et al. Use of zinc acetate to treat copper toxicosis in dogs. J Am Vet Med Assoc 1992;201:564.

[9] Johnson S. Portal hypertension. Part I. Pathophysiology and clinical consequences. Compend Contin Educ Pract Vet 1987;9:741.

[10] Johnson S. Portal hypertension. Part II. Clinical assessment and treatment. Compend Contin Educ Pract Vet 1987;9:917.

[11] Strombeck D, Guilford W. Small animal gastroenterology. Davis (CA): Stonegate Publishing Co., 1990.

[12] Boer H, Nelson R, Long G. Colchicine therapy for hepatic fibrosis in a dog. J Am Anim Hosp Assoc 1984;185:303.

[13] Rogers W, Ruebner B. A retrospective study of probable glucocorticoid-induced hepatopathy in dogs. J Am Vet Med Assoc 1977;170:603.

[14] Badylak S, Van Vleet J. Sequential morphologic and clinicopathologic alterations in dogs with experimentally induced glucocorticoid hepatopathy. Am J Vet Res 1981;42: 1310.

[15] McNeil PE. The underlying pathology of the hepatocutaneous syndrome: a report of 18 cases. In: Ihrke PJ, Mason IS, White SD, editors. Advances in veterinary dermatology, vol. 2. New York: Pergamon Press; 1993. p. 113.

[16] Hosgood G. Arteriovenous fistulas: pathophysiology, diagnosis, and treatment. Compend Contin Educ Pract Vet 1989;11:625.

[17] Willard M, Baley M, Hauptman J, et al. Obstructed portal venous flow and portal vein thrombosis in a dog. J Am Vet Med Assoc 1989;194:1449.

[18] Tyler J. Hepatoencephalopathy. Part I. Clinical signs and diagnosis. Compend Contin Educ Pract Vet 1990;12:1069.

[19] Tyler J. Hepatoencephalopathy. Part II. Pathophysiology and treatment. Compend Contin Educ Pract Vet 1990;12:1260.

[20] Magne M. Primary epithelial hepatic tumors in the dog. Compend Contin Educ Pract Vet 1984;6:506.
[21] Center SA. The jaundiced cat. In: Proceedings of the Feline Medicine Symposium. 1997. p. 41.
[22] Thornburg L. Fatty liver syndrome in cats. J Am Anim Hosp Assoc 1982;18:397.
[23] Biller D, Kantrowitz B, Miyabayashi T. Ultrasonography of diffuse liver disease. J Vet Intern Med 1992;6:71.
[24] Meyer D, French T. The liver. In: Cowell R, Tyler R, editors. Diagnostic cytology of the dog and cat. Goleta (CA): American Veterinary Publications; 1989. p. 189.
[25] Post G, Patnaik A. Nonhematopoietic hepatic neoplasms in cats: 21 cases(1983–1988). J Am Vet Med Assoc 1992;201:1080.
[26] Center S. Feline liver disorders and their management. Compend Contin Educ Pract Vet 1986;8:889.

ELSEVIER
SAUNDERS

Vet Clin Small Anim
35 (2005) 635–653

VETERINARY
CLINICS
Small Animal Practice

Thyroid Disorders in the Geriatric Patient

Susan A. Meeking, DVM

Internal Medicine and Emergency/Critical Care, Animal Medical Center,
510 East 62nd Street, New York, NY 10021, USA

Feline hyperthyroidism

Hyperthyroidism is the most common endocrinopathy of geriatric cats. The clinical signs associated with hyperthyroidism are the result of increased production, secretion, and circulation of the active thyroid hormones thyroxine (T_4) and triiodothyronine (T_3) because of an abnormally functioning thyroid gland. In 98% of these cases, hypersecretion of thyroid hormones is caused by benign adenomatous hyperplasia or thyroid adenoma. The clinical signs associated with this condition are generally treatable with appropriate therapy. Thyroid carcinoma is the cause of hyperthyroidism in only 1% to 3% of hyperthyroid cats.

Clinical features

Since first being recognized in 1979, there have been many studies to investigate the risk factors associated with the development of hyperthyroidism. Recent studies have shown that increased age, a preference for fish or liver and giblets canned food, a canned food diet (especially as >50% of the diet and use of food from pop-top cans), excessive dietary iodine intake, and use of kitty litter increase the risk of a cat developing hyperthyroidism. Siamese and Himalayan breeds were at a significantly lower risk of developing hyperthyroidism. Neutering, number of cats in a household, frequency of vaccination, topical ectoparasitic treatments, insecticides, and herbicides were not identified as risk factors for hyperthyroidism [1–5]. Some authors have hypothesized that goitrogenic compounds in commercial canned food combined with the decreased ability to metabolize goitrogens through glucuronidation pathways have increased the prevalence of

---

E-mail address: susan.meeking@amcny.org

hyperthyroidism in cats over the last few decades as the consumption of canned food increased [6].

Increased awareness of this disorder and routine thyroid screening in older cats have led to earlier detection and thus less severe manifestation of clinical signs before diagnosis compared with the past 20 years.

Hyperthyroidism is the most common endocrinopathy in older cats, with the mean age at diagnosis just less than 13 years of age and less than 5% of hyperthyroid cats being younger than 8 years of age [6]. There has been no reported gender association with the disease and no breeds reported to be more susceptible than others. As discussed previously, Siamese and Himalayan breeds are less likely than all other breeds to develop hyperthyroidism.

The initial clinical signs associated with hyperthyroidism are often overlooked by the owner, who fails to notice the slow progression of changes or notices changes but attributes them to normal aging or to other conditions the pet may have already been diagnosed with, such as chronic renal failure (CRF). The owners often complain of any combination of weight loss, polyphagia, polyuria and/or polydipsia (PU/PD), hyperactivity, gastrointestinal signs (eg, vomiting, diarrhea, increased volume of stool), skin changes (eg, patchy alopecia, matting, dry coat, greasy coat, thin skin), and respiratory signs (eg, panting, cough, dyspnea). Less often, owners identify decreased appetite, decreased activity level, weakness, tremors or seizures, or heat intolerance in their pet.

A palpable thyroid nodule is present in 90% of hyperthyroid cats but can also be found in cats that are not hyperthyroid; thus, it is not pathognomic for the condition. Many of those cats progress to become hyperthyroid and should be monitored frequently [7]. Cardiac abnormalities can include tachycardia (heart rate >240 beats per minute [bpm]), systolic murmur, gallop rhythm, and premature beats. Occasionally, hyperthyroid cats may be presented in congestive heart failure with dyspnea and muffled heart sounds. Hyperthyroid cats are often hyperactive and agitated during physical examination. Other observations may include thin body condition, muscle wasting, dehydration, weakness, small kidneys, and ventroflexion of the neck as well as retinopathies detectable through fundic examination, such as retinal hemorrhage, detachment, or acute blindness [8].

Diagnosis

In geriatric cats, routine health monitoring should include a complete blood cell count (CBC), biochemistry panel, urinalysis (UA), T_4 level, and blood pressure (BP) measurement. In cats with cardiac or respiratory signs, chest radiographs, an electrocardiogram (ECG), and an echocardiogram may also be indicated.

The CBC of hyperthyroid cats may include increased packed cell volume (PCV), macrocytosis, stress leukogram (leukocytosis, neutrophilia, lymphopenia, and eosinopenia), or megathrombocytosis, or it may be unremarkable.

The serum biochemistry panel of hyperthyroid cats often reveals an increase in liver enzymes, with 90% of hyperthyroid cats having mild to moderate elevation in the activity of alkaline phosphatase (ALP) and/or alanine aminotransferase (ALT). Recent studies have show that although serum from normal cats has only the liver isoenzyme of ALP, most hyperthyroid cats have circulating liver and bone ALP isoenzyme [9]. Elevation in liver enzyme activity usually returns to normal with successful management of hyperthyroidism. Azotemia (increased blood urea nitrogen [BUN] and creatinine) occurs in approximately 25% of hyperthyroid cats. Other biochemical changes associated with hyperthyroidism can include an increase in parathyroid hormone (PTH) and plasma phosphate and a decrease in ionized calcium, creatinine, and fructosamine [10–12]. The clinical significance of these biochemical values may be difficult to interpret in hyperthyroid cats with concurrent nonthyroidal illness, such as renal failure or diabetes mellitus.

There are no consistently reported changes in the UA of hyperthyroid cats, but this test is an important part of screening for common nonthyroidal diseases, such as diabetes mellitus, urinary tract infection, and CRF, as well as for differentiation of prerenal and renal causes of azotemia in geriatric cats.

Definitive diagnosis of hyperthyroidism requires demonstration of increased thyroidal radioisotope uptake or increased concentration of circulating thyroid hormones. Quantitative thyroid scans are expensive and require specialized equipment and technical skills; therefore, they are rarely performed. The diagnosis of hyperthyroidism is almost exclusively made based on thyroid hormone assays. Measurement of T_4, free T_4 (f T_4), and T_3 can be performed in cats, whereas no species-specific assay for thyroid-stimulating hormone (TSH) has been developed, precluding its use in feline medicine.

Measurement of T_4 is a reliable method of assessing thyroid function in cats and has become part of standard feline blood panels for older cats. An elevated total T_4 value, along with physical examination and historical changes consistent with hyperthyroidism, is diagnostic for feline hyperthyroidism. A recent study found that T_4 levels are higher than the reference range in more than 90% of hyperthyroid cats without concurrent nonthyroidal illness, whereas T_3 levels were increased in only 67% of hyperthyroid cats [13]. The remaining hyperthyroid cats had T_4 and T_3 levels within the reference range. Cats with historical and physical examination findings suspicious for hyperthyroidism but with high normal or borderline T_4 values should have the T_4 value repeated and possibly have an fT_4 level evaluated. These cats may have early or mild hyperthyroidism that may progress with time. Nonthyroidal illness suppresses serum T_4 levels in all cats, which may result in T_4 values within the normal range in a hyperthyroid cat. Repeating of T_4 levels once the nonthyroidal illness is resolved should reveal T_4 levels compatible with hyperthyroidism.

Measurement of fT_4 levels by equilibrium dialysis in cats with high normal or borderline T_4 values can assist in the diagnosis of hyperthyroidism. Measurement of fT_4 is more sensitive than measurement of total T_4 in cats with a high suspicion of being hyperthyroid but is less specific and may occasionally be elevated in cats without hyperthyroidism.

The T_3 suppression test previously described in many reports is not described here; it is not often used by the general practitioner because of the accuracy of other testing methods and the level of client compliance needed to complete the test adequately. This test is only recommended when repeated T_4 and fT_4 values are unable to confirm a suspected diagnosis of hyperthyroidism.

Systemic hypertension (persistent BP ≥ 160 mm Hg) is common in hyperthyroid cats. Clinical manifestations of systemic hypertension include ocular, cardiovascular, neurologic, and renal effects. Common retinal changes correlated with hypertension, such as edema, hemorrhage, and detachment, are associated with a decrease in or acute loss of vision. Hypertension and its associated retinal changes can be improved in many cats through treatment of the underlying disease and the use of antihypertensive drugs, such as amlodipine [8].

Thoracic radiographs are recommended for any hyperthyroid cat presented with cardiac or respiratory abnormalities. Many hyperthyroid cats have some degree of cardiomegaly on thoracic radiographs. A small number of cats have pleural effusion, pulmonary edema, or pericardial effusion requiring immediate therapy. Normal radiographs do not exclude underlying cardiomyopathy. ECGs and echocardiograms are recommended for those cats with radiographic evidence of cardiac silhouette abnormalities, pleural effusion, pericardial effusion, pulmonary edema, or cardiac abnormalities on physical examination.

ECG changes found in cats with thyrotoxicosis include, in order of prevalence, sinus tachycardia, increased R-wave amplitude in lead II, right axis deviation, atrial premature contractions, left axis deviation, widened QRS complexes, atrial tachycardia or fibrillation, and ventricular premature contractions. These abnormalities are less commonly recognized now than they were when the disease was first recognized in the 1980s. ECG changes often resolve with treatment of hyperthyroidism.

An echocardiogram of hyperthyroid cats is helpful in characterizing the structural and functional changes to the heart. The four described categories of cardiac changes in hyperthyroidism are hyperdynamic function of the myocardium, hypertrophic cardiomyopathy, congestive cardiomyopathy, and no abnormalities found [14]. Repeated echocardiographic studies are recommended to monitor progression of cardiac disease over time in affected cats or with development or change in cardiovascular abnormalities on physical examination.

Treatment

Medical inhibition of thyroid synthesis, surgical thyroid ablation, and radioactive iodine therapy are the currently accepted methods of hyperthyroid treatment. Each option has its advantages and disadvantages, and the type of appropriate treatment must be decided based on the patient's and client's needs.

Concurrent nonthyroidal illness (eg, CRF) in hyperthyroid cats is important when developing a treatment plan. As previously discussed, CRF and other nonthyroidal illnesses can mask hyperthyroidism by lowering serum thyroid hormone levels. At the same time, hyperthyroidism can affect the interpretation of the severity of CRF by increasing the glomerular filtration rate (GFR) and causing a reduction in the severity of azotemia or even masking underlying renal disease. Treatment of hyperthyroidism should decrease the GFR and can reveal or even worsen chronic renal disease.

Oral antithyroid drugs used for the treatment of hyperthyroidism include methimazole, carbimazole, and propylthiouracil. Compared with other modalities of treatment, oral antithyroid drugs have the advantages of being inexpensive, frequently being successful in management of the disease, having small tablet sizes, and having reversible activity as well as not requiring surgery, anesthesia, or hospitalization. The disadvantages include drug-related side effects, the requirement for daily administration of medication, the development of iatrogenic hypothyroidism, and the fact that treatment is not permanent.

Methimazole is currently the drug of choice for medical management of hyperthyroidism in cats. Methimazole can be used in three ways: to assess renal function after treatment for hyperthyroidism, to prepare a hyperthyroid cat for surgery or radioactive iodine treatment by improving clinical signs associated with hyperthyroidism, and for the primary long-term treatment of hyperthyroidism. The treatment protocol should be aimed at controlling the hyperthyroidism while minimizing side effects. Clinical and hematologic changes associated with methimazole administration may include vomiting, anorexia, depression, facial excoriation, eosinophilia, leukopenia, lymphocytosis, agranulocytosis, thrombocytopenia, and hepatopathy. An initial dose of 2.5 mg administered twice daily for 2 weeks is recommended [6]. This dose can be decreased in any cat with a high likelihood of developing side effects. If the initial dose is tolerated, the daily dose should be increased to 7.5 mg divided over two or three doses for an additional 2 weeks. Evaluation of the cat after the initial 4 weeks of treatment should include a history, physical examination, CBC, biochemistry panel, and T_4 level. Based on the pharmacokinetics of the drug, the T_4 level should be assessed 4 to 6 hours after drug administration. If the T_4 value is outside the normal range or the cat is showing signs of side effects, the dose of methimazole should be increased or decreased by increments of 2.5 mg/d every 2 weeks as needed. Most cats are regulated with 5.0 to 7.5 mg divided twice daily. Cats should be monitored every 2 to 4 weeks for the first 3 months of treatment, because this is the period during which they are most likely to experience side effects. After this period, they should be evaluated every 3 to 6 months. Other treatment options should be considered for cats experiencing adverse side effects. Administering oral medication two or three times daily to uncooperative cats can lead to decreased owner compliance and difficulty in regulating thyroid levels. Recently, methimazole has become available in a transdermal formulation through compounding pharmacies. The gel is placed in the pinna of the cat but still requires administration two to three times daily. Side effects are similar to those of oral methimazole, except fewer gastrointestinal side effects are reported with transdermal administration and some cats experience crusting and erythema of the pinna where the drug is applied. Efficacy and pharmacokinetic studies on transdermal methimazole have been inconclusive, and products may be variable between batches and sources [15,16].

Carbimazole is not available in North America but is available in the United Kingdom and Western Europe in place of methimazole. It is converted to methimazole in the body, and its use is similar to that of methimazole, except for a slight variation in the dosage. Carbimazole is reported to have fewer side effects than methimazole.

Propylthiouracil is not currently recommended for the treatment of hyperthyroidism because of the large number of cats developing side effects, such as anorexia, vomiting, lethargy, immune-mediated anemia, and thrombocytopenia.

Radioactive iodine is concentrated in thyroid tissue, and the emitted radiation destroys the surrounding functioning thyroid cells. Because only active thyroid cells are destroyed and atrophied thyroid cells and other surrounding tissues (ie, parathyroid glands) are unaffected, most treated animals do not become hypothyroid or hypoparathyroid. Radioactive iodine therapy is readily available in most areas of North America and is an excellent option for first-line therapy of hyperthyroid cats. The advantages of this treatment modality include one-time treatment for most cats, resulting in a cure; no administration of medication necessary; and no anesthesia or surgery required. Disadvantages include prolonged hospitalization for excretion of radioactivity, need for specialized facilities and technical training, need for second treatment in a small number of cats, and risk to human beings in contact with radioactivity. Radioactive iodine can be administered by many routes, including intravenous or subcutaneous injection or in an oral form. Subcutaneous administration has become the method of choice because of the ease of administration and safety for personnel involved. Some authors recommend treatment with oral antithyroid medication before radioactive iodine administration to assess renal function in the treated cat before permanent treatment is administered.

Radioactive iodine must only be used in specially equipped facilities with properly trained staff. Clients must be properly educated about care of the pet and protection of themselves from radiation after release of the pet from the hospital. This treatment option is successful, resulting in 95% of treated cats being euthyroid 3 months after treatment. A small number (<5%) of severely affected hyperthyroid cats may need additional treatment.

Hyperthyroid cats should undergo medical treatment (methimazole) for hyperthyroidism as well as careful screening for concurrent nonthyroidal illness before thyroidectomy. Thyroid hormone (T_4) values should be within the normal range, and clinical signs of thyrotoxicosis should be resolved before anesthesia and surgery so as to minimize surgical risk. Propanolol or atenolol can be used during surgery in cats with severe tachycardia or supraventricular tachyarrhythmias to slow heart rate, increase stroke volume, and thus increase cardiac output. The reader is referred to surgery textbooks for details of the surgical technique. Disadvantages of surgical treatment of hyperthyroidism include the necessity of anesthesia, expense, possible damage of the recurrent laryngeal nerve, Horner's syndrome, transient or permanent hypoparathyroidism, and failure to improve the cat's clinical signs or relapse of hyperthyroidism. The advantages of surgical treatment of hyperthyroidism include possibility of a permanent cure, and thus no need for daily medication, and simplicity of the procedure, enabling most well-equipped and reasonably experienced practitioners to perform the surgery.

Prognosis

The long-term prognosis for hyperthyroid cats depends on the severity of the condition at the time of diagnosis, concurrent disease, age, and gender. Although all three treatment modalities have been proven successful, the use of appropriate case selection for each type of treatment is important to obtain the best outcome, including client satisfaction. Clients should be encouraged to screen for and treat this disease in older cats, because the outcome is favorable and most cats respond well to at least one method of treatment.

Canine hypothyroidism

Hypothyroidism is the most commonly diagnosed endocrinopathy of dogs. Accurate diagnosis of this disease is based on clinical signs, multiple blood tests, and response to therapy. Definitive diagnosis of hypothyroidism is a constant challenge for the veterinary practitioner. It is a disease characterized by low levels of circulating thyroid hormones, resulting in decreased cell metabolism in many tissues in the body. There are three major categories of hyperthyroidism based on the location along the hypothalamic-pituitary-thyroid gland axis responsible for decreased thyroid hormone circulation.

Primary hypothyroidism is caused by thyroid destruction, resulting in thyroid dysfunction. Causes include lymphocytic thyroiditis, idiopathic follicular atrophy, dietary iodine deficiency, neoplasia, infection, or iatrogenic destruction (eg, thyrotoxic drugs, thyroidectomy, radioactive iodine therapy). More than 95% of hypothyroid dogs have primary hypothyroidism.

Secondary hypothyroidism is caused by decreased TSH secretion by the pituitary gland. This can be caused by congenital malformation of the pituitary gland; destruction of the pituitary gland by neoplasia or infection; or suppression of TSH secretion caused by drugs, hormones, concurrent illness, or malnutrition. This is a rare condition in dogs.

Tertiary hypothyroidism is caused by decreased secretion of thyrotropin-releasing hormone (TRH) from the hypothalamus. This condition has not been reported in dogs.

In general, dogs with primary hypothyroidism have pathologic changes to the thyroid gland and are nonresponsive to stimulation by TSH and TRH, whereas dogs with secondary or tertiary hypothyroidism have atrophied thyroid glands and are responsive to TSH and TRH administration.

Primary hypothyroidism

The most common causes of hypothyroidism in geriatric dogs are lymphocytic thyroiditis and idiopathic thyroid atrophy. Both of these conditions result in destruction of normal thyroid tissue and decreased circulation of thyroid hormones.

Lymphocytic thyroiditis is a progressive disease characterized by infiltration of the thyroid gland by lymphocytes, plasma cells, and macrophages and, eventually, fibrosis of the thyroid gland. The destruction of the thyroid gland is slow, with onset of clinical signs and biochemical changes consistent with hypothyroidism appearing over 1 to 3 years [17]. Lymphocytic thyroiditis is an immune-mediated process characterized by the presence of autoantibodies to thyroid antigens, such as thyroglobulin, T_4, T_3, and others. Binding of thyroid autoantibodies to thyroglobulin, follicular cells, or colloid antigens can activate the complement cascade and antibody-dependent cell-mediated cytotoxicity, resulting in thyroid destruction. This condition is believed to have a genetic link, because prevalence is increased in some breeds of dogs as well as in some lines within certain breeds [17]. Repeated vaccination of dogs has been shown to increase thyroglobulin antibodies, possibly increasing the likelihood of developing immune-mediated thyroid destruction [18]. Combinations of immune-mediated endocrine deficiency disorders, such as hypothyroidism, hypoadrenocorticism, diabetes mellitus, and hypoparathyroidism, have been reported in dogs but are rare [19].

Idiopathic thyroid atrophy is characterized by loss of normal thyroid tissue and replacement with adipose tissue. It is thought that thyroid atrophy with concurrent residual inflammatory changes can be seen as the final stage of lymphocytic thyroiditis. This is supported by a recent report that the mean age at diagnosis of idiopathic thyroid atrophy was older than the mean age at diagnosis of lymphocytic thyroiditis [20]. Idiopathic thyroid atrophy is a diagnosis of exclusion, because there are no blood tests available to diagnose this condition.

Secondary hypothyroidism

Secondary hypothyroidism is uncommon in dogs. It is difficult to diagnose, because TSH assays are not sensitive enough to differentiate between normal and low values. Although this condition is rare, it may be more likely to arise in geriatric patients than in younger patients because of the increased likelihood of concurrent disease and administration of medication that may suppress TSH secretion through thyrotroph suppression. This is the most common cause of secondary hypothyroidism in dogs and is usually reversible if the underlying mechanism of suppression is identified and corrected. Pituitary tumors can also cause secondary hypothyroidism if they are invasive and cause destruction of normal thyrotrophs. Dogs with this condition may exhibit additional pituitary-related endocrinopathies. Congenital pituitary malformation is an unlikely cause of secondary hypothyroidism in geriatric patients.

Clinical features

Breed incidence of hypothyroidism is difficult to assess, although it has been reported on extensively. Criteria for diagnosis and breed prevalence may affect the reported incidence of this disease in a particular breed. It is reported that hypothyroidism is common in Doberman Pinschers, Golden Retrievers, Labrador Retrievers, Cocker Spaniels, German Shepherds, Dachshunds, Poodles, Rottweilers, Spaniels, Terriers, Boxers, and mixed breeds, although there are many conflicting reports regarding the specific breeds predisposed. Dogs are most likely to develop clinical signs between 2 and 6 years of age. There may be breed variation in the age of onset of clinical signs. There is no reported gender predilection for this disease.

Owners of hypothyroid dogs many not be aware of the changes occurring in their dog because of the slow progression of the disease. They may also attribute the changes to normal signs of aging. Common complaints include mental dullness, lethargy and weakness, skin and coat changes, and weight gain.

Because of the multisystemic effects of thyroid hormones, there is a wide range of clinical signs for this disease. In general, the severity of clinical signs correlates with the duration of untreated hypothyroidism. Hypothyroid dogs have a decrease in general metabolism that can manifest clinically as mental dullness, lethargy, weight gain, exercise intolerance, unwillingness to exercise, and heat seeking. These clinical signs generally reverse with appropriate thyroid supplementation [21].

There are many skin and coat changes associated with hypothyroidism. The specific findings vary between animals, breeds, and severity of disease. The classic dermatologic finding is bilaterally symmetric nonpruritic truncal alopecia. Other dermatologic changes can include a dry and scaly coat, rat tail, lichenification, hyperpigmentation, myxedema, *Malassezia* dermatitis, recurrent pyoderma, otitis externa, seborrhea, patchy alopecia, inability to regrow hair after clipping, increased shedding, and alopecia sparing the head and extremities. Hair coat changes are generally related to the fact that most of the hair follicles remain in telogen in hypothyroid dogs. Myxedema of the head is responsible for the "tragic expression" often described in hypothyroid dogs. Most dermatologic changes associated with hypothyroidism do not manifest as pruritic conditions. Pruritus in hypothyroid dogs with dermatologic signs is often indicative of secondary bacterial, yeast, or parasitic infections.

Neuromuscular signs associated with hypothyroidism can result from segmental demyelination, axonopathy, mucopolysaccharide accumulation, cerebral atherosclerosis, or hyperlipidemia. Neuromuscular signs can include facial nerve paralysis, weakness, knuckling or dragging feet, vestibular signs, seizures, ataxia, and circling. It is a common misconception that hypothyroidism can cause laryngeal paralysis and esophageal motility dysfunction. A cause-and-effect relation between these disorders has not been proven; further, these conditions do not respond to treatment for hypothyroidism.

Reproductive abnormalities associated with hypothyroidism are controversial. Previously, it has been reported that hypothyroidism caused decreased libido, testicular atrophy, and decreased sperm production in male dogs. One study failed to reproduce these findings in Beagles with induced hypothyroidism [22]. The association of female reproductive dysfunction and hypothyroidism has not been well studied in veterinary medicine. Although uncommon, it has been reported that hypothyroid bitches may exhibit prolonged interestrus periods, failure to cycle, silent estrous, prolonged bleeding, or inappropriate lactation and mammary development. Reproductive dysfunction in geriatric pets is likely caused by conditions other than thyroid dysfunction.

Cardiovascular abnormalities related to hypothyroidism include bradycardia, arrhythmias, decreased myocardial contractility, and decreased stroke volume. These changes are usually mild but may become significant in the face of aggressive fluid therapy or anesthesia. Cardiovascular changes are usually reversible with long-term treatment for hypothyroidism [23].

Ocular changes are rare but may include corneal lipid deposits, corneal ulceration, uveitis, lipid effusion into aqueous humor, keratoconjunctivitis sicca, secondary glaucoma, and Horner's syndrome.

Gastrointestinal signs are not commonly associated with hypothyroidism, although constipation and diarrhea have been reported. Megaesophagus is another condition previously believed to be associated with hypothyroidism. It has been reported in dogs with hypothyroidism, but a cause-and-effect relation has not been established and clinical signs associated with megaesophagus do not improve with treatment for hypothyroidism.

Myxedema coma is a syndrome seen in severely affected hypothyroid animals. This syndrome is characterized by severe weakness, bradycardia, hypothermia, and inappropriate mentation that can progress to coma. These dogs are also presented with nonpitting edema of the face and neck, hypotension, and hypoventilation. This condition is often fatal because of failure to recognize the cause of clinical signs, and thus failure to institute appropriate treatment, including intravenous or oral administration of thyroid hormone and supportive care.

Dogs with secondary hypothyroidism are presented with the same complaints and physical examination findings as dogs with primary hypothyroidism. These dogs may have additional abnormalities attributable to diseases causing decreased TSH secretion. These can include neurologic signs and signs of other endocrinopathies related to the presence of a pituitary tumor or clinical signs related to any other disease causing thyrotroph suppression.

Diagnosis

Diagnosis of hypothyroidism is complex and is often based on physical examination findings, laboratory tests, and, occasionally, response to treatment. Diagnostic tests for dogs suspected of being hypothyroid include a CBC, biochemical panel, UA, and T_4 (fT_4 and total) and TSH levels.

The CBC of hypothyroid animals may show normochromic, normocytic, nonregenerative anemia. This is found in less than 50% of hypothyroid animals. This anemia is caused by decreased plasma erythropoietin concentration and lack of bone marrow stimulation. There is a generalized decreased demand for red blood cells because of decreased oxygen consumption with decreased metabolism as a result of hypothyroidism. Leptocytes may be seen because of increased cholesterol loading of cell membranes. The leukocyte count is often normal, unless there is a concurrent infection. Platelet counts are normal to increased with normal to decreased platelet size.

Biochemical changes in hypothyroid dogs include fasting hypercholesterolemia, hyperlipidemia, and hypertriglyceridemia as a result of decreased lipid metabolism. Rarely, increased ALT, aspartate aminotransferase (AST), ALP, and creatinine kinase may be seen.

The results of UA of hypothyroid dogs are usually unremarkable. Imaging studies, such as radiography and ultrasonography, may be indicated based on physical examination findings and for the pursuit of diagnosis of concurrent conditions or causes of the euthyroid sick syndrome.

Routine testing of thyroid function for dogs suspected of being hypothyroid should include evaluation of fT_4, total T_4, and TSH concentrations or a combination of these tests as needed. Assessment of T_3, free T_3 (fT_3), and reverse T_3 (rT_3) levels is not routinely recommended for the assessment of thyroid function in dogs.

Total T_4 and fT_4 levels can be used individually as screening tests for hypothyroidism or as part of a panel of thyroid function tests. Serum total T_4 or fT_4 levels well within the normal range indicate that the animal is not hypothyroid. If one or both of these values are in the low normal or below normal range, the animal may be hypothyroid; however, further evaluation is often needed to eliminate the euthyroid sick syndrome. Free T_4 levels measured by equilibrium dialysis are highly sensitive and specific for detection of hypothyroidism. There is a gray zone in the interpretation of these tests, because an overlap exists between the values of normal animals and hypothyroid animals. Individual T_4 values must be evaluated together with the history, physical examination findings, and other clinical pathologic data to determine the likelihood of hypothyroidism in each pet. If, after consideration of the data, it is still unclear whether the animal is truly hypothyroid, further evaluation of thyroid function is indicated.

Serum TSH levels are often increased in primary hypothyroidism as well as in euthyroid dogs with concurrent illness. Increased TSH levels may be detectable earlier in the disease process than low T_4 levels. In some hypothyroid animals, TSH levels remain in the normal range. For these reasons, TSH levels must be interpreted concurrently with T_4 levels as well as with historical, physical examination, and clinical pathologic findings. In animals with normal T_4 and fT_4 and increased TSH without clinical signs of hypothyroidism, it is recommended that testing be repeated in 3 to 6 months. TSH levels cannot be used to diagnose secondary hypothyroidism, because current test techniques are not sensitive enough at low levels to distinguish between low and normal TSH levels.

There are many factors that can affect the results of thyroid function tests. These factors make the correct interpretation of thyroid function tests challenging. Circulating T_4 levels decrease as dogs age, although the levels stay within the normal values but may be in the gray zone. Age has not been shown to affect T_3, fT_4, or TSH levels. Body size and breed of dog affect circulating T_4 levels. There is an inverse relation, with small dogs having a higher baseline T_4 than large dogs. Sight hounds are reported to have a lower baseline T_4 and fT_4 than other breeds [24]. The effect of gender and time of the female cycle on circulating thyroid hormone levels is unclear at this time. Random daily fluctuations in circulating thyroid levels in healthy, euthyroid sick, and hypothyroid dogs can lead to confusing test results. In cases in which the results do not support other findings, veterinarians should consider repeating the tests and re-evaluating the results. Many diseases can suppress circulating thyroid hormone levels through suppression of the hypothalamus or pituitary gland, resulting in depressed TSH secretion, decreased synthesis of T_4, decreased concentration or binding ability of circulating proteins, and inhibition of conversion of T_4 to T_3. This condition is euthyroid sick syndrome. The severity of illness correlates to the degree of thyroid hormone suppression. fT_4 levels tend to be suppressed to a lesser extent than total T_4 levels. Serum TSH levels can be normal or increased with euthyroid sick syndrome. In human and veterinary medicine, there are many drugs that have been shown to have effects on thyroid hormone levels in circulation [6]. The effects of many other drugs have yet to be determined. Drug-related effects should always be considered in the interpretation of a thyroid hormone function test, especially if the test results do not correlate with the other findings. Common drugs that can decrease T_4 or T_3 include diazepam, glucocorticoids, furosemide, penicillin, anticonvulsants, and nonsteroidal anti-inflammatory drugs [25–27]. Halothane, insulin, and narcotic agents are among the drugs shown to increase serum T_4 or T_3 levels. Any drug that an animal is being given at the time of thyroid hormone function testing should be considered to have an effect on thyroid function unless proven otherwise.

The decision to treat a dog for hypothyroidism should be made after consideration of historical, physical examination, and clinicopathologic data, including T_4 level. This is least complicated when all results are compatible with a diagnosis of hypothyroidism. Unfortunately, this is often not the case. Additional thyroid function testing (eg, fT_4, TSH) is indicated when physical examination and historical findings do not strongly support a diagnosis of hypothyroidism but the T_4 level is low, if severe concurrent systemic disease is present, and if drugs known to affect thyroid testing are being used. If multiple test results are not conclusive, response to a trial period of thyroid supplementation can be evaluated. If the animal responds and clinical signs improve, it can be concluded that the animal had hypothyroidism or thyroid-responsive disease.

Thyroid supplement administration suppresses pituitary TSH secretion and causes atrophy of pituitary thyrotrophs and thyroid gland atrophy. Testing of thyroid function in an animal that has received thyroid supplementation requires discontinuation of thyroid supplement for a period of 6 to 8 weeks, depending on the previous dose and length of treatment, to allow the pituitary-thyroid axis to regain function.

Treatment

As discussed previously, thyroid supplement is used to treat hypothyroidism in animals with confirmed hypothyroidism and as trial therapy in animals suspected of being hypothyroid with discordant test results. Oral synthetic levothyroxine is the treatment of choice for both situations. The recommended initial dose is 0.02 mg/kg administered every 12 hours, up to a maximum dose of 0.8 mg. Initial therapy should be continued for 6 to 8 weeks before evaluation of therapy. Although clinical signs resolve at different rates, all are reversible. Improvement in mental alertness is often seen in the first week of treatment, whereas regrowth of hair and reversal of dermatologic and reproductive changes can occur over many months. If a significant improvement in clinical signs is not observed after 8 weeks of therapy, the animal must be re-evaluated. Common complications include misdiagnosis of hypothyroidism, presence of concurrent nonthyroidal disease, poor owner compliance with administration of levothyroxine, expired levothyroxine, inappropriate dose or frequency of administration of levothyroxine, use of generic levothyroxine, and decreased intestinal absorption of levothyroxine.

Therapeutic monitoring should be performed after the initial 6 to 8 weeks of therapy, when there is minimal or no response to treatment, or if signs of thyrotoxicosis occur. Serum T_4 and TSH levels should be evaluated 4 to 6 hours after administration of levothyroxine when twice-daily dosing is used and just before administration and 4 to 6 hours after administration when once-daily dosing is used. When appropriate therapy is instituted after administration of levothyroxine, T_4 levels should be in the high to high normal range and TSH levels should be in the normal range. If T_4 values are significantly increased higher than the normal range or signs of thyrotox-icosis (eg, panting, nervousness, aggression, PU/PD, polyphagia, weight loss) are observed, a decrease in dose or once-daily administration should be considered. If T_4 levels are still low, an increase in dose should be considered. T_4 levels before administration of levothyroxine evaluate trough values of circulating thyroid hormone. If trough values are low or low normal and the animal has failed to improve clinically, an increase in dose should be considered. If therapeutic monitoring is performed in an animal that seems to have failed to respond to treatment and the values obtained are appropriate, investigation of other causes of clinical signs should be pursued. Therapeutic monitoring should occur 2 to 4 weeks after adjusting the dose of levothyroxine.

Synthetic T_3 therapy should be considered in dogs with confirmed hypothyroidism when appropriate levothyroxine therapy has failed to improve clinical signs and therapeutic monitoring reveals low serum T_4 levels and high TSH levels. The most common reason for this problem is decreased intestinal absorption of levothyroxine. The initial dose of oral liothyronine is 4 to 6 µg/kg administered every 8 hours. Therapeutic monitoring of serum T_3 levels should be performed just before and 2 to 4 hours after administration. T_3 values should be in the normal range when the dog is receiving appropriate treatment.

Prognosis

The prognosis for geriatric dogs with primary hypothyroidism receiving appropriate treatment is excellent. This disease should have no effect on life expectancy or quality of life when treated appropriately. The prognosis for geriatric dogs with secondary hypothyroidism is much more guarded, because the most common cause of this condition is a space-occupying mass that has the potential to invade other areas of the brain, specifically the brain stem.

Canine thyroid tumors

Clinical features

Canine thyroid tumors account for 1% to 4% of canine neoplasia and 10% to 15% of canine head and neck tumors [28,29]. In contrast to thyroid tumors in cats, clinically evident thyroid tumors in dogs are most often nonfunctional and malignant. Canine thyroid adenomas are often small and nonfunctional, and thus not detected except at necropsy, where they comprise 30% to 50% of thyroid tumors detected [6]. Thyroid tumors can originate from the thyroid glands or from ectopic thyroid tissue located anywhere from the base of the tongue to the thorax. Thyroid carcinomas are locally invasive and highly metastatic, with the most common locations of metastasis being the lungs, liver, and regional lymph nodes (especially retropharyngeal) [30]. Thyroid tumors are most common in older dogs, with no gender predilection, and Labrador Retrievers, Boxers, Golden Retrievers, and Beagles are reportedly predisposed, although this may be related to breed popularity [6,28].

Affected dogs may be presented with a palpable ventral cervical mass, dyspnea, dysphagia, cough, voice change, regurgitation, intermandibular and ventral cervical edema (precaval syndrome), and weight loss. Dogs with functional thyroid masses may exhibit signs similar to hyperthyroid cats, including PU/PD, polyphagia, panting, restlessness, heat intolerance, and weakness. Many small thyroid masses may be incidental findings, with the owners reporting no clinical signs.

Diagnosis

Physical examination of affected dogs may be unremarkable other than palpation of a ventral cervical mass and observation of problems noted by the owner. Dogs with a functional thyroid mass may be cachetic and tachycardic. Palpation of the mass should help to characterize the size and invasiveness of the mass as well as to detect other abnormalities that could indicate metastasis or other conditions affecting the prognosis for the pet.

Imaging, cytology, or biopsy of the cervical mass leads to the diagnosis in most cases. Ultrasonography of the cervical region is recommended for all dogs presented with a palpable cervical mass or clinical signs related to soft tissue cervical disease. The technique and interpretation of cervical ultrasound have recently been described in detail [6]. Ultrasonography can help to identify the tissue of origin of a cervical mass as well as to characterize the invasiveness of the mass, blood supply to the mass, and association and effects on adjacent structures. Radioactive pertechnetate scans may also be used to image thyroid masses and ectopic thyroid tissue.

Cytology of a cervical mass obtained through fine-needle aspiration (FNA) is easily performed, is noninvasive, and can increase suspicion of the diagnosis of a thyroid tumor. It is recommended that a coagulation profile be obtained before aspiration or biopsy of suspected thyroid masses. FNA should be performed with ultrasound guidance to avoid associated vasculature. If FNA of the mass is nondiagnostic, a surgical core biopsy can be obtained and submitted for histopathologic evaluation. This would require sedation or anesthesia but allows for collection of a larger piece of the mass, which is more likely to be diagnostic and can then be used for immunohistochemistry if necessary. Ultimately, histopathologic evaluation is necessary for a definitive diagnosis of the tumor.

Minimum database blood work is recommended for dogs presented with a suspected thyroid tumor, because they are usually older (>8 years) and a search for concurrent disease and organ dysfunction is also indicated. Affected dogs may need to undergo anesthesia, and the blood work can help to assess the patient's anesthetic risk. There are no consistently reported changes on the CBC, biochemical profile, and UA that are correlated to thyroid tumors.

Thoracic and abdominal imaging should be performed as part of the staging procedure for thyroid tumors. Signs of pulmonary and heart base metastasis can be detected by thoracic radiography, although normal radiographs do not exclude the possibility of microscopic metastasis. Radiographs of the cervical region may identify the suspected or palpated mass, characterize the severity of displacement of other cervical structures, or reveal evidence of invasion of the mass into the larynx and trachea. Abdominal radiographs may reveal an abnormal hepatic silhouette, which has been correlated to hepatic metastasis in some cases, although abdominal ultrasonography is more sensitive for detecting metastasis [6]. Radiographic and ultrasonographic findings are important when discussing treatment options and prognosis with the owner.

Thyroid function tests (eg, T_3, T_4) in dogs with thyroid neoplasia most often suggest that the dog is euthyroid. In 55% to 60% of dogs, there is enough normal thyroid tissue remaining so that the animal's thyroid function remains normal, whereas 30% to 35% are hypothyroid because of destruction of normal thyroid tissue by the expanding tumor or as a preexisting condition unrelated to the tumor [31]. Ten percent of dogs with thyroid tumors are hyperthyroid, which is almost always associated with thyroid malignancy.

Treatment

Treatment of thyroid tumors consists of a combination of surgical resection, chemotherapy, radioactive iodine therapy, and radiation therapy, depending on the progression of the disease in the individual patient [32].

Surgical resection is the recommended treatment for thyroid masses that are freely movable, and thus less likely to be invading surrounding structures. Surgery may also be recommended in some thyroid tumors that are not freely movable so as to debulk the mass before pursuit of other treatment options and to make the patient more comfortable. Surgery-related complications causing death are reported 25% of the time in dogs with freely movable thyroid masses. Histopathologic evaluation of the tissue removed at surgery, including evaluation of margins, is imperative for developing further treatment plans for the patient.

External beam radiation therapy is recommended palliative therapy for dogs with nonresectable thyroid tumors and after incomplete surgical resection of thyroid tumors. In a study of 25 dogs with nonresectable thyroid carcinomas and no evidence of metastasis receiving radiation therapy, the mean progression-free survival time (PFST) was 45 months, with the PFST greater than 150 weeks for 72% of the dogs in the study [33]. In comparison, survival time for dogs with similar disease receiving no treatment was between 2 and 38 weeks after diagnosis.

Radioactive iodine therapy is only recommended for the treatment of functional thyroid tumors with a prolonged iodine trapping capacity, which can be determined by a radioactive iodine tracer study.

Various chemotherapy protocols have been used to treat thyroid carcinomas. Chemotherapy alone has not resulted in increased survival times. Chemotherapy has been shown to have a role as an adjunctive therapy after incomplete surgical resection, after incomplete destruction of thyroid tissue with external beam radiation therapy, and in dogs with demonstrated metastatic disease.

Prognostic factors

The histomorphologic malignancy grade of thyroid neoplasms has been found to be the only significant prognostic factor. Occurrence of metastasis is closely related to the volume of the primary neoplasm. Metastasis was present in 14% of dogs with tumors less than 23 cm^3 at necropsy, 74% of dogs with tumors between 23 cm^3 and 100 cm^3, and 100% of dogs with tumors greater than 100 cm^3 [34]. This demonstrates the importance of early detection and treatment for thyroid tumors.

The long-term prognosis for dogs with thyroid adenoma surviving surgical resection is good to excellent, with surgery often being curative. The long-term prognosis for dogs with thyroid carcinoma is guarded to poor because of the invasive nature of the tumors, high risk of metastasis associated with large size of tumors at the time of diagnosis, and expense of surgery and adjunctive therapy.

Summary

Thyroid disorders are common in older pets. They often present a diagnostic challenge, and reaching a definitive diagnosis can be difficult or impossible in some cases. It is important for the veterinary practitioner to be familiar with the historical, physical examination, and clinicopathologic data findings in each of these diseases and to become comfortable with the treatment, monitoring, and prognosis associated with thyroid diseases in geriatric pets.

Acknowledgment

The author acknowledges Dr. Deborah Greco for giving her the opportunity to write this article and for her assistance throughout the process.

References

[1] Martin K, Rossing M, Ryland L, et al. Evaluation of dietary and environmental risk factors for hyperthyroidism in cats. J Am Vet Med Assoc 2000;217(6):853–6.
[2] Chastain C, Panciera D, Waters C. Evaluation of environmental, nutritional, and host factors in cats with hyperthyroidism. Small Anim Clin Endocrinol 2000;10(1):7.
[3] Edinboro C, Scott-Moncrieff C, Janovitz E, et al. Epidemiological study of relationships between consumption of commercial canned food and risk of hyperthyroidism in cats. J Am Vet Med Assoc 2004;224(6):879–86.
[4] Chastain C, Panciera D, Waters C, et al. Evaluation of dietary and environmental risk factors for hyperthyroidism in cats. Small Anim Clin Endocrinol 2001;11(2):7.
[5] Kass P, Peterson M, Levy J, et al. Evaluation of environmental, nutritional, and host factors in cats with hyperthyroidism. J Vet Intern Med 1999;13(4):323–9.
[6] Feldman E, Nelson R. Canine and feline endocrinology and reproduction. 3rd edition. Philadelphia: WB Saunders; 2004 p. 155–6, 197, 132, 222, 226, 228.
[7] Graves T, Peterson M. Occult hyperthyroidism in cats. In: Kirk R, Bonagura J, editors. Current veterinary therapy XI. Philadelphia: WB Saunders; 1992. p. 334–7.
[8] Maggio F, DeFrancesco T, Atkins C. Ocular lesions associated with systemic hypertension in cats: 69 cases (1985–1998). J Am Vet Med Assoc 2000;217(5):695–702.
[9] Foster D, Thoday K. Tissue sources of serum alkaline phosphatase in 34 hyperthyroid cats: a qualitative and quantitative study. Res Vet Sci 2000;68(1):89–94.
[10] Barber P, Elliott J. Study of calcium homeostasis in feline hyperthyroidism. J Small Anim Pract 1996;37(12):575–82.
[11] Graham P, Mooney C, Murray M. Serum fructosamine concentrations in hyperthyroid cats. Res Vet Sci 1999;67:171–5.
[12] Reusch C, Tomsa K. Serum fructosamine concentrations in cats with overt hyperthyroidism. J Am Vet Med Assoc 1999;215(9):1297–300.
[13] Peterson M, Melian C, Nichols R. Measurement of serum concentrations of free thyroxine, total thyroxine, and total triiodothyronine in cats with hyperthyroidism and cats with non thyroidal disease. J Am Vet Med Assoc 2001;218(4):529–36.
[14] Jacobs G, Panciera D. Cardiovascular complications of feline hyperthyroidism. In: Kirk R, Bonagura J, editors. Current veterinary therapy XI. Philadelphia: WB Saunders; 1992. p. 756–9.
[15] Hoffmann G, Marks S, Taboada J, et al. Transdermal methimazole treatment in cats with hyperthyroidism. J Feline Med Surg 2003;5(2):77–82.
[16] Hoffman S, Yoder A, Trepanier L. Bioavailability of transdermal methimazole in a pluronic lecithin organogel (PLO) in healthy cats. J Vet Pharmacol Ther 2002;25(3):189–93.

[17] Nachreiner R, Refsal K, Graham P, et al. Prevalence of serum thyroid hormone autoantibodies in dogs with clinical signs of hypothyroidism. J Am Vet Med Assoc 2002; 220(4):466–71.

[18] Scott-Moncrieff J, Azcona-Olivera J, Glickman N, et al. Evaluation of antithyroglobulin antibodies after routine vaccination in pet and research dogs. J Am Vet Med Assoc 2002; 221(4):515–21.

[19] Greco D. Polyendocrine gland failure in dogs. Vet Med (Praha) 2000;95(6):477–81.

[20] Graham P, Nachreiner R, Refsal K, et al. Lymphocytic thyroiditis. Vet Clin North Am Small Anim Pract 2001;31(5):915–33.

[21] Greco D, Rosychuk R, Ogilvie G, et al. The effect of levothyroxine treatment on resting energy expenditure of hypothyroid dogs. J Vet Intern Med 1998;12(1):7–10.

[22] Johnson C, Olivier N, Nachreiner R, et al. Effect of ^{131}I-induced hypothyroidism on indices of reproductive function in adult male dogs. J Vet Intern Med 1999;13(2):104–10.

[23] Stephan I, Nolte I, Hoppen H. The effect of hypothyroidism on cardiac function in dogs [in German]. Dtsch Tierarztl Wochenschr 2003;110(6):231–9.

[24] Gaughan K, Bruyette D. Thyroid function testing in greyhounds. Am J Vet Res 2001;62(7): 1130–3.

[25] Daminet S, Croubels S, Duchateau L, et al. Influence of acetylsalicylic acid and ketoprofen on canine thyroid function tests. Vet J 2003;166(3):224–32.

[26] Daminet S, Ferguson D. Influence of drugs on thyroid function in dogs. J Vet Intern Med 2003;17(4):463–72.

[27] Gulikers K, Panciera D. Influence of various medications on canine thyroid function. Compend Contin Educ Pract Vet 2002;24(7):511–22.

[28] Harari J, Patterson J, Rosenthal R. Clinical and pathological features of thyroid tumors in 26 dogs. J Am Vet Med Assoc 1986;188:1160–4.

[29] Birchard S, Roesel O. Neoplasia of the thyroid gland in the dog: a retrospective study of 16 cases. J Am Anim Hosp Assoc 1981;17:369–72.

[30] Lurye J, Behrand E. Endocrine tumors. Vet Clin North Am Small Anim Pract 2001;31(5): 1095–110.

[31] Mooney C. Canine thyroid tumours and hyperthyroidism. In: Torrence A, Mooney C, editors. BSAVA manual of small animal endocrinology. 2nd edition. Cheltenham, United Kingdom: British Small Animal Veterinary Association; 1998. p. 219–22.

[32] Panciera D, Lanz O, Vail D. Treating thyroid and parathyroid neoplasia in dogs and cats. Vet Med (Praha) 2004;99(2):154–68.

[33] Theon A, Marks S, Feldman E, et al. Prognostic factors and patterns of treatment failure in dogs with unresectable differentiated thyroid carcinomas treated with megavoltage irradiation. J Am Vet Med Assoc 2000;216(11):1775–9.

[34] Leav I, Shiller A, Rijnberk A, et al. Adenomas and carcinomas of the canine and feline thyroid gland. Am J Pathol 1976;83:61–93.

ELSEVIER
SAUNDERS

Vet Clin Small Anim
35 (2005) 655–674

VETERINARY
CLINICS
Small Animal Practice

Orthopedic Problems in Geriatric Dogs and Cats

Brian S. Beale, DVM

*Gulf Coast Veterinary Specialists, 1111 West Loop South, Suite 160,
Houston, TX 77027, USA*

Disorders of the joints

Osteoarthritis

Osteoarthritis (OA) is a common cause of pain and dysfunction in geriatric dogs. Clinical signs of pain can vary greatly among individual dogs and are not always obvious (Table 1). The patient may commonly demonstrate only a change in behavior if painful. Examples include reluctance to jump into the car or climb stairs, lagging behind in walks, and slow to rise. Other clinical signs seen with OA may include stiffness of gait, lameness, joint thickening, joint pain, joint swelling, and crepitus. Marked pain may be evident in severely affected dogs. A decreased range of motion is seen as the condition becomes more chronic. OA has been reported to occur in 90% of geriatric cats [1]. Cats suffering from OA can show the typical signs described previously, but their clinical signs may be subtle. Decreased activity level and a more reserved lifestyle may be the only observed signs.

Diagnosis

Diagnosis of OA can be made by correlation of history, physical examination, and radiographic findings. A thorough systematic orthopedic examination is essential and can be performed in 5 to 10 minutes. The examination should include palpation (feeling for swelling or heat) and manipulation of each joint (flexion, extension, collateral stress, abduction, and adduction) of the forelimbs and hind limbs. The muscle bellies and long bones should be palpated for pain or swelling. Radiographic changes include joint capsular distention, osteophytosis, narrowed joint spaces, and

E-mail address: drbeale@gcvs.com

Table 1
Common clinical signs of osteoarthritis

	Dogs	Cats
Mild osteoarthritis	Stiffness, decreased activity, limping	Decreased activity
Moderate osteoarthritis	Limping, pain, muscle atrophy, stiffness, difficulty rising	Decreased activity, reluctance to jump
Severe osteoarthritis	Limping, loss of range of motion, vocalization, muscle atrophy, pain, difficulty rising, crepitus, lethargy	Decreased activity, reluctance to jump, limping, muscle atrophy

subchondral erosion in severe cases. If OA is secondary to joint instability, adjacent soft tissues may hypertrophy, causing radiographic and palpable thickening. Arthrocentesis and synovial fluid analysis can be used to support a diagnosis of OA. A mild increase in mononuclear cells and neutrophils is seen, generally less than 3000 cells/mL. Imaging techniques, such as MRI, CT, and nuclear scintigraphy, can help to define the underlying cause of OA. Arthroscopy allows thorough evaluation of the joint in a minimally invasive manner, also permitting accurate documentation and a better understanding of the arthritic process.

Goals for treatment of osteoarthritic pain

Management of osteoarthritic pain can be complex. The goal of treatment is to eliminate underlying causes of OA (often requiring surgery), to reduce pain and inflammation, to improve joint function, and to slow or halt the arthritic process. It is usually necessary to manage the osteoarthritic patient with a combination approach as outlined in Box 1.

Treatment

Treatment for osteoarthritic pets should be tailored to the individual. A cookbook approach to treatment leads to less than optimal results in some patients. Treatment may include weight loss, environmental modification, controlled exercise and physical therapy, pharmacologic therapy, or surgery (Fig. 1). In cases of secondary OA, the underlying cause must be identified in

---

Box 1. Five steps of osteoarthritis treatment

1. Weight optimization
2. Exercise modification
3. Environment modification
4. Drugs (nonsteroidal anti-inflammatory drugs)
5. Chondroprotectants

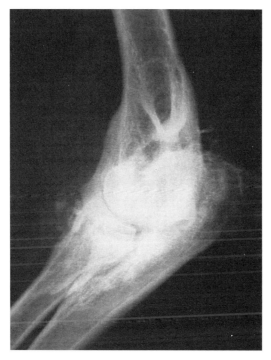

Fig. 1. Elbow osteoarthritis (OA) caused by a fragmented coronoid process is common in geriatric large-breed dogs. Medical treatment with nonsteroidal anti-inflammatory drugs and disease-modifying agents may help to relieve discomfort. Arthroscopic removal of loose fragments can also benefit dogs that have advanced OA.

an attempt to minimize the long-term effects. This may imply removal of an osteochondral fragment or stabilization of a stifle after rupture of a cranial cruciate ligament.

Weight loss, when indicated, ameliorates clinical signs of OA as a result of decreased forces being placed on joint surfaces. In fact, weight loss may help to reduce the dose or frequency of symptomatic therapy using nonsteroidal anti-inflammatory drugs (NSAIDs). Weight reduction before surgery reduces postoperative stress placed on the surgical repair but is not mandatory. Often, exercise is difficult until a predisposing cause of OA is eliminated. Enforced rest and restricted activity provide an opportunity for transient episodes of inflammation to resolve, in addition to decreasing stress placed on surgical repair. Controlled moderate exercise should be instituted long term to help avoid loss of range of motion because of joint capsule fibrosis, to maintain or build muscle mass, and to promote the physiologic health of articular cartilage.

Pharmacologic management of OA is important for three reasons: to decrease inflammation, to provide analgesia, and to improve function. Consideration should be given to drugs that inhibit the release or activity of prostaglandins, leukotrienes, neutral metalloproteases (eg, stromelysin, collagenase), serine proteases, oncoproteins, interleukins, and tumor necrosis factor. NSAIDs and glucocorticoid drugs are common examples. Other products, such as the slow-acting disease-modifying osteoarthritic agents (SDMOAs), are purported to only inhibit mediators of inflammation within the joint but may also stimulate metabolic activity of synoviocytes and chondrocytes. These products are available in injectable and oral forms.

Nonsteroidal anti-inflammatory drugs

NSAIDs are widely used as a means of reducing prostaglandin synthesis (primarily PGE_2) through inhibition of cyclooxygenase (COX). Aspirin and phenylbutazone have historically been the most commonly used agents in dogs. In dogs, aspirin has been recommended to be administered with food at a dose of 25 mg/kg of body weight every 8 hours. Phenylbutazone can be given at a dose of 10 to 22 mg/kg of body weight divided three times a day in dogs. When the higher dose is selected, it is decreased after 48 hours to the lowest effective level, not to exceed a total daily dose of 800 mg regardless of patient body weight. Aspirin and phenylbutazone are not commonly used now because of the availability of superior and safer drugs (COX-1–sparing NSAIDs). Because of the potential for gastric ulceration, NSAIDs should be used be used cautiously in dogs with pain and orthopedic problems. Although many references have suggested dosages for naproxen, meclofe-namic acid, piroxicam, flunixin meglumine, and ibuprofen, they seem to have increased ulcerogenic potential; therefore, their use is discouraged. In general, NSAID use should be avoided if possible in patients having underlying liver or kidney disease or in those patients susceptible to gastrointestinal ulceration.

Carprofen

Carprofen (Rimadyl), an NSAID product from Pfizer Animal Health, is approved for treatment of pain and inflammation associated with OA and for the control of postoperative pain associated with soft tissue and ortho-pedic surgery in dogs. Carprofen is available for oral use in caplet and chewable tablet formulations in 25-, 75-, and 100-mg sizes. Injectable carprofen became available in 2003, and its use for preemptive analgesia and rapid pain control has become common. Carprofen is licensed for subcutaneous use, but extralabel intravenous administration is commonly performed.

Carprofen is routinely used for preemptive and postoperative analgesia. When used for control of surgical pain, the first dose of carprofen can be administered approximately 2 hours before the procedure and then continued after surgery according to the needs of the individual animal. The recommended dose is 4.0 mg/kg. If used preemptively, the drug can be administered at the time of premedication or induction of anesthesia. The effect on bleeding at surgery does not seem to be a clinical problem. A short-lived mild inhibition has been seen experimentally, but bleeding times are normal when evaluated in clinical patients. Coagulation test results, including prothrombin time (PT), APTT, and ACT, are also normal after administration of injectable carprofen.

Gastroduodenal protection occurs because of carprofen's enhanced COX-2 activity. Most NSAIDs in the past have primarily been COX-1 inhibitors, which lead to widespread PGE_2 inhibition, including that found in the gastrointestinal tract, joints, and kidneys. COX-2 inhibitors have their predominant effect on COX in the joint. Carprofen is given orally at a dose of 2.2 mg/kg every 12 hours or 4.4 mg/kg every 24 hours. The flexibility of giving Rimadyl once or twice a day is an added advantage, allowing owners to choose the option that best fits their schedule. Plasma and serum concentrations of carprofen are consistent throughout the treatment period. Serum concentrations peak at 2 hours, whereas synovial concentrations peak between 3 and 6 hours. The synovial concentration of carprofen ranges between 1 and 10 μg/mL during the treatment period in normal and osteoarthritic joints. A significant reduction of PGE_2 from chondrocytes occurs at all concentrations in this range. An idiosyncratic side effect has been reported in dogs on carprofen; rare dogs were reported to have reversible hepatotoxic effects leading to icterus and elevation of alkaline phosphatase and hepatic transaminases. The incidence of this and other side effects is low (less than 1%). Recent studies have shown carprofen to have little effect on kidney and platelet function. Carprofen has recently been found to support cartilage metabolism and proteoglycan synthesis. Carprofen has been anecdotally reported to have success in treatment of osteoarthritic and postoperative pain in cats at a dose of 12.5 mg administered orally every 5 days. No severe adverse reactions have been reported at this dose. The use of carprofen in cats is extralabel; this drug is not approved for use in cats, and no clinical research data are available to substantiate the anecdotal regimen mentioned previously. Cats have been found to be sensitive to the NSAID class of drugs because of differences in liver metabolism of this type of drug.

Deracoxib

Deracoxib (Deramaxx) is a recently released NSAID from Novartis Animal Health approved for use in dogs for postoperative pain and inflammation. The product is available as a chewable tablet. The recommended dose in dogs is 3 to 4 mg/kg administered orally once daily for 7 days or 1 to 2 mg/kg administered orally once daily for chronic use. The chronic dose should be used if treating for OA. Deracoxib has a highly favorable COX-2:COX-1 ratio and has a much higher affinity for the COX-2 receptor site compared with the COX-1 receptor site. The expected side effects are similar to those of other NSAIDS, primarily gastrointestinal disturbances. Cardiovascular side effects have been seen in people taking coxib class drugs, but this does not seem to be a major problem in dogs. Deracoxib should not be used in cats.

Etodolac

Etodolac (Etogesic) is a Fort Dodge product used for treatment of OA in dogs. The drug is available as a nonchewable tablet and is administered at a dose of 10 to 15 mg/kg every 24 hours. Etodolac has been found to be an effective treatment for ameliorating the clinical signs of OA. Side effects with etodolac are typical of those seen with the NSAID class of drugs, with gastrointestinal ulceration being the most common problem.

Meloxicam

Meloxicam (Metacam), a recently released NSAID manufactured by Boehringer-Ingelheim, has been approved for treatment of postoperative pain in dogs. Oral and injectable forms are available. The oral form is a suspension that can be applied to the pet's food or administered directly into the mouth. The dose for dogs is 0.1 mg/kg administered orally once daily. A loading dose of 0.2 mg/kg can be given the first day. The oral liquid is calibrated at one drop to 1 lb of body weight to simplify administration. This is particularly useful for patients having a small body size. The injectable form (5 mg/mL) is administered intravenously or subcutaneously at a rate of 0.2 mg/kg. This is equivalent to giving 1 mL for every 55 lb of body weight for the first dose. If a subsequent dose is given, it should be reduced to half the dose. The oral form can be used after 24 hours at a dose of 0.1 mg/kg administered once daily. Meloxicam is approved in the United States for a single subcutaneous dose before surgery at a rate of 0.3 mg/kg. Meloxicam has been used in cats in Europe at a dose of 0.1 mg/kg administered orally once a day for 2 days and then 0.025 mg/kg administered two to three times a week for chronic use.

Tepoxalin

Tepoxalin (Zubrin) was recently released by Schering Plough as an oral treatment for pain and inflammation associated with OA. The drug is formulated as a rapidly disintegrating tablet that dissolves in the mouth within 4 seconds. Tepoxalin inhibits COX-1, COX-2, and 5-lipoxygenase (LOX). The COX pathway produces prostaglandins, whereas the LOX pathway leads to production of leukotrienes, both of which play a role in OA. Theoretically, inhibition of both pathways may lead to a better ability to reduce the pain of OA; however, it remains to be seen whether this dual-mode inhibition provides an advantage over the strict COX inhibitors in the clinically affected dog with OA. The dose is 10 mg/kg administered once a day. A loading dose of 20 mg/kg can be used on the first day.

Glucocorticoids

Glucocorticoids have traditionally been used to treat degenerative joint disease (DJD) only when more conventional means of therapy have been ineffective. Glucocorticoids effectively reduce inflammation by inhibiting chemotaxis of neutrophils; decreasing microvasculature permeability; inhibiting COX, thereby decreasing prostaglandin production; inhibiting lipoxygenase, thereby decreasing leukotriene production; inhibiting interleukin-1 release; inhibiting oxygen free radical generation; inhibiting metalloproteinases; and stabilizing lysosomal membranes. The use of glucocorticoids for treatment of DJD would seem to be ideal because of their generalized inhibition of inflammatory mediators and cytokines; however, chronic use of these drugs has been found to delay healing and initiate damage to articular cartilage. Prednisone is given orally at an initial dose of 1 to 2 mg/kg once daily in dogs and 4 mg/kg once daily in cats. The potential systemic side effects of glucocorticoids are well documented; therefore, low-dose (0.5–2.0 mg/kg in dogs and 2.0–4.0 mg/kg in cats) alternate-day therapy is the goal if long-term therapy is instituted. Intra-articular injection of triamcinolone hexacetonide at a dose of 5 mg in dogs suggested a protective effect not only under prophylactic conditions but under therapeutic conditions in an experimental DJD model. The sparing effect on cartilage seemed to be a result of decreased production of stromelysin, interleukin-1, and oncoproteins. At best, treatment of DJD with corticosteroids is controversial and should be used for a short period only.

Chondroprotective agents

Chondroprotective agents are a class of drugs used to slow progression of and treat chronic DJD. These drugs should not only be anti-inflammatory but should support anabolic (repair) processes in cartilage, bone, and synovium essential for normalization of joint function. This class of drugs includes the glycosaminoglycans. Examples of these drugs include glycosaminoglycan polysulfate ester (GAGPS), pentosan polysulfate, and sodium hyaluronate.

Adequan (Luitpold Pharmaceuticals, Shirley, NY) is a GAGPS that is purported to provide chondroprotection as a result of the inhibition of various destructive enzymes and prostaglandins associated with synovitis and DJD. Chondrostimulatory effects are also purported as a result of increased synoviocyte secretion of hyaluronate and enhanced proteoglycan, hyaluronate, and collagen production by articular chondrocytes. Although most experimental and clinical studies support the premise that GAGPS possesses properties of chondroprotection and chondrostimulation, some studies have found GAGPS to have no beneficial effect or to actually have a detrimental effect on cartilage metabolism.

A recent clinical study in dogs with hip dysplasia found the greatest improvement in orthopedic scores at a dose of 4.4 mg/kg (2 mg/lb) given intramuscularly every 3 to 5 days for eight injections. The improvement in orthopedic score was not statistically significant, however. Another study found that twice-weekly intramuscular administration of GAGPS at a dose of 5.0 mg/kg from 6 weeks to 8 months of age in growing pups susceptible to hip dysplasia resulted in less coxofemoral subluxation. The longevity of relief provided by GAGPS is unknown. Most studies have evaluated its effect in the short term only. Anecdotal reports of the duration of amelioration of clinical signs range from days to months. It is also not known whether the complete series of injections is needed once clinical signs return or whether a shorter regimen would suffice. The recommended dose for Adequan in dogs and cats is 2 mg/lb administered intramuscularly every 5 days for eight treatments.

Side effects of GAGPS in dogs include short-term inhibition of the intrinsic coagulation cascade as well as inhibition of platelet aggregation. Also, GAGPS has been found to inhibit neutrophils and complement, which may predispose to infections, especially when injected intra-articularly under contaminated conditions.

Sodium hyaluronate has been touted to promote joint lubrication, increase endogenous production of hyaluronate, decrease prostaglandin production, scavenge free radicals, inhibit migration of inflammatory cells, decrease synovial membrane permeability, protect and promote healing of articular cartilage, and reduce joint stiffness and adhesion formation between tendon and tendon sheaths. In the past, sodium hyaluronate has generally been recommended for mild to moderate synovitis and capsulitis rather than OA. Recently, the drug has gained popularity for use in the treatment of OA. Sodium hyaluronate is usually administered intra-articularly. Hyaluronate was used in experimental dogs at a dose of 7 mg per joint administered intra-articularly once weekly, with success in slowing DJD.

Nutraceuticals

These preparations are actually promoted as nutritional supplements rather than pharmaceutic agents. These products are also referred to as chondroprotectants by some. Manufacturers have labeled these products as nutraceuticals. Unfortunately, most of these products have little controlled experimental or clinical research in dogs to substantiate their effectiveness; however, several studies are presently underway. In addition, little regulation of these products is available or enforced. Oral glycosaminoglycan, glucosamine, free-radical scavenger, and herbal products are currently being marketed. Most glycosaminoglycan compounds contain varying amounts of chondroitin sulfates. Dosages vary between products; therefore, manufacturer recommendations should be followed. These products are used alone or often in combination with NSAIDs. Few side effects have been reported with these products.

Cosequin (Nutramax Laboratories, Baltimore, MD) is marketed as a glycosaminoglycan enhancer capable of providing raw materials needed for the synthesis of extracellular matrix of cartilage. Unlike most nutraceuticals, Cosequin has been evaluated in a variety of studies. Cosequin contains glucosamine, which has been described as the building block of the matrix of articular cartilage. It has been described as a preferential substrate and stimulant of proteoglycan biosynthesis, including hyaluronic acid and chondroitin sulfate. Cosequin also contains chondroitin sulfate, mixed glycosaminoglycans, and manganese ascorbate for the purpose of promoting glycosaminoglycan production. Orally administered glucosamine hydrochloride has been associated with relief of clinical signs of DJD and chondroprotection in clinical and experimental studies in people, horses, and dogs. Although glucosamine has a slower onset of relief of clinical signs associated with DJD as compared with ibuprofen, two clinical trials found it to have equal long-term efficacy. No significant side effects have been reported with Cosequin.

Methyl-sulfonyl-methane (MSM) is a white, crystalline, water-soluble, odorless, and tasteless compound that is a derivative of dimethyl sulfoxide (DMSO). MSM has been suggested as an agent for the management of pain and inflammation and as an antioxidant. The rationale behind its use, according to the manufacturer and others, is the possibility of a dietary sulfur deficiency. The product (MSM, Flex-A-Gan 2) is available with recommended doses in capsule and powder forms for use in small and large animals. Similar to most other nutraceuticals, there are no controlled experimental or clinical studies available to support the use of this product for the management of DJD in dogs.

Fatty acid supplementation and optimizing fatty acid content in the diet may be beneficial in reducing the clinical signs of OA by reducing the production of inflammatory types of prostaglandins. These compounds serve as a substrate for COX rather than arachidonic acid, leading to less inflammatory prostaglandins. Fatty acids can be classified as ω-6 (N6) and ω-3 (N3). The optimal ratio of N6:N3 fatty acids for canine diets ideally is less than 5:1, and new diets are now emerging with a ratio less than 1:1. The ω-3 fatty acids eicosapentaenoic acid (EPA) and docosahexaenoic acid (DHA) have been recommended, but EPA has recently been proven to be more effective. Further investigation is needed in this area.

Fracture management

Fractures of the extremities in senior dogs and cats can be challenging because of the tendency for comminution and the slower healing process of bone. It is always a race between a fracture healing and an implant failing. Steps can be taken to tip the scale in the direction of early fracture healing. These steps include the following:

1. Minimally invasive surgical approach
2. Preservation of soft tissue attachments to bone fragments

3. Use of cancellous bone grafts
4. Rigid method of fracture stabilization
5. Early return to function

It is always important to obtain an accurate history before stabilizing fractures. A complete physical examination and appropriate diagnostic tests should be performed. Pathologic fractures are more likely to be seen in the geriatric dog and cat and should be identified before surgery to ensure proper client education and communication.

Surgical approach

Closed reduction and stabilization is the optimal method of treatment when possible. Unfortunately, this method is rarely possible in the senior patient because of the severity of fractures seen, long time until bony union, and tendency for patients to develop bandage sores. Open surgical approaches can be traditional or minimally invasive. The minimally invasive approach has been described as an "open, but don't touch" approach (Fig. 2). The acronym, OBDT, is used to describe this technique. The advantages to using an OBDT technique are preservation of vascular supply to the fracture site, and thus quicker healing; shorter intraoperative time; less postoperative pain; and early return to function. Methods of stabilization that work well with an OBDT approach include the interlocking nail, plate-rod hybrid, and external fixation. Traditional surgical approaches and methods of fracture stabilization can also

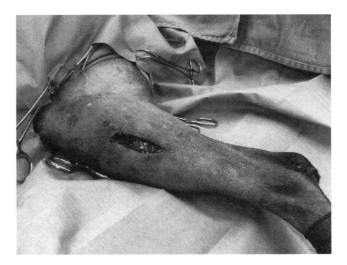

Fig. 2. Bone healing is delayed in older dogs and cats. Fractures should be treated using a minimally invasive surgical approach to preserve blood supply to the fracture site and enhance production of early bone callus. This type of fracture management is often called biologic osteosynthesis.

be used effectively in senior patients, but anatomic reconstruction of the fracture and placement of cancellous bone grafts are recommended.

Bone grafts

Numerous sites for harvest of cancellous bone graft have been described in the dog, but the most practical are the greater tubercle of the humerus, wing of the ilium, and medial proximal tibia. The humerus provides the greatest amount of cancellous bone, but the ilium and tibia provide sufficient amounts for most applications. All these sites are readily accessible, have easily recognizable landmarks, have little soft tissue covering, and provide relatively large amounts of cancellous bone. The greater trochanter can also be used if other sites are not available; however, the yield of cancellous bone is markedly less. Occasionally, multiple sites are required to harvest sufficient quantities of bone to fill large bone defects or during arthrodesis.

Minimal instrumentation is required for harvest of cancellous bone graft. Basic surgical instruments are used to approach the site selected for harvest. A hole is drilled through the near cortex using a drill bit, trephine, or trocar-pointed pin. A curette is used to scoop the graft out of the metaphyseal cancellous bone. The cancellous bone should be scooped out in large clumps if possible. Use a curette that can be comfortably manipulated in the medullary cavity. I prefer to use a relatively large curette, because this speeds harvest and reduces trauma to the graft. Closure is performed routinely in two to three layers. Recently, a technique was described using an acetabular reamer to harvest large amounts of corticocancellous bone graft from the lateral surface of the wing of the ilium.

The graft collected should be handled gently. It is desirable to collect the graft immediately before use. This increases the osteogenic properties of the graft. As graft is harvested, it should be placed on blood-soaked gauze until transfer to the recipient site. Extreme care should be taken to store the graft properly; do not accidentally discard the graft because of misidentification of the gauze as being used. The graft should be atraumatically packed into the recipient site. Lavage of the site should be avoided after the graft is placed.

Fracture stabilization

Interlocking nails

Interlocking nails are particularly useful for stabilization of fractures in the senior dog and cat. An interlocking nail system (Innovative Animal Products, Rochester, MN) is available for repair of fractures involving the femur, humerus, and tibia of small animals. Interlocking nails are useful in simple diaphyseal fractures, comminuted fractures, or fractures of the metaphyseal region, which are often difficult to plate. They have also been used successfully in infected fractures, correctional osteotomies, and nonunions. Interlocking nails offer a second alternative for many fracture types previously repairable with bone plates only. They also can be used for many applications where an intramedullary pin and adjunctive external fixator would be used; an example of this is a simple transverse femur fracture.

The nail is actually a revised Steinmann pin that has been modified by drilling one or two holes proximally and distally in the pin, which allows the placement of screws through the holes (Fig. 3). The nail and screws can be applied in a closed or open fashion because of the incorporation of a specific guide system that attaches to the nail. The specific equipment needed to place the nail includes a handchuck, extension device, aiming device, drill sleeve, drill guide, tap guide, drill bit, tap, depth gauge, and screwdriver. The cost of the system is reasonable, and each nail is approximately half the cost of a comparative bone plate. The nails are available in diameters of 4.7, 6, and 8 mm and in varying lengths. The 4.7-mm nail uses a 2.0-mm screw.

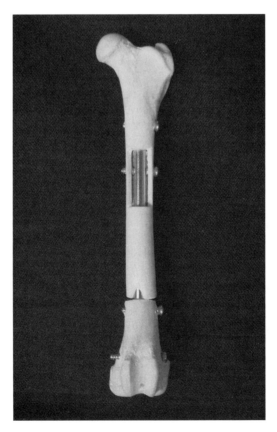

Fig. 3. Interlocking nails can be used to stabilize many fractures of the humerus, femur, and tibia in geriatric pets. The interlocking nail is a modified Steinman pin that allows screws to be placed through the bone and the pin. This type of implant provides good stability against bending, rotational, and axial forces.

The 6-mm nail comes in forms that accommodate a 2.7- or 3.5-mm screw. The 8-mm nail comes in forms that accommodate a 3.5- or 4.5-mm screw.

The interlocking nail neutralizes bending, rotational, and axial compressive forces because of the incorporation of transfixation screws that pass through the pin and lock into the bone. This is in contrast to a single intramedullary Steinmann pin, which only neutralizes bending forces. The interlocking nail has a similar bending strength compared with bone plates but is slightly weaker in neutralization of torsional forces. The screws also prevent pin migration, a common complication seen with Steinmann pins.

When using an interlocking nail, the largest diameter nail that can be accommodated by the medullary cavity at the fracture site should be selected. In most large dogs, an 8 mm nail and 3.5- or 4.5-mm screws can

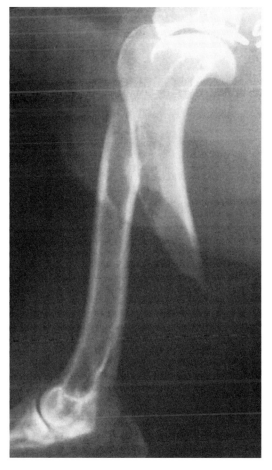

Fig. 4. A fracture of the proximal humerus requires surgical fixation in this geriatric patient. Small comminuted fragments are present at the fracture site.

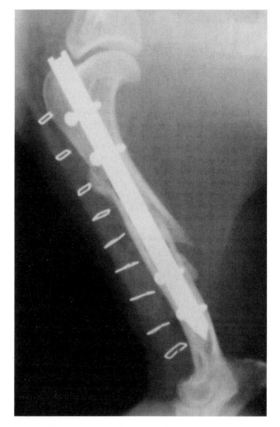

Fig. 5. This comminuted fracture of the humerus in a 12-year-old dog was stabilized with a minimally invasive surgical approach and an interlocking nail.

be used in the femur and humerus (Figs. 4–6). In medium-sized dogs, the 6-mm nail and 2.7- or 3.5-mm screws are typically used. In small dogs and cats, the 4-mm nail and 2.0-mm screws are typically used. The tibia of medium- and large-sized dogs usually accommodates a 6-mm nail, but an 8-mm nail can be used in some large dogs. A 4.0-mm nail can be used in small dogs and some cats for repair of tibial fractures.

Plate-rod hybrid

Fixation of comminuted fractures with an intramedullary pin and a bone plate combination (plate-rod hybrid) does not require reconstruction of the comminuted fragments (Fig. 7A, B and 8A, B). Rather, the area of comminution is bridged or buttressed with a plate-rod combination without manipulation or reduction of the fracture fragments. This type of repair can be used to stabilize comminuted fractures of the humerus, femur, and tibia of dogs and cats.

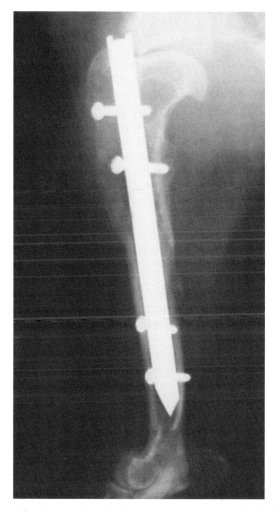

Fig. 6. Early bone callus is seen at 6 weeks after surgery. Preservation of soft tissue attachments to the bone fragments encourages early callus formation.

The intramedullary pin (rod) neutralizes bending forces, and the plate protects against rotational and axial compressive forces. Traditional bone plates are used in most dogs. Veterinary cuttable plates (VCPs) provide adequate strength and stiffness in cats and small dogs when used in combination with an intramedullary pin as well as providing additional holes for screw placement. The addition of the intramedullary pin protects the plate from cyclic bending forces, which can lead to early plate fatigue and screw loosening. This is particularly important in the area of comminution, where plate holes must often be left open.

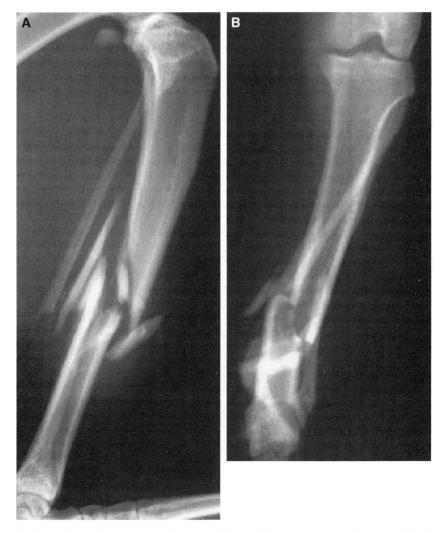

Fig. 7. (*A*, *B*) A highly comminuted fracture of the midtibia requires surgical fixation in this 11-year-old mixed-breed dog. Small comminuted fragments are present at the fracture site. Minimal soft tissues surround this area of the tibia; therefore, preservation of these tissues should be attempted to maintain optimal blood supply to the fragments.

When using a plate-rod combination, the diameter of the pin selected should accommodate approximately 30% to 40% of the medullary cavity at the diaphyseal isthmus. The length of pin should be sufficient to permit seating in the proximal and distal metaphyseal bone if possible. The size of plate selected is often dictated by the size of screw that can be placed in the bone. Ideally, at least two bicortical screws should be placed proximally and

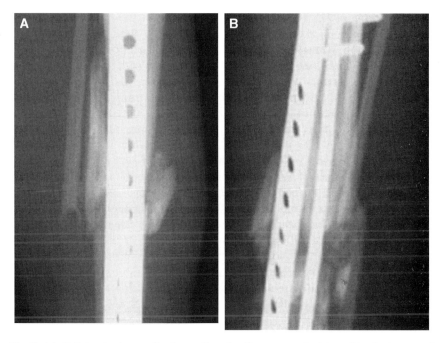

Fig. 8. (*A, B*) Extensive bone callus is seen 8 weeks after surgery. A plate-rod implant was used to stabilize the fracture. The open screw holes are protected by the intramedullary pin. This implant can be applied in a minimally invasive manner and is quite rigid.

distally, although this is not always possible. Adequate room must be present to allow screw purchase past the intramedullary pin. To accomplish screw placement, the screws must be angled away from the intramedullary pin or the plate must be offset slightly. Monocortical screws are used if bicortical screws cannot be placed.

Application of a plate-rod hybrid is similar for most comminuted fractures of the humerus, femur, and tibia. A lateral approach is generally made to the humerus and femur, and a medial approach is usually made to the tibia. An attempt should be made to minimize dissection of soft tissues, thus encouraging more rapid healing. Because of the strength and rigidity of plate-rod repair and the goal of preserving blood supply to bone fragments, complete rebuilding of the bony cylinder with cerclage wires is undesirable. The goal of the dissection is to gain just enough visualization to ensure proper placement of the intramedullary pin and plate. The appropriate pin is selected and placed in a routine fashion. Pins may be placed retrograde or normograde, depending on the bone involved and fracture location. The pin is driven just past the end of the fragment. The fracture is reduced, and the pin is driven into the medullary cavity of the opposing main fragment. Spatial realignment (rotation and length) of the limb is established as the pin is seated into the fragment. A bone plate is contoured and applied to the tension surface of the bone, bridging the area of comminution. Consideration should be given when positioning the plate to allow screw placement with minimal interference with the intramedullary pin. Bicortical screws are placed where possible. Ideally, at least two bicortical screws are placed in the proximal and distal fragments. Additional bicortical or monocortical screws are placed as permitted by the location of fracture fragments and location of the underlying intramedullary pin. Occasionally, markedly displaced fragments do not become incorporated into the healing callus. These fragments can be partially reduced with "lasso" sutures using 2-0 or 3-0 absorbable suture. Sutures are passed around the fragment as well as the bone and plate without compromising blood supply. The suture is gently tightened and secured when the fragment is drawn closer to the other fragments. This technique brings isolated fragments into the vicinity of the main fragments and may increase the likelihood of their participation in the healing process. After placement of the plate-rod hybrid, fracture stability is checked and a cancellous bone graft is placed if desired.

External fixators

External fixators are useful for the management of fractures in the senior dog and cat. The traditional type of external fixator is linear in nature, but circular external fixators are also available and are particularly useful in some fractures. External fixators can be used with a closed or open reduction of the fracture (Fig. 9). This is often the method of choice in open fractures or fractures associated with extensive soft tissue damage. Many published articles and short courses are available to train the veterinary surgeon in the proper use of these devices. External fixators are extremely versatile and well suited for the general small animal practice. They can be used for primary and adjunctive stabilization. External fixators, such as bone plates, can be used to counteract axial, bending, and torsional forces. External fixators are composed of fixator pins that are secured by a combination of connecting clamps and connecting bars. Alternatively, fixator pins may be secured with acrylic (polymethylmethacrylate), which decreases cost and allows flexibility in pin alignment. Fixator pins are available in smooth and partially threaded varieties. Partially threaded pins have superior holding power; therefore, the chance of premature loosening of the fixator is decreased. Positive-contrast pins, also called enhanced threaded pins (IMEX Veterinary, Longview, TX; Synthes Ltd, Paoli, PA; and Gauthier Medical, Rochester, MN), are stronger than traditional threaded pins, because the threads are tooled on the surface of the shaft rather than cut into the shaft. Fixator pins are placed at appropriate angles and spacing using a low-speed (150 rpm) high-torque power drill. Predrilling with a drill bit is recommended to reduce bone trauma resulting in premature pin loosening. External fixators used as the sole method of

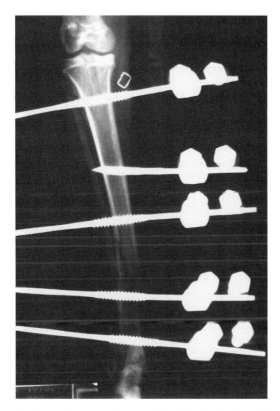

Fig. 9. Geriatric patients may have poor bone quality. Closed reduction of fractures and use of an external fixator with threaded fixator pins is a good option in this type of patient.

fracture fixation are usually type II or III. When used as adjunctive fixation, type I fixators are most commonly used. Fixators used as adjunctive fixation can actually be "tied-in" to intramedullary pins used as the primary fixation, thereby increasing the stability of the total implant system.

Postoperative period

The postoperative period is often not given the level of attention that is deserved to optimize recovery from repair of orthopedic problems in senior dogs and cats. Perioperative analgesia is important for an early return to function, to enhance healing, and to reduce the length of hospital stay The use of NSAIDs and narcotics helps to achieve this goal. Bandaging and restricted activity may be necessary after surgery, and pet owners need to be educated on the importance and expectations of their use. Physical therapy exercises may be needed to prevent fracture disease, encourage early return to function, and obtain maximum return to function.

Further readings

Anderson MA. Oral chondroprotectant agents Part 1. Compend Contin Educ Pract Vet 1999; 21(7):601–9.
Beale BS. Use of nutraceuticals in osteoarthritic dogs and cats. Vet Clin N Am Small Anim Pract 2004;34(1):271–90.
Brinker WO, Piermattei DL, Flo GL, editors. Handbook of small animal orthopedics and fracture repair. 3rd edition. Philadelphia: WB Saunders; 1997.
Horstman CL, Beale BS, Conzemius MG, et al. Biological osteosynthesis versus traditional anatomic reconstruction of 20 long-bone fractures using an interlocking nail:1994–2001. Vet Surg 2004;33:232–7.
Hulse DA, Johnson AL. Fundamentals of orthopedic surgery and fracture management. In: Fossum TW, editor. Small animal surgery. 1st edition. St. Louis: Mosby; 1997. p. 705–65.
Hulse D, Hyman W, Nori M, et al. Reduction in plate strain by addition of an intramedullary pin. Vet Surg 1997;26:451–9.
Johnson AL, Egger EL, Eurell JC, et al. Biomechanics and biology of fracture healing with external skeletal fixation. Compend Contin Educ Prac Vet 1998;20(4):487–502.
McLaughlin R, Roush J. Medical therapy for patients with osteoarthritis. Vet Med 2002;97(2): 135–44.
McNamara PS, Johnston SA, Todhunter RJ. Slow-acting, disease-modifying osteoarthritic agents. Vet Clin N Am Small Anim Pract 1991;27(4):863–7 951–2.
Palmer RH. Biological osteosynthesis. Vet Clin N Am Small Anim Pract 1999;29(5):1171–85.
Reems MR, Beale BS, Hulse DA. Use of a plate-rod construct and principles of biological osteosynthesis for repair of diaphyseal fractures in dogs and cats: 47 cases (1994–2001). J Am Vet Med Assoc 2003;223:330–5.
Wallace JM. Meloxican. Compend Contin Educ Pract Vet 2003;25(1):64–5.

Reference

[1] Hardie EM, Roe SC, Martin FR. Radiographic evidence of degenerative joint disease in geriatric cats: 100 cases (1994–1997). J Am Vet Med Assoc 2002;220(5):628–32.

ELSEVIER
SAUNDERS

Vet Clin Small Anim
35 (2005) 675–698

VETERINARY
CLINICS
Small Animal Practice

Behavior Problems in Geriatric Pets

Gary Landsberg, DVM[a],*, Joseph A. Araujo, BSc[b,c]

[a]Doncaster Animal Clinic, 99 Henderson Avenue, Thornhill, Ontario L3T2K9, Canada
[b]Department of Pharmacology, University of Toronto, Toronto, Ontario, Canada
[c]CanCog Technologies, 24 Lippincott Street, Toronto, Ontario M5T 2R5, Canada

Aging pets often suffer a decline in cognitive function (eg, memory, learning, perception, awareness) likely associated with age-dependent brain alterations. Clinically, cognitive dysfunction may result in various behavioral signs, including disorientation; forgetting of previously learned behaviors, such as house training; alterations in the manner in which the pet interacts with people or other pets; onset of new fears and anxiety; decreased recognition of people, places, or pets; and other signs of deteriorating memory and learning ability [1]. Many medical problems, including other forms of brain pathologic conditions, can contribute to these signs. The practitioner must first determine the cause of the behavioral signs and then determine an appropriate course of treatment, bearing in mind the constraints of the aging process. A diagnosis of cognitive dysfunction syndrome is made once other medical and behavioral causes are ruled out.

Distribution of behavior problems in older pets

The case load of senior pets referred to veterinary behaviorists provides some idea of the most common behavior concerns among the owners of older pets. In one study including 62 dogs aged 9 years or older, the following behavioral problems were exhibited: separation anxiety (29%), aggression toward people (27%), house soiling (23%), excessive vocalization (21%), phobias (19%), waking at night (8%), compulsive or repetitive behaviors (5%), and intraspecies aggression (5%) [2]. A more recent study including 103 dogs older than 7 years of age indicated a similar distribution of behavioral problems but also attributed a substantial number of cases

---

* Corresponding author.
E-mail address: gmlandvm@aol.com (G. Landsberg).

doi:10.1016/j.cvsm.2004.12.008

(7%) to cognitive dysfunction [3]. The recent inclusion and, possibly, the limited awareness of cognitive dysfunction as a cause of behavioral signs in the senior pet likely have resulted in an underestimation of its prevalence. The primary presenting complaint in 83 senior cats seen at three behavior referral practices (including 25 cases from Dr. Landsberg's referral practice, 33 cases from Dr. Horwitz's referral practice, and 25 cases from a study by Chapman and Voith [4]) was house soiling (inappropriate elimination or marking) in 73% of cases. Intraspecies aggression (10%), aggression to people (6%), excessive vocalization (6%), restlessness (6%), and over-grooming (4%) were the next most common reasons for referral. Although these studies provide some insight into the most serious behavior concerns of the owners of senior pets (ie, those requiring referral to a veterinary behaviorist), these cases may not be representative of the more common and subtle behavior changes of older pets that are not sufficiently serious, dangerous, or intolerable to necessitate referral. In fact, some of the behavioral signs that arise in senior pets may not seem sufficiently significant for the owners to even mention them to their veterinarian.

In a study of 180 dogs from 11 to 16 years of age that had no underlying medical illnesses, owners were asked to report any signs of cognitive dysfunction, including disorientation, altered sleep-wake cycles, decreased responsiveness to stimuli, less interest in interacting with the owners, decreased activity levels, or increased house soiling [5]. Twenty-eight percent and 68% of the owners of 11- to 12-year-old dogs and 15- to 16-year-old dogs reported at least one sign consistent with cognitive dysfunction, respectively. Furthermore, 10% and 36% of the owners of 11- to 12-year-old dogs and 15- to 16-year-old dogs reported signs in two or more categories, respectively. At a follow-up interview 12 to 18 months later, 22% of dogs that did not have any signs of impairment at the first interview developed at least one sign, whereas 48% of dogs that had impairment in one category were likely to have impairment in two or more categories [6]. In a more recent pet owner survey commissioned by Hill's Pet Nutrition, 75% of the owners of dogs aged 7 years and older reported at least one change in behavior consistent with cognitive dysfunction, but only 12% of these owners reported the change to their veterinarian [7].

In a prospective study of aged cats presented to veterinary clinics for routine annual care, 154 owners of cats aged 11 years and older were asked to report any signs of cognitive dysfunction. The questionnaire included questions about alterations or deficits in special orientation, social interactions, responsiveness to stimuli, activity, sleep-wake cycles, anxiety or irritability, and house soiling. Although 43% of the cats showed signs consistent with cognitive decline, 19 of the cats were removed from consideration because of underlying medical conditions that possibly caused the clinical signs. Thus, 35% of cats were determined to have cognitive dysfunction. A greater percentage of the older cats were affected; 50% of 46 cats older than 15 years of age had an average of 2.5 signs per cat compared with 28% of the 11- to 15-year-old cats with 1.8 signs per affected cat. In 11- to 15-year-old cats, altered social interactions were most commonly reported. By contrast, the most common signs in cats older than 15 years of age were alterations in activity levels, including aimless activity and excessive vocalization during the day [8].

Cognitive dysfunction as a clinical entity in dogs is reported to arise with increasing frequency beginning at the age of 11 years [1,2,5,6]. Recent experimental evidence suggests that a decline in cognitive function may occur much earlier than typically reported in the clinic, likely because of the limited diagnostic measures available currently (ie, owner reports of clinical signs, absence of objective test measures). Although these initial signs may be subtle and relatively innocuous, they may progress to a point where they have a significant impact on the pet's quality of life and the owner's ability to continue to care for the pet. One Australian survey of veterinary practices indicated that 23% of 90 dogs and 9% of 57 cats were euthanized because of senility [9].

Causes of behavior problems in the aging pet

Medical causes

The aging process is associated with progressive and irreversible changes that could affect a pet's behavior. Any painful or uncomfortable condition (eg, arthritis, dental disease) can lead to increased irritability or fear of being handled. If mobility is affected, the pet may become increasingly aggressive or might have more difficulty in accessing its elimination area. Organ failure, tumors, degenerative conditions, immune diseases, endocrinopathies, and sensory decline are more common in the aging pet and can have profound effects on behavior. Any disease of the central nervous system (eg, tumor) or its circulation (eg, anemia, hypertension) also can affect behavior. For example, behavior changes in hypothyroid dogs can range from lethargy to aggression [10], whereas cushingoid dogs may exhibit altered sleep-wake cycles, house soiling, excessive panting, and polyphagia. By contrast, hyperthyroid cats may be more active, irritable, or reactive to stimuli. The effects that medical conditions can have on behavior are presented in Table 1.

Behavioral threshold: combined factors

Senior pets often present with multiple medical conditions, which may result in increased behavioral signs. Multiple medical factors may "push" the pet beyond a threshold to where a behavior problem is exhibited. This might be analogous to dermatology cases in which multiple stimuli may be required before a pet is presented with pruritus. Medical conditions might also "lower" the threshold at which a behavioral problem is exhibited (ie, level of tolerance). For example, a pet that is fearful of children may begin

Table 1
Common medical conditions in older pets and their effects on behavior

System–organ	Examples of behavioral signs/behavioral implications
Neurologic	Diseases directly or indirectly affecting the central nervous system may lead to changes in temperament and mentation; signs might include those consistent with cognitive dysfunction, personality changes, repetitive behavior, or anxiety.
Neoplasia	Signs vary with tumor type
Seizure disorders	Motor or behavioral and/or psychomotor: usually episodic with an aura and/or a postictal episode with normal function between events
Cranial nerve function	Altered response to stimuli
Toxins	Exogenous: higher risk in pets with polyphagia, compulsive chewing or licking (eg, lead, pesticides, illicit drugs), or endogenous (eg, liver or kidney failure)
Circulatory and/or respiratory and/or hematopoietic	Decreased oxygenation to central nervous system leading to signs ranging from cognitive dysfunction to specific signs related to regions involved
Endocrine	Signs related to hormonal effects (eg, excesses of cortisol, thyroxine sex hormones)
Degenerative pathologic findings affecting neurotransmitter function and receptors	Decline in cognitive function, altered mentation and personality changes: altered receptor function and neurotransmission; French authors describe additional brain pathologic findings leading to involutive depression and hyperaggressiveness
Neuromuscular, peripheral neuropathy	Weakness, decreased mobility, house soiling, anxiety, altered responsiveness to stimuli; irritable, and pain-induced aggression
Musculoskeletal	Mobility, irritability, aggression, house soiling, altered responsiveness to stimuli, decreased social interaction, and increased attention seeking; weakness and/or decreased mobility; increased pain, irritability, aggression, and house soiling
Gastrointestinal	
Inflammatory and/or malabsorption	Irritability, house soiling, night waking, appetite, nutritional effects
Constipation	Irritability, house soiling
Dental	Pain-related aggression, decreased interest in food, irritability
Hepatobiliary disease	Potential for toxic effects on central nervous system; hepatic encephalopathy
Endocrine	
Hyperthyroidism (feline)	Irritability, activity, appetite, marking, aggression
Hyperadrenocorticism	Panting, polyphagia, restlessness, waking, altered elimination habits, cognitive dysfunction syndrome signs
Diabetes mellitus	House soiling, irritability, polyphagia, lethargy

Urogenital	
Renal failure	House soiling, irritability, and/or central nervous system signs if uremic
Urinary tract infection and/or urolithiasis, prostate	House soiling, irritability
Testicular tumors	Thecoma: testosterone effects; mark, mount, aggression
	Sertoli cell: feminizing effects; aggression
	Granuloma cell: aggression, estrus signs
Ovarian tumors	
Cardiovascular and/or circulatory and/or respiratory and/or hematopoietic	If altered central nervous system tissue perfusion and/or oxygenation: altered mentation or personality, decreased exercise tolerance, decreased activity, signs consistent with cognitive dysfunction syndrome
Dermatologic and/or skin	Increased irritability: mobility (eg, with footpad and/or nail involvement)
Special senses	Altered response to stimuli: less or more reactive; may be more confused, irritable, or anxious or have altered-sleep wake cycle, especially if multiple senses involved
Vision	Decreased response to stimuli: altered sleep-wake cycle; decreased ability to perform previously learned tasks; altered response to people and/or other pets
Hearing	Decreased and/or altered response to stimuli, including owners and/or strangers and/or other pets; perhaps more reactive, sensitive, anxious, or unpredictable
General and/or multiple organ effects	
Pain	Multiple possible causes (eg, dental disease, anal sacculitis, otitis, arthritis, disk disease): may lead to avoidance, aggression, decreased activity, restless behavior, or house soiling
Obesity	Lethargy, less mobile, less active leading to further cognitive decline; obesity can also have an impact on health, well-being, and longevity
Weight loss, muscle wasting	Decreased activity and/or response to stimuli, lethargy, irritability; if polyphagic, could lead to food stealing, possessiveness, night waking, pica, house soiling
Dehydration, decreased response to thirst	Constipation: house soiling, irritability.
Decreased immune competence, neoplasia	Increased susceptibility to infection, immune disease and tumors: signs related to organ system involved
Hypothermia, decreased thermoregulation	Less interactive, lethargy, anxiety, attention seeking, heat seeking, reluctant to go outdoors, altered sleep-wake cycle
Nutritional balance	Although most pet foods provide adequate nutrition for the senior pet, some home-made recipes and even some commercial foods may not address the needs of the senior pet; insufficient digestibility and nutritional imbalances that might not have an impact on the younger pet may be unhealthy for the senior pet; an improved nutritional state might prevent, improve, or slow the decline of many medical conditions

to bite as it becomes uncomfortable, becomes less mobile, or begins to develop visual or auditory decline. Varying degrees of cognitive decline associated with brain aging may also lead to alterations in the manner in which a pet perceives or responds to stimuli. Therefore, the treatment, or partial control, of underlying medical factors may not entirely eliminate the behavioral problem.

Primary behavior problems

Changes in the pet's environment may also contribute to the emergence of behavior problems. Schedule changes, a new member of the household (eg, baby, spouse), a new pet, or environmental modifications (eg, renovations, new household) all may influence a pet's behavior. Furthermore, medical or degenerative changes may cause the pet to be more sensitive or less adaptable to change. As problems emerge, undesirable responses may be rewarded inadvertently. In addition, as owners become increasingly frustrated, they may add to the pet's anxiety, especially if punishment is used to deter the behavior.

Diagnosis and treatment of behavior problems of the senior pet

The diagnosis and treatment of behavior problems are beyond the scope of this article and are well reviewed in many of the veterinary behavior texts available to the practitioner. In fact, many of the behavior problems of older pets may arise from the same causes (and require the same treatment) as those in younger pets. Because the older pet may be more affected by medical problems, including brain aging, and may be more sensitive and less able to adapt to changes and stressors in its environment, we have chosen to focus on some of the diagnostic and treatment considerations that might be specific to the older pet.

Diagnosis

Medical causes and factors

Virtually any medical condition can affect behavior. As age increases, it becomes increasingly important to look at the pet as a whole and to determine the effect of each organ system on the pet's health and behavior. This approach may differ somewhat from the approach taken toward a younger pet with health or behavior problems, where a group of signs are more likely to be attributed to a single medical problem.

Older pets have a declining immune system and are at higher risk for neoplasia and degenerative diseases, including many conditions that can be quite painful, such as arthritis and dental disease. Organ function and the special senses also become increasingly impaired with age. Pain and sensory impairment have profound effects on behavior and may be underreported, especially in cats. In one canine study, owners reported signs attributed to visual impairment in 41% of 11- to 12-year-old dogs and 68% of 15-to 16-year-old dogs. Owner estimates of hearing impairment ranged from 48% of 11- to 12-year-old dogs to 97% of 15- to 16-year-old dogs [6]. These signs could be caused by impairment of the sensory organ itself or cognitive dysfunction, where sensory transmission and processing are impaired.

Behavior and memory circuits are mainly located in the forebrain, such as in the limbic system and hippocampus. Therefore, a change in personality or mood, inability to recognize or respond appropriately to stimuli, and loss of previously learned behavior might be indicative of any type of forebrain involvement. In some cases (but not all), there may be other concurrent clinical signs, such as cranial nerve involvement, seizures, motor deficits, or emesis. Alterations in consciousness, awareness, and responsiveness to stimuli can arise from any disease process that involves the brain stem or forebrain but may also arise if there are deficits in the sensory system that provides input into these brain areas. Behavioral signs may also be caused by health issues that do not specifically affect the central nervous system or cognitive function. For example, any disease that affects elimination (eg, frequency, volume, control) could lead to house soiling. Some of the common medical conditions in older pets and their effects on behavior are presented in Table 1. For more details on screening the well and sick senior pet, the reader is directed to review the recently published guidelines of the American Animal Hospital Association (AAHA) task force on senior care.

Primary behavior problems

As part of any diagnostic workup, the first step is to determine what medical conditions might be causing or contributing to the behavioral signs and what impact they might have on the treatment of the problem. Therefore, should any behavioral signs or alterations in behavior arise, a physical examination, including a full neurologic assessment, as well as appropriate screening and diagnostic testing is required initially. The behavioral history also is a critical element in diagnosis to ensure that all signs are recognized and all inciting and contributing factors are considered. The history may reveal a significant change in the environment (eg, moving into a new home, change in owner's schedule) or new consequences (eg, particularly fearful event). In addition, some problems may have been present long before the pet became elderly, yet the behavior has only recently become a problem for the owners. For example, the pet that is potentially aggressive to strangers or children might not exhibit problems until a new spouse or child moves into the home. Of course, the older pet might be more sensitive and less able to adapt to changes in its environment.

Treating behavior problems in geriatric pets

The treatment of behavior problems, regardless of age, generally requires a combination of behavior modification as well alterations to the pet's environment. With the onset of health problems, some of which may be irreversible, it may become increasingly difficult to teach new tasks or to undo the effects of previous learning. Therefore, clear information regarding the prognosis and the limits of what may be achieved needs to be provided to the owner so as to determine what treatment regimen would be most practical and acceptable for the problem(s) at hand.

Aggression to human beings

Aggression in senior pets may arise as a result of medical problems that lead to pain, altered perception, altered recognition of stimuli (eg, sensory decline, cognitive dysfunction), or altered mentation that might arise from diseases affecting the central nervous system (see Table 1). Older pets, whether as a result of cognitive decline or other health issues, may be more irritable, anxious, and fearful, and thus increasingly aggressive toward individuals who are unfamiliar. Pets with pain or sensory decline also may begin to react more fearfully or aggressively toward novel stimuli. In addition, stimuli that were formerly acceptable to the pet may no longer be tolerated (eg, petting, brushing, teeth cleaning, lifting). Therefore, identifying and treating all underlying medical problems might result in improvement (eg, reducing pain). In addition, all stimuli possibly leading to aggression must be identified. Although avoiding potentially aggression-evoking stimuli could be the best and most practical option, the use of a reward-based retraining program may help to eliminate fear and increase desirable responses. Punishment of any type must be avoided. A leash and head halter in dogs (leash and harness in cats) can help to ensure safety and control as well as to improve communication with a pet whose sight or hearing is in decline. Clicker training also can be especially useful for older pets that are not significantly hearing impaired. Desensitization and counterconditioning techniques are needed to resolve anxiety and fear associated with the specific stimuli. Drugs for cognitive dysfunction might be indicated, but antidepressants, such as fluoxetine, and anxiolytics, such as buspirone or benzodiazepines, also could be useful, depending on the cause of the aggression.

Intraspecific aggression

Aggression between dogs in the home may arise as the younger dog matures and the older dog ages. With increasing age, the older pet may begin to respond differently to the younger pet because of cognitive decline, sensory decline, or mobility issues, which, in turn, could lead to anxiety and aggression on the part of the younger pet. Similarly, the senior pet may be unable to recognize or respond to the signals of the younger pet, leading to further anxiety and aggressive interactions. Although desensitization and counterconditioning should be the primary focus of treatment, the age and health of the older pet may limit what can be accomplished. Therefore, increased supervision (perhaps with a leash and harness or a leash and head halter) and environmental alterations that prevent undesirable interactions may be necessary as well. If cognitive dysfunction is an issue, medical treatment should be useful. Fluoxetine may also be useful for stabilizing mood, whereas anxiolytics could be considered on rare occasions.

House soiling

For house soiling that arises in senior pets, medical issues must first be addressed. Any disease process that increases urine output or frequency can lead to house soiling, especially if the owner cannot change his or her schedule (dogs) or increase the frequency of litter box cleaning and the number of litter boxes (cats) to accommodate the increased need to eliminate. Similarly, bowel diseases that lead to altered frequency or increased discomfort can lead to inappropriate defecation. Close attention to history should help to determine whether marking, incontinence, or cognitive dysfunction is an issue. Another important consideration in the history is whether there is any indication of increased fear or anxiety that could lead to house soiling or increased marking behavior. In addition to treating the underlying medical problem, dogs may require more frequent trips outdoors. If the pet eliminates indoors when the owner is at home, reinforcing of outdoor elimination in addition to increased supervision is required. Environmental alterations, such as confining the pet during departures, allowing for an indoor soiling area, or adding a dog door, may be considered also. For cats, a wide array of environmental modifications, especially with respect to the height and type of litter box, might help to address issues like polyuria or decreased ability to access and use the litter box (eg, arthritis, visual deficits). These can include adding new litter boxes, more frequent litter box cleaning, changing litter type to one with reduced clumping, alterations to the litter box so that it is larger or has lower sides, improving access and lighting to the litter box, or merely preventing access to problem areas. Although Feliway (Veterinary Product Laboratories, Phoenix, AZ) or drug therapy, such as fluoxetine or buspirone, might be useful if there is a marking component, it has little or no effect on litter avoidance and location preferences.

Separation anxiety, fear, and phobias

A change in the pet's daily routine can have a greater impact on the senior pet, which is more sensitive to change and less able to adapt. In addition, medical problems like cognitive dysfunction, sensory decline, organ failure, and endocrinopathies may result in increased fear and anxiety as well as altered responses to stimuli. In turn, the owner's response, whether it is increased frustration and punishment or the use of affection and treats in an attempt to calm the pet down, can further serve to aggravate the problem. Although the prognosis may be poorer for the senior pet with fear and anxiety, some improvement should be possible if underlying medical problems can be controlled at least in part and the owner institutes appropriate behavior modification techniques. Treatment of separation anxiety and noise phobias generally requires the same steps as with the younger pet. In particular, environmental adjustments to help the pet and owner cope, training relaxation, providing a predictable daily routine, teaching the owner to ensure a calm and settled response before attention or reinforcers are given (learn to earn), and desensitization and counterconditioning to departure stimuli can be used. Head halter control also can help to train and calm fearful or anxious dogs. Drug therapy is often advisable when the pet is fearful, anxious, or phobic, but special attention to the selection, benefits, and risks of pharmacologic intervention is required in the senior pet. Pets with cognitive dysfunction might be treated with selegiline, which should not be combined with antidepressants. Pheromones and some natural compounds, such as melatonin, may be useful for some problems, with little or no chance of adverse effects. Sedating and anticholinergic drugs can have additional risks in the elderly, whereas pets with renal or hepatic compromise require cautious use of drugs excreted by the kidneys or metabolized by the liver, respectively. For example, compared with clomipramine or amitriptyline, fluoxetine is neither sedating nor anticholinergic; buspirone is a nonsedating anxiolytic; and oxazepam, lorazepam, and clonazepam are benzodiazepines that might be considered in pets with hepatic compromise because they have no active intermediate metabolites. Dose information is presented in Table 2.

Excessive vocalization and nocturnal restlessness

Elderly pets are particularly prone to untimely and excessive vocalization as well as to waking at night. Although cognitive dysfunction and medical

Table 2
Drug dosing guidelines

Drug	Dog	Cat
Selegiline	0.5–1.0 mg/kg q 24 hours (mornings)	0.5–1.0 mg/kg q 24 hours (mornings)
Nicergoline	0.25–0.5 mg/kg q 24 hours (mornings)	1.25 mg q 24 hours (mornings)
Propentofylline	3 mg/kg bid	12.5 mg q 24 hours
Oxazepam	0.2–1.0 mg/kg bid	0.2–0.5 mg/kg bid
Lorazepam	0.02–0.1 mg/kg prn	0.02–0.1 mg/kg bid
Clonazepam	0.1–0.5 mg/kg bid–tid	0.1–0.2 mg/kg sid–bid 0.02 mg/kg sid–qid (sleep disorders)
Buspirone	1.0–2.0 mg/kg bid–tid	2.5–5.0 mg per cat bid
Fluoxetine	1.0–2.0 mg/kg q 24 hours	0.5–1 mg/kg q 24 hours
Melatonin	0.1 mg/kg sid–tid	0.5 mg

Abbreviations: bid, twice daily; prn, as needed; q, every; qid, four times daily; sid, once daily; tid, three times daily.

Note that the only products licensed for veterinary use in this table are selegiline for dogs and propentofylline and nicergoline for dogs in some countries outside North America. Therefore, most doses are only based on anecdotal guidelines, and side effects and contraindications are not established for off-label use.

problems may be a cause of night waking or altered sleep-wake cycles, the pet's daily routine and owner responses may also be major contributing factors. Pets that sleep more during the day and have a decrease in daily activity and mental stimulation may be awake and more active through the night. Owner responses may then further aggravate the problem when trying to calm, quiet, or settle the pet by reinforcing the behavior. Conversely, the owner who is frustrated and upset by the pet's behavior and uses punishment to try to settle the pet may further increase the pet's anxiety. In addition to any medical treatment that might be indicated, owners must ensure that they do not reinforce the undesirable responses; they must provide a stimulating daily routine to ensure that the pet regularly rests, naps, and sleeps through the night. This may be difficult because of the pet's decreasing interest and physical ability to engage in daily activities; however, alternatives to running and playing could include short walks; short reward-based training sessions; and a variety of new stimuli, such as manipulation and chew toys. In addition to therapies that help to re-establish normal sleep-wake cycles, such as night time sleep aids, day time stimulants, or antidepressants, drugs and complimentary forms of therapy for cognitive dysfunction might be useful.

Repetitive and compulsive disorders

An increase in restlessness as well as in stereotypic or repetitive behaviors is reported in senior pets. Unless there is an identifiable change in the pet's environment, the onset of these problems in older pets likely is indicative of cognitive dysfunction syndrome or some other underlying medical cause. In addition to medical treatment, treatment for compulsive disorders generally requires that the pet be given a more predictable daily routine with sufficient outlets to keep it occupied (eg, social play, object play) during times it is not resting or sleeping. Because the older pet may be less active and interactive, it can be challenging for the owner to ensure that the pet is provided with sufficient novel and stimulating activities, but the absence of sufficient enrichment may, in fact, compound the problem. Selegiline and dietary therapy should be considered if the signs are consistent with cognitive dysfunction syndrome, but for compulsive disorders, fluoxetine might be the first drug of choice because it is neither sedating nor anticholinergic.

Cognitive dysfunction syndrome

Cognitive dysfunction is a neurodegenerative disorder of senior dogs and cats that is characterized by gradual cognitive decline over a prolonged period (18–24 months or longer) [1,11–13]. Initially, the characterization of cognitive dysfunction was established in the laboratory by comparing the performance of young and elderly dogs on a variety of cognitive tasks using a standardized test box (Fig. 1) [1,14–19]. Similar to human beings, aged

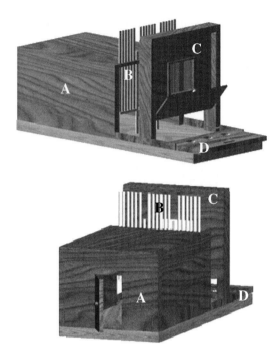

Fig. 1. An illustration of the standardized test apparatus used for canine cognitive testing. The top panel shows the side on which the tester is located, and the bottom panel shows the rear of the apparatus. For the duration of cognitive testing, the dog remains in a wooden chamber (*A*), from which the dog enters through a hinged door in the rear. Adjustable metal bars (*B*) provide an area through which the dog can use its head to access the response area. A wooden partition (*C*) separates the tester from the dog. The tester is able to view the dog at all times through a one-way mirror located in the partition. The tester can present a tray (*D*) to the dog by raising a hinged door on the wooden partition and sliding the tray into the response area. Depending on the cognitive task, various objects may be located over any of the three wells in the tray; the dog is required to displace the correct object to obtain a food reward in the corresponding well. The tester withdraws the tray and closes the hinged door between trials or during delays. (Courtesy of J. Costa, Toronto, Ontario, Canada.)

dogs typically do not demonstrate decline in simple learning, such as when they are repetitively rewarded for approaching one of two distinct objects [20,21]. After a dog learns this simple discrimination task, the reward contingencies are reversed so that the previously rewarded object is no longer rewarded and the dog must learn to respond selectively to the object that was not rewarded in the simple learning task (Fig. 2). When this reversal phase is implemented, aged dogs require significantly more attempts to learn to respond consistently to the rewarded object than young dogs [14,20]. This impairment might be analogous to executive function impairments observed in human aging and Alzheimer's disease [14]. Spatial memory also can be examined by assessing a subject's ability to recall the location of a food reward after a delay of 5 seconds or more (Fig. 3);

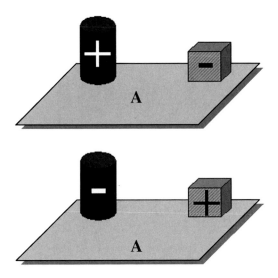

Fig. 2. An example of an object discrimination task. The dog is presented with one of two objects on the sliding tray (*A*; see Fig. 1). As an example of a simple learning task (*upper panel*), the dog would be rewarded for responding to the cylinder (+) but not for responding to the cube (−). Once the dog selectively responds to the cylinder, it then can be tested on a reversal learning task (seen in the lower panel). For the reversal learning task, the dog must modify its response pattern and selectively respond to the cube (+) but not to the cylinder (−). During both tests, the location of the objects is randomized between trials and an unobtainable food reward is presented with the nonrewarded object to prevent the use of olfactory-based responses.

subsequently, the dog's memory can be taxed to a greater extent by increasing the delay [17,19]. Using memory tasks, old dogs can be separated into three groups (unimpaired, impaired, and severely impaired), which may correspond to the three human subgroups of successful aging, mild cognitive impairment (MCI), and dementia [17,21]. Although the age of onset may be 11 years or greater before clinical signs become apparent in dogs, recent findings suggest that cognitive decline can be detected as early as 6 years of age in the laboratory environment. In particular, spatial memory ability declines early in dogs (Fig. 4) [22,23]. Thus, many parallels are observed between canine cognitive aging and human aging and Alzheimer's disease. Specifically, the disease process can be detected long before clinical signs appear using sophisticated cognitive testing procedures, and spatial memory and executive function are impaired early in the disease process.

To determine whether a dog or cat might be showing signs of cognitive dysfunction, veterinarians must rely almost entirely on owner-reported history. Only with careful questioning is it likely that signs would be detectable in the earliest stages of development. By contrast, subtle changes might be more noticeable in animals that have had a high level of training (eg, agility training, service work).

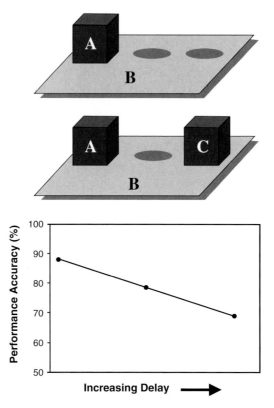

Fig. 3. A schematic of the spatial memory task. During the initial phase (*upper panel*), the dog is presented with an object (*A*) on the sliding tray (*B*; see Fig. 1). After the dog displaces the object and obtains the food reward in the well beneath the object, the tray is withdrawn for a delay. After the delay (*middle panel*), the dog is presented with two objects identical to that in the initial phase; one object is in the same location as the initial phase, and the other is located over one of the remaining two food wells. The dog is rewarded for responding to the object in the novel location (in this case, object *C*). For all spatial memory testing, the locations of the objects are randomized between trials and an unobtainable food reward is presented with the nonrewarded object to prevent the use of olfactory-based responses. The lower panel shows a representative graph of the data obtained using this task; as the delay increases, performance accuracy decreases.

Cognitive dysfunction may cause behavioral changes in the following categories:

1. Spatial disorientation and/or confusion
2. Altered learning and memory (eg, house soiling, learned commands, trained tasks)
3. Activity: purposeless, repetitive, or decreased
4. Altered social relationships
5. Altered sleep-wake cycles (eg, night waking)

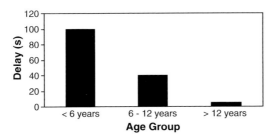

Fig. 4. Representative data of maximal memory across age groups on a spatial memory task. The maximal memory is the longest delay a dog can perform at successfully when tested using an incremental delay procedure over a given number of days (typically 40 days). Dogs younger than 6 years of age can perform successfully at much longer delays (eg, 100 seconds) than dogs older than 6 years of age (eg, 40 seconds). Many dogs older than 12 years of age cannot perform at extremely short delays (eg, 5 seconds).

6. Increased anxiety or restlessness
7. Altered appetite and/or self-hygiene
8. Decreased perception and/or responsiveness

Diagnosis

The history, physical, and neurologic examinations, along with the results of screening tests, lead to a diagnosis or determine if further tests are indicated (eg, radiographs, ultrasound, MRI, brain stem auditory evoked response [BAER]). Ensuring that the owner has provided a complete list of all presenting signs (behavioral and medical), including any behavioral changes in comparison to when the pet was younger (<7 years), provides a framework for determining what medical problems might be responsible for the signs. The findings of the physical examination, previous health problems, and concurrent medication help to guide the practitioner toward what diagnostic tests are initially necessary. The results of these initial tests may then necessitate further diagnostics (eg, radiographs, ultrasound, MRI, BAER) or a therapeutic treatment trial (eg, pain management medication) to achieve a more accurate diagnosis and to determine if the clinical signs resolve. Ruling out all other possible medical conditions that may cause or contribute to the presenting signs leads to a diagnosis of cognitive dysfunction.

Aging and its effect on the brain

A number of anatomic changes can be identified in older dogs and cats; however, it is unclear which of the changes are responsible for which signs. With increasing age, there is a reduction in brain mass, including cerebral and basal ganglia atrophy; an increase in ventricular size, meningeal calcification, demyelination, and glial changes (including an increase in the size and number of astrocytes); increasing amounts of lipofuscin and apoptic bodies; neuro-axonal degeneration; and a reduction in neurons [24,25]. There is also an increased accumulation of diffuse β-amyloid plaques and perivascular infiltrates in dogs, cats, and human beings with cognitive dysfunction (Fig. 5). In dogs and cats, the plaques are diffuse and lack a central core, although in Alzheimer's disease, the amyloid distribution includes neuritic plaques and concurrent neurofibrillary tangles [12,13]. No clear evidence for early tangle formation has been found in aged dogs, although there may be evidence of early neurofibrillary tangle formation in cats [26].

Numerous vascular and perivascular changes have been identified in older dogs, including microhemorrhage or infarcts in periventricular vessels. Arteriosclerosis of the nonlipid variety may also be seen in the older dog or cat (as a result of fibrosis of vessel walls, endothelial proliferation, mineralization, and β-amyloid deposition). This angiopathy may compromise blood flow and glucose use. Functional changes that may occur in the aging brain include depletion of catecholamine neurotransmitters, an increase in monoamine oxidase B (MAOB) activity, and a decline in cholinergic integrity [27–29]. Cholinergic decline is well established in human aging and Alzheimer's disease [30] and may play a significant role in the early spatial memory decline observed in dogs [31].

Role of β-amyloid in cognitive decline

β-Amyloid is undetectable in young dogs and cats but is extensive in the oldest dogs and cats. Although the exact role of β-amyloid accumulation in the development of cognitive dysfunction is yet to be determined, it is neurotoxic and can lead to compromised neuronal function, degeneration of synapses, cell loss, and depletion of neurotransmitters and is correlated with the severity of cognitive dysfunction [13,32]. In dogs, errors in learning tests, including discrimination, reversal, and spatial learning, were strongly associated with increased amounts of β-amyloid deposition, indicating a correlation between cognitive dysfunction and β-amyloid accumulation, but a causative role has not been established [33].

Role of reactive oxygen species in cognitive decline

A small amount of oxygen that is used by the mitochondria for normal aerobic energy production is converted to reactive oxygen species (also known as free radicals), such as hydrogen peroxide, superoxide, and nitric oxide within the mitochondria. As mitochondria age, they become less efficient and produce relatively more free radicals and less energy compared with younger mitochondria [34,35]. Increased monoamine oxidase (MAO) activity may also result in increased liberation of oxygen free radicals. Normally, antioxidant defenses, including enzymes like superoxide dismutase (SOD), catalase, glutathione peroxidase and free radical scavengers like vitamins A, C, and E, eliminate free radicals. If the balance of detoxification and production is tipped in favor of overproduction, as is the

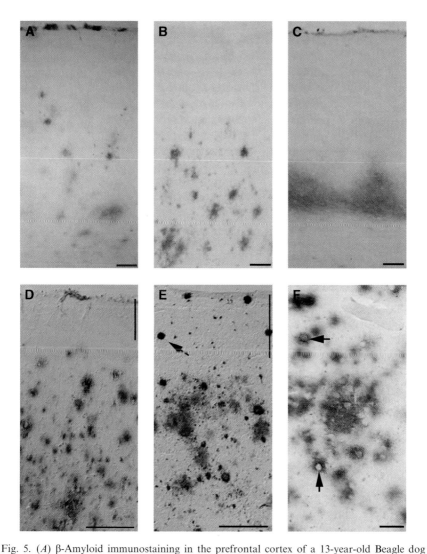

Fig. 5. (*A*) β-Amyloid immunostaining in the prefrontal cortex of a 13-year-old Beagle dog demonstrates diffuse β-amyloid plaques in layers III to VI. (*B*) A section from the frontal cortex of a nondemented 90-year-old woman illustrates a similar pattern of plaque deposition as that seen in the aged dog. The distribution of β-amyloid is in the deeper cortical layers in both cases. (*C*) An 18-year-old Siamese cat exhibits a diffuse cloud of β-amyloid immunostaining in the cortex adjacent to the white matter. (*D*) In a cognitively impaired 12-year-old Beagle dog, β-amyloid immunostaining in the prefrontal cortex is extensive and affects layers II to VI. The molecular layer is free of Aβ deposition (indicated by the vertical line). (*E*) β-Amyloid immunostaining in the frontal cortex of an 86 year-old man with Alzheimer's disease shows a similar extent of β-amyloid deposition as that seen in the dog. The diffuse plaques are similar in size between the dog and the man, but dogs do not develop compact plaques (*arrow* in *E*). (*F*) A higher magnification photograph of the impaired dog in D, which illustrates the presence of intact cells (*arrows*) within the plaques. Bars in A through E = 200 μm. Bar in F = 50 μm. (*From* Head E, Milgram NW, Cotman CW. Neurobiological models of aging in the dog and other vertebrate species. In: Hof PR, Mobbs CV, editors. Functional neurobiology of aging. San Diego: Academic Press; 2001, p. 457–68; with permission.)

case with increasing age, the excess of free radicals can react with DNA, lipids, and proteins, leading to cell damage, dysfunction, mutation, neoplasia, and cell death. The brain is particularly susceptible to the toxic effects of free radicals because of its large metabolic needs, and evidence of increased brain oxidative damage has been reported in dogs [36].

Vascular insufficiency and cognitive decline

There may be a link between vascular insufficiency, decreased perfusion (eg, decreased cardiac output, anemia, arteriosclerosis, blood viscosity changes, vasospasm), and the signs of brain aging. In a subset of dogs, decreased regional cerebral blood volumes have been reported, which could be related to age-dependent cognitive dysfunction [37].

Treatment

The first step is to treat any underlying medical problem. Many age-related disease processes cannot be resolved; however, it may be possible to slow the disease-related decline (eg, dietary intervention for renal failure) or to control the clinical signs (eg, pain relief for arthritis). Even when medical problems can be resolved, the behavior problem might persist because of learning and conditioning. For example, the cat that begins to avoid its litter box because of feline lower urinary tract disease (FLUTD) may develop new surface or location preferences. Behavior problems that persist after medical problems are treated require behavior counseling.

Although behavioral modification and environmental adjustments may be needed to control specific behavior problems, cognitive decline should also be treated with a combination of nutritional therapy, drugs, and environmental management. Studies have shown that continued enrichment in the form of training, play, exercise, and novel toys can help to maintain cognitive function (ie, "use it or lose it") [38]. Keeping a regular and predictable daily routine may help to reduce anxiety, maintain temporal orientation, and keep the pet active during daytime hours so that it sleeps better through the night. Making gradual changes to the pet's household or routine can also help the senior pet to adapt better. As sensory acuity, sensory processing, and cognitive function decline, adding new odor, tactile, and sound cues (if the pet is not significantly hearing impaired) might help the pet to navigate its environment better and maintain some degree of environmental familiarity and comfort.

Nutritional and dietary therapy

One strategy in the treatment of cognitive dysfunction in animals is dietary therapy. This involves supplementing the diet of senior pets with antioxidants to improve antioxidant defenses and reduce the toxic effects of free radicals. A variety of studies suggest that high intake of fruits, vegetables, and vitamins E and C decreases the risk of cognitive decline [38,39].

A new senior diet (Hill's Prescription diet Canine b/d, Hill's Pet Nutrition, Inc., Topeka, KS) that is supplemented with antioxidants, mitochondrial cofactors, and essential fatty acids is now available. The supplemented diet improved performance on a number of cognitive tasks when compared with a nonsupplemented diet in a longitudinal cognitive study. Improved performance was observed as early as to 2 to 8 weeks after the onset of therapy [11] and continued for longer than 2 years [22,23,40,41]. In a double-blind clinical trial of 142 dogs, there was a significant improvement in cognitive signs in the group on the fortified diet (Hill's Prescription diet Canine b/d) compared with the control group [42] over 60 days. Another recent study also found that performance on a landmark task was improved by the antioxidant diet in aged Beagles and that blood concentration of vitamin E was positively correlated with improved performance [43].

Environmental enrichment and previous cognitive experience

In addition to the effects of the fortified diet, the effect of enrichment (cognitive and environmental) and previous cognitive experience were also assessed in the previously mentioned longitudinal cognitive studies in dogs. In one study, the effects of diet and environmental enrichment (exercise, novel toys, and ongoing testing) were investigated. After following these dogs for longer than 2 years, the dogs in the control group (no enrichment and no supplemented diet) showed a dramatic decline in cognitive function, whereas those in the enriched diet group or the environmental enrichment group performed better than controls on discrimination and reversal learning tasks. The combined effect of the enriched diet and the enriched environment provided the greatest improvement, however [15,40]. In a second study, aged Beagles with previous cognitive experience were compared with naive dogs. Previous cognitive experience had a positive impact on performance, which was further improved with the antioxidant-fortified diet [43]. These findings suggest that novel and continuous stimulation may aid in the reduction or prevention of cognitive dysfunction.

Drug therapy

Selegiline is a selective and irreversible inhibitor of MAOB in the dog [27]. Although the mechanisms by which selegiline produces clinical improvement in dogs with cognitive dysfunction syndrome are not clearly understood, enhancement of dopamine and perhaps other catecholamines in the cortex and hippocampus is presumed to be an important factor [44]. Selegiline increases brain 2-phenylethylamine (PEA), which is a neuro-modulator that enhances dopamine and catecholamine function and may itself enhance cognitive function [45]. Selegiline may also contribute to a decrease in free radical load in the brain by inhibiting MAOB and increasing free radical clearance by enhancing the activity of enzymes like SOD [46].

Because alterations in neurotransmitter function can lead to behavior changes, such as increased irritability, decreased responsiveness to stimuli, fear, agitation, and altered sleep-wake cycles (as well as depression in human beings), antidepressants and anxiolytics might also be considered for some older pets. Because the elderly are particularly susceptible to the effects of anticholinergic drugs, it is prudent to consider therapies with less anticholinergic effects and those that are less sedating. Furthermore, anticholinergic drugs can cause increased cognitive impairment in aged dogs [31]. When benzodiazepines are considered for anxiety or inducing sleep in the senior pet, oxazepam and lorazepam, which have no active intermediate metabolites, might be safest. Recent studies suggest that cholinergic augmentation with the use of acetylcholinesterase inhibitors may have beneficial effects on cognitive dysfunction in dogs [47]; however, it is cautioned that acetylcholinesterase inhibitors currently approved for use in human beings may not demonstrate an appropriate pharmacokinetic profile for use in senior pets. Modafinil and adrafanil also may provide some benefit to certain cognitive impairments, likely through a noradrenergic mechanism. In laboratory tests, adrafanil at a dose of 20 mg/kg increased exploratory behavior and improved learning but impaired memory performance [48–50]. Consequently, adrafanil may be useful for treating particular behavioral signs, such as reduced activity, but not others.

Other treatment strategies include anti-inflammatory drugs (particularly nonsteroidal anti-inflammatory drugs [NSAIDS]) and hormone replacement therapy. Estrogen may have an anti-inflammatory effect and an antioxidant effect and may increase cerebral blood flow. Estrogen-treated female dogs made significantly fewer errors in size-reversal learning tasks than estrogen-treated male dogs or placebo-treated male and female dogs. Estrogen-treated aged female dogs made more errors in spatial memory tasks than estrogen-treated male and control dogs, however [51]. Testosterone therapy might be another consideration, because in a recent study of a small group of dogs, intact aging male dogs showed less evidence of cognitive impairment than neutered dogs [52]. Other drugs not presently licensed for use in North America that may show promise include nicergoline, an α_1- and α_2-adrenergic antagonist that may increase cerebral blood flow and enhance neuronal transmission, and propentofylline, which inhibits platelet aggregation and thrombus formation.

There are no drugs licensed for the treatment of cognitive dysfunction in cats, but there are anecdotal reports of successful use of some canine medications. The possibility of improving signs, however, must be weighed against the potential risks, which are not well established in cats. Selegiline is reported to be useful in senior cats for improving clinical signs of cognitive dysfunction, such as disorientation, increased vocalization, decreased affection, and repetitive or restless activity. In addition, in a small non–placebo-controlled study of 27 cats averaging approximately 4 years of age, selegiline was reported to be effective in improving a variety of behavioral signs ranging from productive signs (eg, aggression, insomnia, bulimia) to deficit signs (eg, anorexia, increased sleep) [53]. Except for occasional cases of gastrointestinal upset, no adverse effects have been reported to date. Nicergoline might be dosed by dissolving a 5-mg tablet in water, giving one quarter of the solution, and discarding the rest, whereas a dose of one quarter of a 50-mg tablet daily might be considered for propentofylline.

Other therapeutic strategies

Medical conditions ranging from endocrinopathies to organ failure can also have varying effects on cognition and may lead to further accumulation and decreased clearance of free radicals. Perhaps the most significant effects on health and life span might best be achieved through weight control.

Naturopathic supplements, nutraceuticals, and homeopathic remedies have been suggested for calming, reducing anxiety, or inducing sleep. These include melatonin, valerian, dog appeasing pheromone (DAP, Veterinary Product Laboratories, Phoenix, AZ), Feliway pheromone sprays, and Bach's flower remedies (Nelsonbach USA Ltd, Wilmington, MA). Phosphatidyl-serine is a phospholipid that constitutes a major building block of the cell membrane. Because the neurons are highly dependent on their plasma membranes, phosphatidylserine may facilitate the activities of the neuron that are dependent on the cell membrane, such as signal transduction, release of secretory vesicles, and maintenance of the internal environment. Ginkgo biloba may improve memory loss, fatigue, anxiety, and depression in the elderly, possibly because of MAO inhibition, free radical scavenging, or enhancement of blood flow. Combination natural products that contain a wide variety of ingredients, including docosahexaenoic acid, flavonoids, carotenoids, L-carnitine, lipoic acid, ginkgo biloba, phosphatidylserine, and other antioxidants (eg, vitamins E and C), are now available from veterinary and human manufacturers. Although many of the aforementioned therapies have not been formally tested in the clinic or laboratory, they may provide an alternative, and relatively safe, treatment in pets that are refractory to standard therapies.

References

[1] Landsberg GM, Hunthausen W, Ackerman L. The effects of aging on the behavior of senior pets. In: Handbook of behavior problems of the dog and cat. 2nd edition. London: WB Saunders; 2003. p. 269–304.
[2] Landsberg GM. The most common behavior problems in older dogs. Vet Med 1995; 90(Suppl):16–24.
[3] Horwitz D. Dealing with common behavior problems in senior dogs. Vet Med 2001;96(11): 869–79.
[4] Chapman BL, Voith VL. Geriatric behavior problems not always related to age. DVM 1987; 18:32.
[5] Nielson JC, Hart BL, Cliff KD, et al. Prevalence of behavioral changes associated with age-related cognitive impairment in dogs. J Am Vet Med Assoc 2001;218(11):1787–91.

[6] Bain MJ, Hart BJ, Cliff KD, et al. Predicting behavioral changes associated with age related cognitive impairment in dogs. J Am Vet Med Assoc 2001;218(11):1792–5.

[7] US marketing research summary. Omnibus study on aging pets. Topeka (KS): Hill's Pet Nutrition, Inc; 2000.

[8] Moffat K, Landsberg G. An investigation into the prevalence of clinical signs of cognitive dysfunction syndrome (CDS) in cats [abstract]. J Am Anim Hosp Assoc 2003;39:512.

[9] McMullen SL, Clark WT, Robertson ID. Reasons for the euthanasia of dogs and cats in veterinary practices. Aust Vet Pract 2001;31(2):80–4.

[10] Aronson L. Systemic causes of aggression and their treatment. In: Dodman NH, Shuster L, editors. Psychopharmacology of animal behavior disorders. Malden, MA: Blackwell Scientific; 1998. p. 64–102.

[11] Milgram NW, Head E, Weiner E, et al. Cognitive functions and aging in the dog: acquisition of nonspatial visual tasks. Behav Neurosci 1994;108(1):57–68.

[12] Cummings BJ, Satou T, Head E, et al. Diffuse plaques contain C-terminal AB42 and not AB40: evidence from cats and dogs. Neurobiol Aging 1996;17(2):4653–9.

[13] Cummings BJ, Head E, Afagh AJ, et al. β-Amyloid accumulation correlates with cognitive dysfunction in the aged canine. Neurobiol Learn Mem 1996;66(1):11–23.

[14] Tapp PD, Siwak CT, Estrada J, et al. Size and reversal learning in the beagle dog as a measure of executive function and inhibitory control in aging. Learn Mem 2003;10(1):64–73.

[15] Milgram NW, Zicker SC, Head EA, et al. Dietary enrichment counteracts age-associated cognitive dysfunction in canines. Neurobiol Aging 2002;23(5):737–45.

[16] Milgram NW, Head E, Muggenburg B, et al. Landmark discrimination learning in the dog; effects of age, an antioxidant fortified food and cognitive strategy. Neurosci Biobehav Rev 2002;26(6):679–95.

[17] Adams B, Chan A, Callahan H, et al. Use of a delayed non-matching to position task to model age-dependent cognitive decline in the dog. Behav Brain Res 2000;108(1):47–56.

[18] Head E, Mehta R, Hartley J, et al. Spatial learning and memory as a function of age in the dog. Behav Neurosci 1995;109(5):851–8.

[19] Chan AD, Nippak PM, Murphey H, et al. Visuospatial impairments in aged canines (Canis familiaris): the role of cognitive-behavioral therapy. Behav Neurosci 2002;116(3):443–54.

[20] Milgram NW, Head E, Weiner E, et al. Cognitive functions and aging in the dog: acquisition of nonspatial visual tasks. Behav Neurosci 1994;108(1):57–68.

[21] Adams B, Chan A, Callahan H, et al. The canine as a model of human brain aging: recent developments. Prog Neuropsychopharmacol Biol Psychiatry 2000;24(5):675–92.

[22] Araujo JA. Age-dependent learning and memory decline in dogs: assessment and effectiveness of various interventions. Presented at the 141st American Veterinary Medical Association Conference. Schaumburg, IL; 2004.

[23] Araujo JA, Studzinski CM, Siwak CT, et al. Cognitive function and aging in beagle dogs. In: Proceedings of the American College of Veterinary Internal Medicine Forum, Minneapolis, 2004. Lakewood (CO): American College of Veterinary Internal Medicine; 2004.

[24] Borras D, Ferrer I, Pumarola M. Age related changes in the brain of the dog. Vet Pathol 1999;36(3):202–11.

[25] Su M-Y, Head E, Brooks WM, et al. MR imaging of anatomic and vascular characteristics in a canine model of human aging. Neurobiol Aging 1998;19(5):479–85.

[26] Head E, Moffat K, Das P, et al. Beta-amyloid deposition and tau phosphorylation in clinically characterized aged cats. Neurobiol Aging, in press.

[27] Milgram NW, Ivy GO, Head E, et al. The effect of L-deprenyl on behavior, cognitive function, and biogenic amines in the dog. Neurochem Res 1993;18(12):1211–9.

[28] Gerlach M, Riederer P, Youdim MBH. Effects of disease and aging on monoamine oxidases A and B. In: Lieberman A, Olanow CW, Youdim MBH, et al, editors. Monoamine oxidase inhibitors in neurological diseases. New York: Marcel Dekker; 1994. p. 21–30.

[29] Araujo JA, Chan ADF, Studzinski C, et al. Cholinergic disruption age-dependently impairs canine working memory while sparing reference memory and spatial perception [abstract]. Washington, DC: Society for Neuroscience; 2002. p. 4.

[30] Bartus RT, Dean RL II, Beer B, et al. The cholinergic hypothesis of geriatric memory dysfunction. Science 1982;217(4558):408–14.

[31] Araujo JA, Chan ADF, Winka LL, et al. Dose-specific effects of scopolamine on canine cognition: impairment of visuospatial memory, but not visuospatial discrimination. Psychopharmacology (Berl) 2004;175(1):92–8.

[32] Colle M-A, Hauw J-J, Crespau F, et al. Vascular and parenchymal beta-amyloid deposition in the aging dog: correlation with behavior. Neurobiol Aging 2000;21(5):695–704.

[33] Head E, Callahan H, Muggenburg BA, et al. Visual-discrimination learning ability and beta-amyloid accumulation in the dog. Neurobiol Aging 1998;19(5):415–25.

[34] Beckman KB, Ames BN. The free radical theory of aging matures. Physiol Rev 1998;78(2):547–81.

[35] Shigenaga MK, Hagen TM, Ames BN. Oxidative damage and mitochondrial decay in aging. Proc Natl Acad Sci USA 1994;91(23):10771–8.

[36] Head E, Liu J, Hagen TM, et al. Oxidative damage increases with age in a canine model of human brain aging. J Neurochem 2002;82(2):375–81.

[37] Tapp PD, Chu Y, Araujo JA, et al. Effects of scopolamine challenge on regional cerebral blood volume. A pharmacological model to validate the use of contrast enhanced magnetic resonance imaging to assess cerebral blood volume in a canine model of aging. Prog Neuropharmacol Biol Psychiatry, in press.

[38] Sano M, Ernesto C, Thomas R, et al. A controlled trial of selegiline, alpha tocopherol, or both for the treatment for Alzheimer's disease. N Engl J Med 1997;336(17):1216–22.

[39] Joseph JA, Shukitt-Hale B, Denisova NA, et al. Long-term dietary strawberry, spinach, or vitamin E supplementation retards the onset of age-related neuronal signal transduction and cognitive behavioral deficits. J Neurosci 1998;18(19):8047–55.

[40] Milgram NW, Head EA, Zicker SC, et al. Long term treatment with antioxidants and a program of behavioral enrichment reduces age-dependent impairment in discrimination and reversal learning in beagle dogs. Exp Gerontol 2004;39(5):753–65.

[41] Cotman CW, Head E, Muggenburg BA, et al. Brain aging in the canine: a diet enriched in antioxidants reduces cognitive dysfunction. Neurobiol Aging 2002;23(5):809–18.

[42] Dodd CE, Zicker SC, Jewell DE, et al. Can a fortified food affect the behavioral manifestations of age-related cognitive decline in dogs. Vet Med 2003;98:396–408.

[43] Ikeda-Douglas CJ, Zicker SC, Estrada J, et al. Prior experience, antioxidants, and mitochondrial cofactors improve cognitive dysfunction in aged beagles. Vet Ther 2004;5:5–16.

[44] Knoll J. L-Deprenyl (selegiline), a catecholaminergic activity enhancer (CAE) substance acting in the brain. Pharmacol Toxicol 1998;82:57–66.

[45] Paterson IA, Jurio AV, Boulton AA. 2 Phenylethylamine: a modulator of catecholamine transmission in the mammalian central nervous system. J Neurochem 1990;55:1827–37.

[46] Carillo MC, Ivy GO, Milgram NW, et al. Deprenyl increases activity of superoxide dismutase. Life Sci 1994;54(20):1483–9.

[47] Araujo JA, Studzinski CM, Milgram NW. Further evidence for the cholinergic hypothesis of aging and dementia from the canine model of aging. Prog Neuropharmacol Biol Psychiatry, in press.

[48] Siwak CT, Gruet P, Woehrle F, et al. Behavioral activating effects of adrafinil in aged canines. Pharm Biochem Behav 2000;66(2):293–300.

[49] Siwak CT, Tapp PD, Milgram NW. Adrafinil disrupts performance on a delayed-matching-to-position task in aged beagle dogs. Pharm Biochem Behav 2003;76(1):161–8.

[50] Milgram NW, Siwak CT, Gruet P, et al. Oral administration of adrafinil improves discrimination learning in aged beagle dogs. Pharm Biochem Behav 2000;66(2):301–5.

[51] Tapp PD, Siwak CT, Head E, et al. Sex differences in the effect of oestrogen on size discrimination learning and spatial memory. In: Overall KL, Mills DS, Heath SE, et al, editors. Proceedings of the Third International Congress on Veterinary Behavioral Medicine. Wheathamstead, UK: Universities Federation for Animal Welfare; 2001. p. 136–8.
[52] Hart BL. Effect of gonadectomy on subsequent development of age-related cognitive impairment in dogs. J Am Vet Med Assoc 2001;219(1):51–6.
[53] Dehasse J. Retrospective study on the use of selegiline (Selgian®) in cats. Presented at the American Veterinary Society of Animal Behavior, New Orleans, 1999.

ELSEVIER
SAUNDERS

Vet Clin Small Anim
35 (2005) 699–712

VETERINARY
CLINICS
Small Animal Practice

Geriatric Veterinary Dentistry: Medical and Client Relations and Challenges

Steven E. Holmstrom, DVM

Animal Dental Clinic, 987 Laurel Street, San Carlos, CA 94070, USA

"My pet is too old for dental procedures performed under anesthesia" is a common statement made by clients with geriatric pets. Is age, per se, really a disease? Although there are medical conditions that go along with aging, the important concept to impart to the client is that age itself is not a disease [1]. If the patient "passes" a complete preoperative workup, proper anesthetics are used, and procedures and monitoring are correct, a favorable outcome should be anticipated. There are some physiologic age-related changes that require understanding and accommodation to [2] Untreated, the dental disease that is present may progress and the quality of life of the patient may suffer.

Ideally, preparation for the geriatric patient begins at an early age, with the practice's education of the clientele about the advantages of proper dental hygiene. This marketing at an early age pays off later for all parties concerned: the patient, the client, and the practice. The patient has a much healthier oral cavity. The client appreciates the better breath that goes along with a healthier oral cavity and faces less expensive veterinary bills as a result. Finally, the practice gains loyal clients.

Introducing veterinary dentistry to your practice

How does all this happen? Where does it start? It starts with the training of the veterinarian and staff. This training and knowledge can be obtained in a variety of different ways. The American Veterinary Dental Society (AVDS; 618 Church Street, Suite 220, Nashville, TN 37219; telephone: 800-332-AVDS) is a source of updated information. Membership in the AVDS includes receipt of the *Journal of Veterinary Dentistry* four times a year. The *Journal of Veterinary Dentistry* has the latest information on veterinary

---

E-mail address: Steve@Toothvet.info

doi:10.1016/j.cvsm.2004.12.009
vetsmall.theclinics.com

dentistry and provides resources for continuing education, such as the Annual Veterinary Dental Forum (AVDF). The AVDF provides lectures and wet laboratories from basic to advanced veterinary dentistry. In addition to the *Journal of Veterinary Dentistry*, there are a number of other texts in veterinary dentistry, some of which are listed as suggested reading at the end of this article. On-line services, such as Veterinary Information Network (VIN; 777 West Covell Boulevard, Davis, CA 95616; telephone: 800-700-4636 or 530-756-4881; telefax: 530-756-6035; e-mail: VINGRAM @vin.com) and Network of Animal Health (NOAH; available at: http:// www.avma.org/noah/noahlog.asp), are available to answer questions and serve as references. Equally important to reinforce the newly learned knowledge are staff training sessions and meetings to make sure that everyone, including clients, is on the "same page." It is important to make sure that clients are following through with the recommendations. Contrary to the belief of the client, compliance often is actually less than the practitioner and staff believe [3]. The American Animal Hospital Association (12575 West Bayaud Avenue, Lakewood, CO 80228; telephone: 303-986-2800; telefax: 303-986-1700; e-mail: info@aahanet.org) has the "Compliance Tool," an Excel spreadsheet to help track client compliance.

At the same time that veterinarian and staff training is going on, proper equipment should be inventoried and obtained if not present. Gas anesthesia, preferably isoflurane or sevoflurane, should be obtained. Minimal monitoring equipment should include a pulse oximeter, electrocardiographic equipment, and blood pressure measurement equipment. Magnetostrictive or piezoelectric ultrasonic scalers speed up the procedure, decreasing anesthesia time. Air-powered equipment should be used for polishing and extracting teeth. Multiple sets of hand scalers, curettes, and probe/explorers should be available. To avoid cross-contamination, these instruments should be gas- or steam-sterilized before use. Additionally, multiple packs of sterilized dental elevators in various sizes and extraction forceps should be available.

In reality, neither knowledge nor equipment is ever complete, because the more dental knowledge one obtains, the more the need for additional dental knowledge and equipment is recognized. Once knowledge and equipment are in place, the practice is ready to start marketing to the public. Generally, there is a lot untapped dental care in most practices. This can make external marketing unnecessary. Concentrating on the patients that the practice has through practice marketing collateral, such as wall charts and handouts, and the message on the telephone answering machine as well as addressing client concerns regarding better health care should fill the dental schedule. Using models and smile books to demonstrate the specific disease and care needed should increase client compliance. It is also helpful to understand the difference between the terms *prophy* and *periodontal therapy*. Prophy is a derivation of the word prophylaxis, which means to prevent disease. All too often, patients are admitted for a prophy with teeth that are in a poor state of health. In addition to the obvious halitosis, there is calculus and there may be gingival inflammation, recession, periodontal pockets, bone loss, and mobile teeth. Clearly, this patient has periodontal disease. This is no longer a prophy case. Contrary to what we are saying, we are not preventing disease in such a case; the patient already has disease. The proper term for this should be *periodontal therapy* or, if surgery is performed, *periodontal surgery*. By taking time to discuss the situation with the client, he or she can understand why more than just a "teeth cleaning" or a "dental examination" is going to be performed.

Client education

Most clients have three "hot buttons." They are fees, anesthesia, and extractions. These need to be discussed during the initial visit at the time of the physical examination and before treatment.

Use of a written "treatment plan" or estimate can be a marketing tool to discuss the entire procedure from beginning to end. This itemized plan can be reviewed with the client and used as an outline. First, the client needs to be informed of the necessity for the anticipated procedures. He or she needs to know that one of the difficulties in veterinary dentistry is the inability to perform a thorough examination of the oral cavity while the patient is awake. This makes anesthesia essential for the complete examination and treatment. A general discussion of potential conditions that may need treatment, the recommended treatment, and the options for treatment should be initiated. The need for preanesthetic blood profiles, chest radiographs, or other tests can be explained. The benefits of intravenous catheterization and fluid therapy, preanesthesia medications, and pain medications can be discussed. The type of anesthesia induction, need for intubation, and gas anesthesia to be used are reviewed. The client should be informed about the procedure itself, including the advantages and disadvantages of the recommended procedure and alternatives. We live in a busy world, and clients often are not available for consultation when a definitive diagnosis is made. This problem can be solved in the treatment plan by asking and giving the client options if the client is not available. These options are as follows: (1) do what you need to do; (2) call first, and if the client cannot be reached, go ahead with the procedure; or (3) if the client cannot be reached, do nothing unless contacted by the client. Additionally, a written treatment plan in the form of a questionnaire can be used to obtain permission for such things as clipping hair for catheters and monitors and establishing how long the patient is likely to be hospitalized, for example.

A client's fears over the second hot button, anesthesia, can be alleviated by a discussion of the facts about modern anesthesia. There have been few studies on the morbidity and mortality of patients given general anesthesia. A study in 1993 that evaluated 8087 dogs and 8702 cats indicated the incidence of complications like abnormal heart rates, abnormal respiratory rates, abnormal mucus membrane color, difficult intubation, excitable recovery, extended recovery, and cardiac arrest to be 2.1% for dogs and 1.3% for cats. Death attributable to anesthesia was reported at 0.11% for dogs and 0.1% for cats. Complications were associated with the use of xylazine and lack of heart rate monitoring (American Society of Anesthesiologists [ASA] classification) [4]. There are risks involved in general anesthesia; however, as the products and technology improve, the incidence of complications decreases. Using modern anesthesia (eg, sevoflurane, isoflurane), anesthesia monitors, pulse oximeters, blood pressure monitors, electrocardiograms, capnographs, and technicians to monitor and log the anesthesia parameters all help to make the anesthesia safer and alleviate client concerns.

The third hot button, exodontics, can be mitigated by assuring the client that if there are alternatives to extractions, they will be recommended and agreeing with the client that extractions are not to be performed without the benefit of evaluation via dental intraoral radiography and considerations of alternatives. None of us likes to euthanize our patients; in the same light, we should consider extraction "tooth euthanasia" or "toothanasia."

Preprocedure evaluation

Before the procedure, the patient should receive a complete physical examination. Routine information, such as the names of the client and patient, species, breed, gender, date of birth, and date of examination, should be recorded in the patient's record. A history should be obtained that includes the chief complaint, diet, any medical history that the patient may have, and any previous dental care. Dental disease is often associated with malodorous breath. Most of the time, halitosis is associated with periodontal disease, but it can also be caused by fractured teeth, other infections, and tumors. "Doggy breath" is not normal, and it indicates disease most of the time.

Obtaining the patient's history is extremely important, because dental procedures require general anesthesia. Physical, metabolic, immune, and endocrine abnormalities and ongoing medical treatment affect decisions when constructing a safe anesthesia protocol. Many of the routine questions, such those about diet, frequency of feeding, chew toys, and play toys, can be asked and recorded by veterinary staff (Table 1). Some of these items can be harmful, and future dental problems may be avoided by client education.

Although a complete examination of the oral cavity in an awake patient may be difficult or impossible, it should still be attempted unless there is evidence that proceeding would cause harm to the client, staff, or examiner. The first step is to note the skull type (brachycephalic, mesocephalic, dolichocephalic, or variation). Next, examine the face and jaw for symmetry, swellings, and any abnormalities of the salivary glands and regional lymph nodes. Lifting the lips, the occlusion and any occlusal wear are noted and the amount of plaque and calculus present in general is

Table 1
Dental history checklist

Diet type	Moist, dry, home-cooked, table scraps
Diet brand	
Frequency of feeding	Daily, twice daily, three times daily, free-fed
Chew toys	None, fence, bones, rocks, firewood, soft nylon, animal products, other
Home oral hygiene	Brushing, oral rinse, food additive, chewable treats, edible treats
Brushing frequency	None, daily, weekly, monthly

recorded. Tooth abnormalities, including missing teeth and supernumerary teeth, carious lesions, and dental trauma, should be noted. The periodontal status is recorded by noting gingival inflammation, gingival edema, significant periodontal pocket depth, gingival recession, gingival hyperplasia, attachment loss, and tooth mobility.

Periodontal health should be evaluated and graded [5]. A healthy periodontium has a knifelike margin. The line of the gingival margin flows smoothly from tooth to tooth. Stage 1 is early gingivitis, where there is a redness of the gingiva at the crest of the gingival margin and a mild amount of plaque and calculus. There is loss of visualization of the fine blood vessels at the gingival margins. The condition is reversible with treatment. Stage 2 is established or chronic gingivitis and is similar to stage 1, but there is an increase in inflammation, including edema and subgingival plaque development. The line of gingival margin topography has started to become irregular but is still unbroken, and gingival recession has not started. The condition is reversible with prophylaxis and home care. Stage 3 is early periodontitis and represents a developing periodontal disease stage, with gingivitis, edema, the beginning of pocket formation, and increasing amounts of plaque and calculus supragingivally and subgingivally. Because of the proximity of inflamed capillaries to the gingival surface, the gingiva bleeds on gentle probing. The gingival topography no longer flows smoothly from tooth to tooth, because there may be mild gingival recession or gingival hypertrophy. Stage 4 is established periodontitis. Some of the signs that may be associated with stage 4 are severe inflammation, deep pocket formation, gingival recession, easily recognized bone loss, pus, and tooth mobility. The gingiva usually bleeds easily on probing.

In addition to dental tissue, the oral cavity in general should be examined for lesions. At this time, as much of the oral cavity as possible should be examined. After the physical and oral examinations are completed, an initial and tentative diagnosis can be established. At this time, client communication becomes crucial. This is a good time to review the findings with the client and to recommend preoperative testing if a database has not already been established. Anesthesia using up-to-date equipment, medications, and monitors should be uncomplicated for the healthy patient. Recognizing and diagnosing the unhealthy patient is where the challenge lies. Minimally, a complete blood cell count, including platelet evaluation, and blood chemistry to evaluate renal and hepatic function should be performed. Additional biochemical analysis should be performed if there are any indications of abnormalities. If the evaluation of the cardiac and pulmonary system reveals any abnormalities, chest radiographs, an electrocardiogram, or ultrasound should be considered. Complicating medical conditions should be treated, or the anesthesia protocol should be modified to fit the patient's condition.

Preoperative instructions should be given to the client. Included are orders not to feed the patient after midnight the day before the procedure. Serious consideration should be given to not withholding water from patients that may be subject to dehydration if deprived of water.

Dental procedure

After admitting the patient on the day of the procedure and performing the preanesthesia evaluation, preoperative medications should be administered and an intravenous catheter placed. Usually, balanced electrolyte solutions, such as lactated Ringer's solution, are used for fluid therapy during anesthesia. Fluid therapy can help to prevent hypotension-induced problems in the perioperative period. Colloids, such as dextran 70 and hetastarch, are administered to patients that are hypoproteinemic or hypotensive under anesthesia [6]. There is no set volume or rate for the administration of fluids that is suitable for all circumstances. Fluid administration should be prescribed according to the patient's requirements and response. General guidelines suggesting that fluid therapy is adequate include strong peripheral pulses, pink mucous membranes with a capillary refill time less than 2 seconds, systolic arterial pressure greater than 100 mm Hg, and a return to consciousness at the end of anesthesia. The rate and volume of fluid administration are dependent on the degree of hypotension or shock, the patient's fluid status as indicated by the packed cell volume and plasma protein concentration, the type of fluid administered, and the response to fluid therapy. The rate of fluid administration for routine anesthesia in an animal that is not hypotensive is usually 5 to 10 mL/kg/h. This rate of fluid administration is higher than the daily amount of fluid required to maintain hydration because it is intended to offset some of the vasodilation and hypotension induced by anesthesia. Hypotensive patients may receive supplementary fluid boluses of 5 to 10 mL/kg over 5 to 10 minutes as required to return arterial pressure to an acceptable level. Another consideration is the medical status of the patient; for example, the rate and volume of fluids administered should be reduced in patients with cardiac disease.

Antibiotics, if indicated, should be administered 1 hour before the procedure. Amoxicillin at a dose of 10–12 mg/kg or clindamycin at a dose of 5 to 11 mg/kg is an appropriate antibiotic to be administered. Contrary to popular practice, in the absence of abscessation, there is no need to start antibiotic therapy days or weeks in advance of the procedure. In addition, patients should be evaluated regarding their actual need for antibiotic therapy. Healthy patients with stage 1 or stage 2 periodontal disease seldom need antibiotic therapy, whereas patients with stage 3 or stage 4 periodontal disease may require antibiotics. This decision should be made on an individual basis, with an evaluation of oral and overall health.

There are several anesthetic agents that can be used for the induction and maintenance of anesthesia [7]. The author prefers PropoFlo (Abbott Animal Health, North Chicago, IL) administered through intravenous catheterization, followed by intubation and maintenance with sevoflurane (SevoFlo; Abbott Animal Health). Sevoflurane does have some advantages over isoflurane, including a better anesthesia index and less respiratory depression at a similar level of anesthesia [8]. Anesthesia monitoring is imperative for a safe anesthesia experience in the critical geriatric patient [9]. A written anesthetic log that records all observations, treatments, and events should be kept. Written orders and records help to ensure the reliability of care, and retrospective assessment of the log helps to identify and document trends in physiologic state. Pulse oximetry provides a convenient, continuous, and noninvasive determination of arterial oxygen saturation. The probe can be placed on the tongue, pad web, hock, prepuce, or vulva, or pulse oximetry can be measured via rectal probe. Blood pressure monitoring accomplished by indirect measurements can be obtained by Doppler blood flow detection or oscillometric techniques. Both of these methods can alert the anesthesia team to hypotensive problems so that they can be corrected. Pulmonary function and ventilation are monitored by monitoring carbon dioxide. Low carbon dioxide values (<35 mm Hg) indicate hyperventilation and can be attributable to pulmonary or nonpulmonary causes. Patients with decreased levels of consciousness or central nervous system disease have decreased respiratory rates. Lung failure is associated with elevated carbon dioxide levels. If the underlying cause cannot be corrected, hypercapnic patients must be mechanically ventilated. Using a capnograph to measure end-tidal carbon dioxide provides a noninvasive method of continuously approximating arterial carbon dioxide partial pressure. A capnograph measures the partial pressure of carbon dioxide in the expired air obtained at the end of expiration. End-tidal carbon dioxide is a good estimate of arterial carbon dioxide in normal lungs but becomes less precise in patients with major pulmonary disease.

Complete prophylaxis

It is important that quality dental care be provided. There are a number of steps that must be accomplished to ensure maximum benefit to the patient. They are the preliminary examination and evaluation, supragingival gross calculus removal, periodontal probing (and periodontal charting), subgingival calculus removal, detection of missed plaque and calculus, polishing, sulcus irrigation and fluoride treatment, periodontal diagnostics, final charting, and, finally, home care.

Step 1: preliminary evaluation

The first step in the dental procedure is a complete evaluation to determine the necessary diagnostic and treatment measures.

Step 2: supragingival gross calculus removal

Supragingival gross calculus is removed. Many types of instruments may be used to perform this step. Hand scalers are used for supragingival removal of calculus. They should not be inserted below the gumline. A pull stroke (a stroke pulling the calculus toward the coronal aspect) is used to remove calculus. Using calculus removal forceps is a fairly quick method to remove supragingival calculus. The longer tip is placed over the crown, and the shorter tip is placed under the calculus ledge. The calculus is cleaved off when the tips are brought together. Sonic or ultrasonic scalers quickly remove the smaller deposits of supragingival calculus. When properly applied, this vibration breaks up calculus on the surface of teeth. Supragingival and subgingival scaling is often performed at the same time. Texts are available that describe the proper use of ultrasonic scalers (American Animal Hospital Association) [10].

Step 3: periodontal probing (and periodontal charting)

A periodontal probe is used to measure the depth of the sulcus or pocket. The measured distance must be carefully evaluated, because the measurement of sulcular or pocket depth is not the same as that of attachment loss. If the gingival margin is located at the normal cementoenamel junction, the probed depth corresponds to attachment loss. If previous recession of the gingiva has occurred, however, and the marginal gingiva has moved coronally, the pocket depth is less than the actual loss of the attached gingiva. If gingival hyperplasia and a pseudopocket are present as a result, the probed depth is greater than the real attachment loss.

Record keeping is an important part of the dental procedure. It is best to use full-page dental charts to allow more room for recording. Because periodontal disease is progressive, charting provides important support for follow-up examinations. Accurate records of pocket measurements, furcation exposure, and mobility establish a baseline that adds meaning to subsequent examinations, which is useful in evaluating treatment and home care.

Step 4: subgingival calculus removal

A curette or ultrasonic scaler with a subgingival tip should be used to remove subgingival calculus. Several companies make specialized ultrasonic inserts that can be used subgingivally. Removal of subgingival calculus is an extremely important part of the procedure. If subgingival calculus remains, the patient is not likely to receive long-term benefits from treatment; bacterial plaque is likely to continue destroying the periodontium, leading first to bone deterioration and, eventually, to tooth loss.

Step 5: detection of missed plaque and calculus

Explorers, air drying, and disclosing solution are three ways to detect missed plaque and calculus. The explorer aids in a tactile evaluation of the tooth surface while checking for subgingival calculus. Air drying makes the deposits appear chalky white. Painting a small amount of disclosing solution (Reveal; Henry Schein, Melville, NY) on the teeth with a cotton-tipped applicator shows plaque and calculus that were missed while scaling. After being irrigated with water, areas where plaque remains on the tooth surface are stained with red or blue pigment, depending on the brand. Clean teeth do not retain the stain.

Step 6: polishing

Polishing with an electrical or air-powered polisher removes any plaque that may have been missed and smoothes the tooth surface. Some practitioners have expressed concern that excessive polishing could cause enamel loss. Risk of enamel loss may be a factor with human patients, whose teeth may be polished 3 or 4 times a year for many years; however, most veterinary patients are lucky to have their teeth cleaned 10 times over their life span.

Given that polishing is necessary to perform a complete prophy, the choice of equipment is important. There are four types of prophy angles: disposable plastic heads, metal heads with disposable prophy cups, metal oscillating angles, and plastic oscillating angles. One advantage of the disposable plastic prophy angles is that they are relatively inexpensive and do not need to be cleaned after use; they are simply discarded. They should not be cleaned and used on multiple patients. The rubber in the prophy cup cannot withstand multiple uses. The teeth are polished with a low-speed handpiece at approximately 3000 to 8000 rpm. The plastic oscillating angles have the advantages of not wrapping hair around the cup in the process of polishing and of being disposable. The use of "personal polishers" that can be purchased at drugstores is not satisfactory.

Step 7: sulcus irrigation and fluoride treatment

Gentle irrigation of the sulcus flushes out trapped debris and oxygenates the intrasulcular fluids. A saline, stannous fluoride, or diluted chlorhexidine solution can also be used. The dilution of chlorhexidine that is used for irrigation of a sulcus is 0.12%. If a pocket with periodontal disease is present, a 0.05% solution with sterile physiologic saline should be used. A blunted 23-gauge irrigation needle with a syringe is effective for this procedure. Acidulated phosphate fluoride foam (Flurafom; Virbac, Fort Worth, TX) at a dilution of 1.23% may be applied to slow the reattachment of plaque after the prophy. This material is applied with a cotton-tipped applicator and allowed to sit on the tooth surface for 3 to 5 minutes. It is then wiped (not washed) from the tooth surface.

Step 8: periodontal diagnostics

Diagnostics should always include periodontal probing (if not already performed) and intraoral radiology. Dental radiographs are a valuable diagnostic tool that has rapidly become standard of care. Radiographs should be taken to evaluate the dental and bony structures for periodontal bone loss, root canal disease, and other conditions. Studies have shown that the diagnostic yield of full-mouth radiographs in feline and canine patients is high and that routine full-mouth radiography is justified [11,12]. Radiographic findings can be numerous. In the healthy patient, the alveolar crestal bone is seen close to the neck of the tooth. In stage 1 or stage 2 periodontal disease, there is no change from that of healthy periodontium. In stage 3, subgingival calculus may be noted, and a rounding of the alveolar crestal bone at the cervical portion of the tooth can be seen on careful examination at the earliest part of stage 3. Up to 30% of the tooth root may be affected by vertical or horizontal bone loss. In stage 4, subgingival calculus and vertical or horizontal bone loss of 30% or greater of the root length are noted. There are two types of pocket formation: suprabony and infrabony pockets. These are differentiated by the location of the bottom of the pocket with respect to the adjacent alveolar bone. Infrabony pockets have the depth of the pocket apical to the level of the alveolar bone and are associated with radiographically identifiable vertical bone loss. Suprabony pockets have the fundus of the pocket superficial to the height of the alveolar bone and are associated with horizontal bone loss radiographically.

Step 9: final charting

Final charting involves a review of the previously performed diagnostic and periodontal charting. This final review should include any additional treatment performed.

Step 10: home care

The last step in the complete prophy is home-care instruction. Given the process of creation of plaque, this is an important step. Twenty minutes after the teeth have been "cleaned," a glycoprotein layer starts to form on the tooth surface. Without disinfectants like chlorhexidine or fluoride, bacterial colonies can form on the tooth surface in as little as 6 to 8 hours.

This is known as plaque. Bacteria attach to the tooth surface via the glycoprotein layer. Attached bacteria die in 3 to 5 days. Calcium from saliva is incorporated into the dead bacteria, and the result is known as calculus or tartar. Home care removes the plaque surface and prevents it from forming into calculus.

Treatment of periodontal disease

Periodontal disease is treated by periodontal therapy or periodontal surgery.

Periodontal therapy

The goal of periodontal therapy is to preserve the dentition in a state of health, comfort, and function. Treatment should alter or eliminate microbiologic pathogens and contributing risk factors, resolve inflammation, arrest disease progression, and create an environment that deters recurrent disease.

In the past, veterinary dental procedures were basically nonsurgical "prophys" or "dentals" that could be called soft tissue management, because the bony defects were not diagnosed or surgically corrected. This therapy consisted mainly of various combinations of the following procedures: oral hygiene instruction (often not followed through by the owner or patient), manual and/or mechanical scaling and root planing, delivery of local and/or systemic chemotherapeutic agents, and elimination of contributing factors. In human dentistry, there have been university-conducted clinical trials that supported the effectiveness of nonsurgical treatment. These trials should be interpreted by clinicians with respect to their practical application, however. The success of treating generalized or localized severe periodontal disease depends on patient compliance with home care and recalls (every 3–4 months). These same patient and client considerations exist in veterinary dentistry. This is further complicated by the need for anesthesia for many of the posttreatment evaluations so as to check all pocket depths and furcations. It may be that visual evaluation shows improvement of marginal or free gingival health but advanced disease is still present deeper in the pockets (and furcations). This leads to further bone loss and eventual loss of teeth. Therefore, before the clinician selects root planing or nonsurgical management as the definitive and only mode of treatment, the severity of the periodontal condition must be assessed. It is critical that the root surface and furcations associated with deep (greater than 4 mm) pockets be meticulously clean. If this cannot occur, extraction or periodontal surgery is the only alternative.

The patient needs to have shallow pockets after therapy for the following reasons:

1. Deep pockets are technically more difficult to clean and may require extended anesthetic time.
2. Deep pockets frequently contain more pathogens and provide an environment facilitating proliferation of anaerobes.
3. Deep pockets usually cannot be monitored unless anesthesia is used.
4. Deep pockets and furcations may need management by the veterinarian every 3 to 4 months, because the bacteria repopulate the pocket in approximately 128 days.
5. Wound healing shows a long epithelial attachment after root planing in deep pockets, which breaks down soon after the prophy, and bacteria invade the pocket once again.

Along with these dilemmas, the goal of decreasing pocket depth must be accomplished while the patient is under anesthesia, preferably in one sitting. This may require multiple modalities, including scaling and root planing for the supragingival and shallow suprabony pockets, and periodontal debridement.

There has been a change in instrumentation theory, which moves away from complete stripping of the dentin surface. This has been caused by the availability of newer thinner instruments. Unlike the wider instrument tips used for supragingival ultrasonic scaling, the newer tips are thinner, easier to use, and can enter the periodontal pocket with less distention of the gingiva; in addition, they minimize harm to the tissues that can occur with the use of curettes. There are also newer antimicrobials and antibiotics used in treatment.

Periodontal debridement is the treatment of gingival and periodontal inflammation. Its goal is to remove surface irritants mechanically while attempting to maintain soft tissues and allow them to return to a healthy noninflamed state at the same time. Formerly, it was thought that calculus and toxins from bacteria were embedded in the cementum. Therefore, it was necessary to remove the cementum. Newer research has shown that molecular growth factors contained within the cementum aid in the reattachment of the periodontal ligament to the root surface. Now, only the removal of plaque and calculus is mandatory.

When properly used, ultrasonic scalers remove the least amount of cementum as compared with sonic scalers or hand instruments. Additionally, ultrasonic scalers provide water lavage, which gives better visualization of the tissues, removes debris from the pocket, improves cleaning of the tissues because they are being irrigated, and results in better wound healing. Ultrasonic scalers are able to clean the root surface more efficiently; the sonic waves produced have a cavitation effect, disrupting the bacterial cell wall. This increases their effectiveness compared with hand instruments, resulting in less treatment and anesthesia time.

Ultrasonic periodontal therapy has several advantages compared with traditional ultrasonic therapy as well as the manual use of a curette. First, because the ultrasonic tip creates less distention of the gingival tissues than a curette, there is less trauma and faster healing. No sharpening of the ultrasonic instrument is required, and because there are no cutting edges, the chance of gingival laceration is reduced, which makes it safer.

There are several manufacturers of ultrasonic tips for the metal stack type ultrasonic machines and several varieties of tips (Dentsply International, York, PA 17405–0872; Parkell, Farmingdale, NY 11735; and Hu-Friedy, Chicago, IL 60618–5982). Generally, it is best to use shorter tips for shallow pockets and longer tips for deeper pockets. Some tips have corkscrew type angles to them. These all advance around crowns and into the furcation.

Additional treatment for periodontal disease includes gingivectomy for hyperplasic tissue (pseudopockets) and some suprabony pockets. Periodontal mucoperiosteal flaps (open flaps) give access to shallow pockets and root planing suprabony pockets. There is a flap for osteoplasty in one- and two-walled infrabony pockets and ledges, flaps with osseous grafting and epithelia exclusion membranes to regenerate three-walled bony defects and root amputations, and apically repositioned flaps to reposition tissue for furcation treatment. Long-term success requires good oral hygiene, shallow pockets, correct tooth alignment, good systemic health, and a nutritionally and abrasively adequate diet. Discussion of these treatments is planned in a future issue of this journal.

Fractured teeth

There are three options for treatment: ignore the fracture, extract the tooth, or endodontic therapy. A common misconception in veterinary medicine is that fractured teeth can be ignored. Unfortunately, bacteria enter the root canal system through the fracture site. Once at the apex, they can spread periapically to the rest of the system. At that point, the tooth has little difference from a foreign body. Tooth extraction is a valid option. The extraction procedure can be traumatic, however, and there is loss of function of the extracted tooth and the tooth it occludes against. The third option is endodontic therapy, where the pulp chamber and root canal are removed. The root canal system is sealed, and the tooth is resorted. This can be much easier on the geriatric patient than a sometimes difficult extraction.

Oral neoplasia

Various benign and malignant neoplasias can occur in the oral cavity. The key point in treating these is taking radiographs and biopsies to get a complete evaluation. In the absence of other systemic disease, the excuse that the "patient is too old" should not be used.

Summary

Quality of life is an important issue for geriatric patients. Allowing periodontal disease, fractured teeth, and neoplasia to remain untreated decreases this quality of life. Age itself should be recognized; however, it should not be a deterrent to successful veterinary dental care.

Recommended Reading

Bellows J. Small animal dental equipment, materials, and techniques. Ames (IA): Blackwell Publishing; 2004.
Holmstrom SE. Veterinary dentistry for the technician and office staff. Philadelphia: WB Saunders; 2000.
Holmstrom SE, Frost P, Eisner ER. Veterinary dental techniques. Philadelphia: WB Saunders; 2004.
Wiggs RW, Lobprise HB. Veterinary dentistry principles and practice. Philadelphia: Lippincott-Raven; 1997.

References

[1] Glowaski MM. Anesthesia for the geriatric patient. Presented at the Tufts Animal Exposition, North Grafton, MA, 2002.
[2] Hartsfield SM. Anesthetic problems of the geriatric dental patient. In: Marretta SM, editor. Problems in veterinary medicine. Philadelphia: JB Lippincott; 1990. p. 26–8.
[3] Grieve GA, Neuhoff KT, Thomas RM, et al. Understanding the compliance gap. In: The path to high quality care. Lakewood: American Animal Hospital Association; 2003. p. 14–5.
[4] Dyson DH, Maxie MG, Schnurr D. Morbidity and mortality associated with anesthetic management in small animal veterinary practice in Ontario. J Am Anim Hosp Assoc 1998; 34:325–35.
[5] Holmstrom SE, Frost P, Eisner ER. Dental prophylaxis and periodontal disease stages in veterinary dental techniques. 3rd edition. Philadelphia: WB Saunders; 2004. p. 175–232.
[6] Hellyer PW. Anesthesia and fluid therapy. Presented at the Western Veterinary Conference, Las Vegas, NV, 2002.
[7] Forsyth SS. Anesthetic induction. Presented at the World Small Animal Veterinary Association World Congress Proceedings, 2003.
[8] Galloway DS, Ko JCH, Reaugh F, et al. Anesthetic indices of sevoflurane and isoflurane in unpremedicated dogs. J Am Vet Med Assoc 2004;225(5):700–4.
[9] Barton L. Monitoring the critical patient. Presented at the Atlantic Coast Veterinary Conference, 2002.
[10] Holmstrom SE. Veterinary dentistry for the technician and office staff. Philadelphia: WB Saunders; 2000. p. 159–69.
[11] Verstraete JM, Kass PH, Terpak CH. Diagnostic value of full mouth radiology in cats. Am J Vet Res 1998;59:692–5.
[12] Verstraete JM, Kass PH, Terpak CH. Diagnostic value of full mouth radiology in cats. Am J Vet Res 1998;59:686–91.

ELSEVIER
SAUNDERS

Vet Clin Small Anim
35 (2005) 713–742

VETERINARY
CLINICS
Small Animal Practice

Nutrition for Aging Cats and Dogs and the Importance of Body Condition

Dorothy P. Laflamme, DVM, PhD

Nestle Purina PetCare Research, Checkerboard Square, St. Louis, MO 63164, USA

The average age of pet dogs and cats continues to increase such that between one third and one half of pet dogs and cats are 7 years of age or older [1]. In the United States, there has been a nearly twofold increase in the percentage of pet cats older than 6 years of age (from 24% to 47%) over the past 10 years [2]. Likewise, in Europe the number of dogs considered to be "senior" (> 7 years of age) increased by approximately 50%, whereas the number of cats older than 7 years of age increased by over 100% between 1983 and 1995 [3].

Aging brings with it physiologic changes. Some changes are obvious, such as whitening of hair, a general decline in body and coat condition, and failing senses (sight and hearing). Other changes are less obvious, however, and these include alterations in the physiology of the digestive tract, immune system, kidneys, and other organs. Of course, pets, like people, do not age consistently, and chronologic age does not always match physiologic age. Although many pets remain active and youthful well into their teens, most dogs start to slow down and may show signs of aging beginning as early as 5 or 6 years of age. The aging process is influenced by breed size, genetics, nutrition, environment, and other factors. As a general rule, dogs and cats 7 years of age or older, which is the age when many age-related diseases begin to be more frequently observed, may be considered to be "at risk" for age-related problems [3]. "Geriatric" screening should be considered as a preventive medicine service conducted to identify diseases in their early stages or to head off preventable diseases. An important part of this evaluation is a thorough nutritional assessment.

Nutritional requirements can change with age. In addition, many diseases common in older dogs and cats may be nutrient-sensitive, meaning that diet can play an important role in the management of the condition. This article

E-mail address: dorothy.laflamme@rdmo.nestle.com

0195-5616/05/$ - see front matter © 2005 Elsevier Inc. All rights reserved.
doi:10.1016/j.cvsm.2004.12.011 *vetsmall.theclinics.com*

discusses the impact of aging on nutritional requirements, reviews patient nutritional evaluation, and then addresses some common nutrition-related problems in older dogs and cats.

Effects of aging on nutritional requirements

Energy needs

Maintenance energy requirements (MERs) are the energy needs required for the normal animal to survive with minimal activity. Individual MERs can vary based on genetic potential, health status, and whether the animal is sexually intact or neutered. In addition to these factors, MERs seem to decrease with age in human beings, rodents, and dogs [4,5]. In one study involving English Setters, Miniature Schnauzers, and German Shepherd dogs, the MERs of 11-year-old dogs were approximately 25% less than those of breed-matched 3-year-old dogs [5]. Others have reported an 18% to 24% decrease in MERs of older dogs across various breeds [4]. The greatest decline seemed to occur in dogs older than 7 years of age [6].

Age-related changes in MERs in cats are more controversial. Some report no change in MERs with age when evaluated in short-term studies [4]. When MERs were evaluated over a longer period (3–12 months), however, a different picture emerged. Based on data from more than 100 cats ranging in age from 2 to 17 years, MERs decreased with age in cats through approximately 11 years of age (Fig. 1) [7]. Based on a subset of these cats for

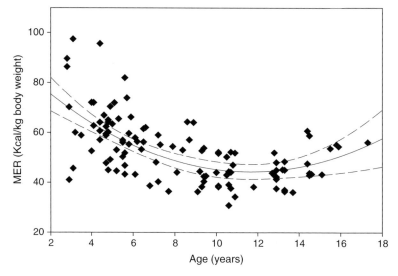

Fig. 1. Effect of age on maintenance energy requirements (MERs) of adult cats. MERs decrease until approximately 11.5 years and then increase. The lines shown represent the second-order regression with a 95% confidence interval: MERs (kcal/kg/d) = 89.576 − [7.771 · Age (years) + 0.334 · Age (years)^2]; r^2 = 0.34; P < 0.001.

which repeated measures were available, MERs decreased approximately 3% per year. By approximately 12 years of age onward, however, MERs per unit of body weight actually increased. This increase was confirmed in another study involving 85 cats between 10 and 15 years of age [8]. MERs increased throughout this age group, with the greatest increases occurring after 13 years of age.

A primary driver of basal metabolic rate, hence MERs, is lean body mass (LBM). The LBM, which includes skeletal muscle, skin, and organs, contains most metabolically active cells and accounts for approximately 96% of basal energy expenditure [9]. With exercise, the contribution of muscle and LBM to energy needs increases further. Across species, including dogs and cats, LBM tends to decrease with age [10,11]. This, plus a decrease in activity, can contribute to the reduction in MERs seen in aging dogs and middle-aged cats.

If energy needs decrease in a pet and energy intake does not decrease accordingly, the animal becomes overweight. It is this last point that drives the market position of many foods for older dogs and cats. Most commercial foods for geriatric pets contain a reduced concentration of dietary fat and calories. Some have dietary fiber added to reduce the caloric density further. These products may be appropriate for the large number of pets that are overweight or likely to get that way. If energy intake is not managed appropriately, dogs and cats may become overweight and subject to associated health risks. Arthritis and diabetes, for example, which are common in older dogs and cats, are aggravated by excess body weight.

Not all older animals are overweight or less active. In fact, although "middle-aged" animals tend to be overweight, a greater proportion of dogs and cats older than 12 years of age are underweight compared with other age groups [12]. This effect is especially pronounced in cats. In addition to an increase in MERs in this age group, which may partly explain weight loss, recent research has identified that older cats may experience a reduction in digestive capabilities.

Earlier research in our laboratory indicated that older cats retain their digestive capabilities [13]. That study was done with young adult and middle-aged cats, however (>8 years of age). The only significant differences in digestive function indicated a slight increase in carbohydrate digestibility in older cats. More recently, however, an evaluation was completed to look at a broader range of ages. Consequently, it was shown that fat digestibility decreases with age in a large number of geriatric cats [11]. The prevalence of compromised fat digestibility increases with age and affects approximately one third of cats older than 12 years of age (Fig. 2) [11]. In addition, approximately 20% of cats older than 14 years of age have a reduced ability to digest protein. Reduced protein digestion or fat digestion could contribute to weight loss in aging cats.

These patients as well as others that are underweight may benefit from a more energy-dense highly digestible product to help compensate for these

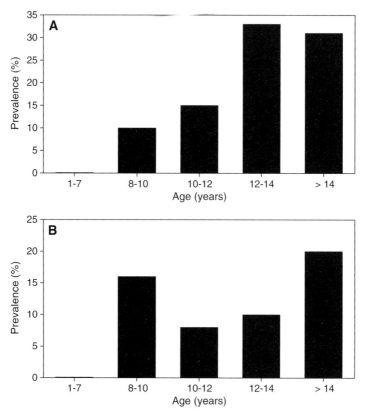

Fig. 2. Prevalence of low fat (*A*) or protein (*B*) digestive function in cats by age. Low fat digestibility was defined as less than 80% digestible compared with normal digestibility of 90% to 95%. Low protein digestibility was defined as less than 77% digestible compared with normal digestibility of 85% to 90%. (*Data from* Perez-Camargo G. Cat nutrition: what's new in the old? Compend Contin Educ Pract Vet 2004;26(Suppl 2A):5–10.)

age-related changes. A nutritional assessment should be completed on each patient to determine its individual needs rather than assuming that all older pets need reduced calorie intake.

Protein needs

Protein is another nutrient of extreme importance for aging pets. In the past, many veterinarians have recommended protein restriction for older dogs in the mistaken belief that this would help to protect kidney function [14]. More recent research has unequivocally demonstrated that protein restriction is unnecessary in healthy older dogs [15–17]. On the contrary, protein requirements sufficient to support protein turnover actually increase in older dogs [18].

In a classic study comparing the protein requirements of young and old Beagles, the older dogs required approximately 50% more protein than young adult dogs to maintain nitrogen balance and maximize protein reserves [18]. In addition, protein turnover was reduced in the older dogs, even at the highest level of protein fed.

The current standard for establishing adult protein (nitrogen) requirements is the nitrogen balance method, which compares nitrogen intake with nitrogen output. Maintenance of LBM or measures of protein turnover provide better indicators of protein adequacy compared with nitrogen balance studies, however. Protein turnover is the cycle of catabolism of endogenous protein and synthesis of new proteins needed by the body at any given time, including hormones, enzymes, immune proteins, and others. When dietary protein intake is insufficient, the body responds by decreasing catabolism and synthesis and mobilizing protein from LBM to support essential protein synthesis. Normal animals can adapt to this low-protein intake and maintain nitrogen balance yet be in a protein-depleted state. In this situation, animals may appear healthy but have a decreased ability to respond to environmental insults, including infections and toxic substances [18]. In addition to the direct effect of inadequate protein intake, aging has a detrimental effect on protein turnover. In one review, 85% of the studies found an age-related decline in endogenous protein synthesis [19]. In otherwise healthy animals, even mild protein deficiency can significantly impair immune function [20,21]. These effects may be more pronounced in the older dog because of the reduced LBM and age-related reduction in protein turnover.

In dogs, it took three times as much protein to maintain protein turnover than that needed to maintain nitrogen balance in old and young dogs, with older dogs needing more protein than young dogs [18]. Approximately 3.75 g of casein protein per kilogram of body weight per day was required for older Beagles compared with 2.5 g/kg/d for young adult Beagles. A more recent study also showed that dogs could maintain nitrogen balance on protein as low as 16% of energy but that protein turnover was maximized in young and old dogs when protein was increased to 32% of energy [22].

Actual protein needs may vary based on individual factors, such as breed, lifestyle, health, and individual metabolism. In addition, calorie intake affects dietary protein need. With lower calorie intake, the percent of calories as protein must increase to maintain the same protein intake. Older dogs tend to consume fewer calories, and thus less food, than younger dogs. Therefore, diets for older dogs should contain a higher percentage of dietary protein, or an increased protein-to-calorie ratio, to meet their needs. Diets containing at least 25% of calories from protein should meet the protein needs of most healthy senior dogs.

Similar data showing an age effect in cats are lacking; however, cats of all ages have high protein requirements. Similar to other species, cats need considerably more protein to maintain LBM than needed to maintain nitrogen balance. Based on assessment of LBM, adult cats need more than 5 g of protein per kilogram of body weight, or approximately 34% of their dietary calories as protein, to support lean body mass and protein turnover [23].

Other nutrients

All dogs and cats have specific needs for vitamins and minerals, which are normally provided by complete and balanced diets. There is little, if any, evidence that the requirements for these nutrients differ in healthy older animals. Patients with subclinical disease associated with a mild malabsorption syndrome or polyuria may have increased losses of water-soluble nutrients, such as B vitamins, or fat-soluble nutrients, such as vitamins A and E, however. As noted previously, approximately one third of geriatric cats have a reduced ability to digest dietary fats. In these cats, there is a significant correlation between fat digestibility and the digestibility of other essential nutrients, including several B vitamins, vitamin E, potassium, and other minerals [24]. Geriatric cats with gastrointestinal disease are more likely to be deficient in cobalamin (vitamin B_{12}) compared with younger cats [25]. Thus, older cats should be carefully evaluated for possible nutrient deficiencies and may benefit from supplemental amounts of these nutrients.

Oxidative damage plays an important role in many diseases of aging, including arthritis and other inflammatory diseases, cancers, neurologic disease, cardiovascular disease, and others [26–33]. There even exists a popular theory suggesting that "aging" is induced by an imbalance between free radical production or exposure and the body's antioxidant defenses [27]. Certainly, a deficiency of antioxidant nutrients can have detrimental effects on in vivo antioxidant function, immune function, and markers of health [26,34,35]. In addition, adequate dietary protein is critical to support endogenous glutathione production, a key antioxidant for disease prevention [33].

Considerable evidence in human beings and animals suggests that dietary antioxidants may provide some protection against oxidative stress and normal aging processes [27,33,35,36]. Numerous studies on antioxidants in dogs or cats have reported beneficial effects on markers of oxidative status [37–41]. It is difficult to show clear cause-and-effect relations between the diseases and antioxidant status, however, because oxidant damage is subtle and difficult to measure and the associated diseases develop slowly over many years [28]. Given the weight of available information, it is reasonable to recommend or provide increased amounts of antioxidant nutrients for aging dogs and cats.

Geriatric nutritional evaluation

Before instituting a dietary change in any patient, especially an older dog or cat, a thorough nutritional evaluation should be completed. This should include an evaluation of the patient, the current diet, and feeding management. The goal of dietary history taking is to identify the presence and significance of factors that put patients at risk for malnutrition. Understanding how the nutritional needs of older animals may change and a thorough evaluation of the individual patient allow an appropriate dietary recommendation. Such recommendations should take into account the needs of the patient and client preferences.

Changes in feeding management should be considered part of total patient management. As with any aspect of medical management, the patient should be re-evaluated at appropriate intervals to ensure achievement of desired results.

Patient evaluation

A complete medical history should be assessed, including vaccination history, heartworm and flea preventive methods, and any prior diseases. A thorough physical examination should be conducted, including body weight and body condition score (BCS), oral examination, digital rectal examination, and evaluation of the skin and hair coat. Thin and brittle hair or dry and flaky skin can have many causes but may be a sign of nutritional deficiencies. A comprehensive geriatric evaluation may include the following blood, urine, and fecal analyses: complete blood cell count (CBC); platelet count; biochemical profile; serum bile acids analysis; and complete urinalysis, including sediment examination, urine protein/creatinine ratio, and fecal flotation. Although these tests are not sensitive nutritional indicators, abnormalities may provide evidence of clinical or subclinical problems that may benefit from dietary modification. For example, anemia, low serum albumin, low potassium, increased serum urea nitrogen, increased triglycerides or cholesterol, or increased serum glucose may indicate problems that could benefit from dietary modification as part of medical management.

Increases or decreases in body condition should trigger further evaluation. If weight loss is evident (from the physical examination or the medical history), further evaluation should determine if this is associated with increased or decreased calorie intake. A detailed dietary history and evaluation are warranted. If the patient shows an increase in or excessive BCS, it is again important to consider current diet and feeding management. Older dogs and middle-aged cats tend to have reduced energy needs. If calorie intake is not adjusted accordingly, weight gain results. Unexplained weight gain should be evaluated for predisposing causes, such as hypothyroidism. Animals that are overweight are likely to benefit from weight reduction.

Dietary evaluation

A complete dietary evaluation must include everything that is consumed. One approach to gathering this information is to have the client complete a written dietary history form (Fig. 3). The diet history should include the normal diet as well as other foods the pet has access to. Commercially prepared

Dietary Information Form   **Date:**   _____

Owner's Name: _____   Pet's Name: _____

Species :   Dog   Cat   Other   Breed: _____   Pet's Gender: M   MC   F   FS

Age: _____   Body Weight*: _____   Body Condition Score: _____   Activity: High   Med   Low   Very Low

Diet History:
What food(s) are currently fed – main meal:

Dry Food: ____never ____ occasional/ small proportion ____about half ____ mostly _____ exclusively

If fed, what brands and amounts are fed most often: _____

Canned Food: ____never _____ occasional/ small proportion ____about half ____ mostly _____ exclusively

If fed, what brands and amounts are fed most often: _____

Home prepared foods ____never ____ occasional/ small proportion ____ half ____ mostly ____ exclusively

If fed, please provide recipes used.

What treats and/or supplements are currently fed?

Commercial treats: ____ No ____Yes. What brands and amounts are fed most often: _____

_____

Fresh foods or table scraps: ____No ____ Yes. What foods and amounts are fed most often: _____

_____

Dietary supplements: ____No ____Yes. What supplements and amounts are fed most often: _____

_____

Have there been recent changes in foods/brands fed? ____ No _____ Yes. If so, when and why?

_____

How is your pet's appetite _____ Good _____ Poor   Any recent changes? _____

How frequently does your pet defecate: _____ 0-1/day ____2 –3 /day ____ 4 or more/day ____ don't know

How would you characterize his/her stool? Mostly: ____firm/hard ____formed but not hard _____ loose

Where does your pet spend most of his time: _____ Indoors ____Outdoors _____About half in and half out

How much time does your pet spend walking, playing or running each day? :   ____ < 30 min/day ____ 30 – 60 min/day

        ____ 1 to 3 hours/day _____ > 3 hours/day ____ mostly inactive but > 3 hours/day once or twice per week

Are there other pets in your household? ____ Yes____ No

Do you have any questions regarding your pet's diet? _____

Fig. 3. Diet history form.

foods should be identified by brand. If needed, manufacturers can be contacted to obtain product information, such as typical calorie and nutrient content, digestibility, and other details. Any changes to the diet should be identified as well as the reason for the change. Because many pet owners provide treats and human table food "samples" for their pets, these also should be identified by types and amounts. Clients may not consider nutritional supplements part of the diet, so they should be asked specifically about these.

Once the nutritional characteristics of the total diet are known, they should be compared with the individual patient's needs. In general, inactive animals or those that are somewhat overweight should be receiving lower calorie foods yet may need foods with an increased nutrient-to-calorie ratio formulated to compensate for increased needs of other nutrients. Feeding such animals a high-calorie food may require an inappropriate reduction in the volume of food, resulting in lack of satiation as well as restriction of essential nutrients. Conversely, feeding a low-calorie food to a pet with high energy needs may require excessive food intake, resulting in loss of body weight or excessive stool volume.

Feeding management evaluation

Knowing what diets are fed does not indicate whether or not they are fed appropriately and eaten acceptably. Clients should be asked how much and how often each of the foods identified previously are fed. Other important questions include the following:

Do pets in a multiple-pet household share a food bowl, or are they fed
   individually?
Are pets fed measured amounts of food or free choice?
How well does the pet accept the food?
Have there been any changes in how the patient is fed or how it eats?

This information is not only important in determining the adequacy of the current dietary situation but in planning a dietary recommendation that achieves good client acceptance and compliance.

Common diet-sensitive conditions in geriatric animals

Few diseases in modern pets are "diet induced." One possible exception to this is obesity, which, although many interactive factors are involved, is ultimately caused by consuming more calories than needed by the dog or cat. Many other diseases are "diet-sensitive," however, meaning that diet can play a role in managing the condition. Examples of diet-sensitive conditions common in aging dogs and cats include chronic renal disease, diabetes mellitus (DM), arthritis, and many others. Information on the management of many of these diseases can be found in other articles in this issue. The remainder of this article focuses first on weight loss and then on the most common nutritional problem in older dogs and cats, which is obesity, and some obesity-related conditions.

Weight loss

Not all older patients are overweight. In fact, a greater proportion of dogs and cats older than 12 years of age are underweight than any other age group [12]. Weight loss is not unusual in older patients and may be associated with increased or decreased intake (Fig. 4). The implications for dietary modifications vary, depending on the specific diagnosis.

If intake is normal or increased but the client has recently been feeding a commercially available senior diet or other diet with reduced calories to a highly active dog or geriatric cat, weight loss could be a normal response. The pet may have high energy needs because of individual metabolism or lifestyle. Alternatively, malabsorption of nutrients may be involved. Approximately one in three geriatric cats experiences fat malabsorption,

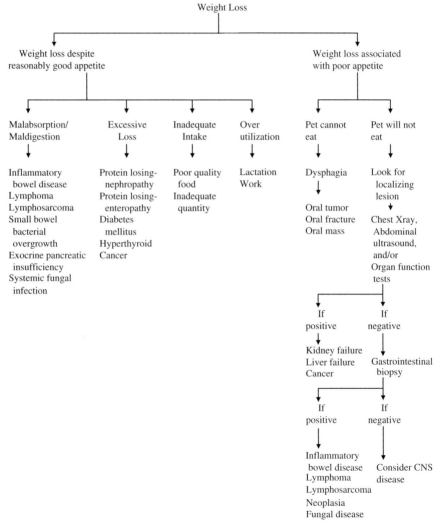

Fig. 4. Diagnostic algorithm for weight loss in geriatric patients. (Courtesy of Nestle Purina PetCare Company, St. Louis, MO.)

and one in five experiences protein malabsorption [11]. If other reasons for weight loss are excluded, the patient should be evaluated for diseases like intestinal or pancreatic diseases, renal disease, or cancer.

Body weight loss seems to be an early indicator of chronic disease in geriatric cats. When body weight data from 258 cats were evaluated retrospectively, a definite pattern emerged between body weight change and death secondary to various diseases [11]. Cats dying from cancer, renal failure, and thyroid disease began to lose weight 2.5 years before death. On average, more than 6% of the body weight was lost in the second year before death, and the average body weight loss in the last year of life was more than 10% for these cats. It is not known if tempering this disease-associated weight loss could delay mortality or reduce morbidity in aging cats, yet it seems logical to consider it.

If weight loss in dogs or cats is caused by pancreatic exocrine insufficiency, lymphangiectasia, or liver disease with fat malabsorption, a high-carbohydrate and low-fat diet may be useful. Bile acids from the liver and pancreatic lipase are important for the normal digestion and absorption of long-chain triglycerides (LCTs), the lipids found in most diets. Absorption of LCTs can drop by 50% to 70% of normal in the absence of bile acids and to near zero in the absence of pancreatic lipase. Even when steatorrhea is not apparent, fat digestion may be somewhat reduced. Hydroxylation of unabsorbed fatty acids by colonic microflora can contribute to secretory diarrhea in these patients.

In dogs that are suspected of fat malabsorption, restriction of LCTs is recommended, although adequate essential fatty acids must be provided (ie, dietary LCTs between 5% and 10% of diet dry matter). Inclusion of medium-chain triglycerides (MCTs) as part of the dietary fat in canine diets may be advantageous, because MCTs provide a concentrated source of energy and can be digested and absorbed fairly well despite a lack of pancreatic lipase or bile acids. They are mostly absorbed into the portal blood rather than lymphatic lacteals, so they are less likely than LCTs to contribute to lymphangiectasia. Because MCTs do not provide essential fatty acids, they should not constitute more than 50% of the dietary fat.

Decreased intake may occur for many reasons. In a multiple-dog household, pack relations can change with age and time. An evaluation of feeding management may indicate that an "alpha" dog has been displaced and is no longer receiving free access to a common food bowl. Poor dental health could prevent an otherwise healthy dog or cat from consuming adequate nutrition. Dry foods help to reduce the build up of plaque and tartar on teeth, but soft foods may be needed after extensive tooth loss. Systemic diseases, such as hepatic, renal, gastrointestinal, or adrenal dysfunction, or central nervous system disorders may affect appetite and should be considered if more obvious explanations are not apparent. If a specific diagnosis cannot be found, symptomatic treatment for weight loss should include consumption of a high-calorie and nutrient-dense food.

Dietary fat helps to make foods more palatable as well as providing needed calories.

If poor appetite is a problem, intake may be encouraged by selecting a palatable diet, moistening dry food with warm water, warming food to body temperature, offering fresh food frequently, and having clients pet and encourage the patient during feeding. Cats usually respond well to acidic diets with high moisture content; however, some prefer dry foods. Bowls used for feeding cats should be wide and shallow so that the sides do not touch the cat's whiskers. Minimize noise and stress during feeding periods. If a recent dietary change precipitated the anorexia, consider offering the previous diet. Nutrient modifications that are beneficial in disease management are less important than providing adequate nutrition. Ensure that the patient's nasal passages are clear, because dogs and cats rely on olfaction in selecting foods. Although uncommon, some geriatric cats do experience permanent hypogeusia.

Chemical appetite stimulants may be helpful for short-term use in overcoming anorexia. Benzodiazepine derivatives are commonly used and are effective in up to 50% of patients. Diazepam may be used in dogs or cats and is most effective when administered intravenously (0.2 mg/kg, with a maximum dose of 5 mg per patient) [42]. Fresh palatable food should be offered immediately, because feeding usually starts within 1 minute and may continue for up to 20 minutes. Oxazepam (2.5 mg per cat) results in eating within 20 minutes after oral dosing. Sedation and ataxia are common side effects to diazepam and oxazepam administration.

Recently, excellent results were reported when anorectic cats and dogs were treated with midazolam and propofol, respectively [43,44]. Anorectic cats began eating within 2 minutes after intravenous administration of midazolam (2–5 µg/kg of body weight), with no apparent evidence of sedation or other side effects. Anorectic dogs given intravenous propofol (1–2 mg/kg of body weight) experienced a brief period of sedation, followed by a strong appetite response. No adverse effects were noted in either study. If adequate ongoing oral intake is not achieved, enteral or parenteral nutritional support should be considered.

Obesity

Approximately one of every four dogs and cats presented to veterinary practices in the United States is overweight or obese [12]. The prevalence peaks between 5 and 10 years of age, affecting nearly 50% of dogs and cats in this age group. Obesity can be defined as an excess of body fat sufficient to result in impairment of health or body function. In people, this is generally recognized as 20% to 25% greater than ideal body weight. This degree of excess body weight seems to be important in dogs as well. A lifelong study in dogs showed that even moderately overweight dogs were at greater risk for earlier morbidity and a shortened life span [45].

In that study, one group of Labrador Retrievers was fed 25% less food than their sibling-pairmates throughout life. The average adult BCSs for the lean-fed and control dogs were 4.6 ± 0.2 and 6.7 ± 0.2, respectively, based on a nine-point BCS system [45]. Thus, the control dogs were moderately overweight and actually weighed approximately 26% more, on average, than the lean-fed group. The lean-fed dogs were well within the ideal body condition of 4 to 5 on this nine-point scale. The difference in body condition was sufficient to create significant differences between the groups in median life span, which was 13 years for the lean-fed dogs compared with only 11.2 years for the control group, a difference of approximately 15%. An impressive correlation between BCS at middle age and longevity in these dogs can be seen in Fig. 5. Dogs with a BCS of 5 or less at middle age were far more likely to live beyond 12 years of age compared with those with a higher BCS. In addition, control dogs required medication for chronic health problems or arthritis an average of 2.1 years or 3.0 years, respectively, sooner than their lean-fed siblings [45].

Obese cats also face increased health risks, including an increased risk of musculoskeletal problems (arthritis), DM, hepatic lipidosis, and early mortality [46].

Recent research has suggested a mechanism for the link between excess body weight and so many diseases. It seems that adipose tissue, once

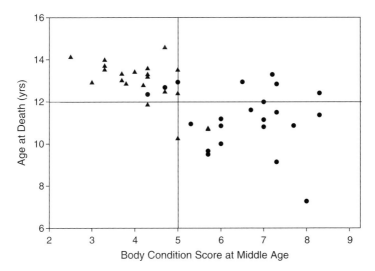

Fig. 5 Effect of body condition on longevity in dogs. The lean-fed dogs (▲) received 25% less food than their control group littermates (•). Body condition score (BCS) was determined annually using a nine-point system. Data shown are the mean BCSs for ages 6 through 8 years for each dog as the independent variable for age of death. Dogs with a BCS of 5 or less at middle age were more likely to live beyond 12 years of age (P < 0.001) compared with dogs with a BCS higher than ideal. For additional details on the test design, see the article by Kealy et al [45]. (Data from Richard D. Kealy, PhD and Dennis F. Lawler, DVM, St. Louis, MO).

considered to be physiologically inert, is an active producer of various hormones, such as leptin, and cytokines. Of major concern is the production of inflammatory cytokines from adipose tissue, specifically tumor necrosis factor-α (TNFα), interleukin (IL)-1β and IL-6, and C-reactive protein [47–50]. The persistent low-grade inflammation secondary to obesity is thought to play a causal role in chronic diseases like osteoarthritis (OA), cardio-vascular disease, and DM [49,51]. In addition, obesity is associated with increased oxidative stress, which also may contribute to obesity-related diseases [52,53].

There are many factors that play a role in creating obesity. Prevention of obesity relies on understanding contributing or associated risk factors and managing them appropriately. Important risk factors for obesity in pets include neutering and inactivity. Neutering can significantly reduce MERs as well as increase spontaneous food intake [54–56]. Controlling food intake can reduce the development of obesity in neutered pets [57].

Despite widespread concern about obesity among pet owners, most do not recognize their own overweight dog as being overweight. As noted previously, obesity is associated with significant health risks; thus, diagnosing and managing obesity is an important part of the nutritional management of aging dogs and cats.

The first step in an effective obesity management program is recognition of the problem. Perhaps the most practical methods for in-clinic assessment of obesity are a combination of body weight and BCS. There are several BCS systems. This author prefers using validated nine-point systems for dogs and cats [58–60]. With these systems, each unit increase in BCS is approximately equivalent to 10% to 15% greater than ideal body weight, so a dog or cat with a BCS of 7 weighs approximately 20% to 30% greater than the ideal weight. By recording body weight and BCS, ideal body weight can be more easily determined. Animals that are becoming obese can be recognized sooner and managed more easily. An illustrated BCS system can provide a useful tool for client education regarding obesity prevention and management.

Once the clinician and owner have recognized obesity in a pet, it is important to develop a management plan that fits the needs of the patient and owner. This must consider client ability and willingness to control calories and enhance exercise for the pet. Numerous options are available, so the keys to success are flexibility in design and regular follow-up with the client. Of utmost importance is the recognition that individual animals can differ greatly in their MERs. Thus, the degree of calorie restriction that induces significant weight loss in one dog or cat may cause weight gain in another. Adjustments in calorie allowance made on a regular basis (eg, every month) help to address these individual differences as well as the reductions in MERs that occur during weight loss.

Use of an appropriate diet for weight loss is important, and there are several criteria to consider. Although it is ultimately calorie restriction that induces weight loss, it is important to avoid excessive restriction of other essential nutrients. Therefore, a low-calorie product with an increased nutrient/calorie ratio should be considered. Further, an important goal for weight loss is to promote fat loss while minimizing loss of lean tissue, which may be influenced by dietary composition.

Fat restriction in weight-loss diets reduces calorie density, which helps to reduce calorie intake. Fat contains more than twice the calories per gram of protein or carbohydrate. In a study of obese human subjects, when carbohydrate replaced dietary fat in ad libitum–fed diets, weight loss was significantly enhanced [61]. In a canine study, dogs fed a low-fat and high-fiber diet lost more body fat compared with dogs fed a high-fat and low-fiber diet [62]. Conversely, several human studies have shown that extremely low-carbohydrate diets can facilitate increased weight loss [63 65]. In this author's experience, such diets alter the selection of foods consumed and greatly reduce intake of sugars and other highly refined carbohydrates, thus reducing calorie intake. Anecdotal reports suggest that this approach also works in overweight cats, but no data as yet support this premise. Conversely, numerous studies have shown that increasing dietary protein, often in exchange for carbohydrates, has beneficial effects for weight management [66–71].

Dietary protein is especially important in weight-loss diets. Providing low-calorie diets with an increased protein-to-calorie ratio significantly increases the percentage of fat lost and reduces the loss of LBM in dogs and cats undergoing weight loss [66,67]. Protein has a significant thermic effect, meaning that postprandial metabolic energy expenditure is increased more when protein is consumed, compared with carbohydrates or fats [72]. In addition to directly contributing to a negative energy balance in support of weight loss, the thermic effect of protein seems to contribute to a satiety effect provided by dietary proteins [73,74]. Finally, a higher protein diet helped to sustain weight maintenance after weight loss in human subjects [75]. This effect is likely to apply to dogs and cats as well.

Other nutraceuticals and herbal compounds continue to be evaluated for use in weight-loss diets. To date, published data on these have been conflicting. Carnitine seems to have received the most attention. Carnitine is produced endogenously from the amino acids lysine and methionine and facilitates β-oxidation of fatty acids. Supplementation with this compound is likely to be of greatest benefit when the intake of dietary protein or other key nutrients is insufficient to promote adequate endogenous production. In semistarved cats and rats undergoing extremely rapid weight loss, L-carnitine reduced hepatic fat accumulation in cats and enhanced lipid metabolism and reduced ketogenesis in rats [76,77]. In human subjects, severe calorie restriction resulted in reduced urinary and plasma carnitine, an effect that was attenuated by increased dietary protein during weight loss [78]. With a few exceptions, studies evaluating carnitine for weight management have shown little benefit [79–82]. In a canine study, dogs retained more LBM when fed a carnitine-supplemented diet but also lost less body weight [83]. Another study in dogs showed no significant difference in body composition changes with carnitine supplementation but implied a benefit for metabolic stimulation [84]. One study demonstrated a significant increase in the rate of weight loss in cats supplemented with carnitine compared with a control group (24% versus 20%, respectively, over an 18-week period) [85].

In addition to diet, feeding management and exercise are critically important to successful weight management. Most clients provide treats for their pets. Rather than requiring that they cease this pleasurable activity, create a "treat allowance" equal to 10% of the daily calories. Clients may be provided with a menu of low-calorie foods or commercial treats that would be appropriate.

Increasing exercise aids in weight management by expending calories. Interactive exercise provides an alternative activity for the pet and owner to enjoy together rather than food-related activities. Activity in cats may be enhanced by interactive play, such as with a toy on a string or a laser light.

Gradual weight loss in dogs, as in people, is more likely to allow long-term maintenance of the reduced body weight [86]. Weight rebound can be minimized by providing controlled food intake and adjusting the calories fed to just meet the needs of the pet for weight maintenance. Clients already accustomed to measuring food and monitoring their pet's weight should be encouraged to apply these behavior modifications to long-term weight management.

Diabetes mellitus

The most significant risk factors for feline DM are age and obesity as well as male gender [3,46,87,88]. Compared with cats less than 7 years of age, cats between 7 and 10 years of age are 8 times more likely to become diabetic and cats older than 14 years of age are 14 times more likely to become diabetic [87]. Obese cats are approximately 4 times as likely to become diabetic compared with cats with optimal body condition [46]. Obesity causes insulin resistance and impaired glucose tolerance in otherwise normal cats [89,90]. One proposed mechanism by which obesity may lead to insulin resistance is by compromising the functionality of the GLUT4 receptor [91,92]. Under normal circumstances, insulin triggers an intracellular cascade resulting in activation of the GLUT4 transport system, which then facilitates glucose entry into the cell. Obesity leads to increased triglycerides in skeletal muscle, which reduce GLUT4 expression and contribute to insulin resistance [91,92]. In addition, TNFα, which is increased in obesity, reduces the expression of GLUT4 [48]. Insulin resistance is a cardinal sign of type II diabetes, the most common form in cats [90,93].

Like cats, obese dogs develop changes in glucose tolerance and insulin resistance. Unlike the scenario in cats, however, this does not seem to progress and obesity does not seem to be a risk factor for development of diabetes in dogs [94,95]. Because obesity is a well-recognized risk factor for type II diabetes, this difference probably relates to the observation that dogs develop immune-mediated type I diabetes rather than type II diabetes. Conversely, obesity can increase the difficulty in regulating glucose in diabetic dogs; thus, obesity remains a concern for these patients.

The primary goal of therapy for DM is to maintain blood glucose concentrations as close to normal as possible through the use of exogenous insulin, diet, and other therapies, along with control or avoidance of concurrent illnesses [96]. Nutritional management is an important factor in the treatment of all diabetic patients. Type I diabetics are insulin dependent. Management is targeted at maintaining a stable and moderate blood glucose concentration through alterations in insulin. Diet serves an adjunct role because it can influence the amount of insulin required and can moderate the postprandial glycemic load [96]. Type II diabetics continue to have some capacity for insulin production. The role of dietary management in type II diabetes is to decrease the need for exogenous insulin while maintaining glycemic control. The dietary considerations for canine and feline diabetics include appropriate calorie intake to reach and maintain ideal body condition, complete and balanced nutrition to provide all essential nutrients, and nutritional modifications to address metabolic disturbances induced by DM. The specific modifications for canine and feline diabetics may differ because of differences in the underlying pathology findings of disease and species differences in normal metabolism.

Rapidly digestible carbohydrates (RDCs) provide abundant starch and sugars and promote an increase in postprandial blood glucose concentrations. In insulin-dependent diabetics, excess RDCs require more exogenous insulin to maintain glycemic control. Therefore, diets that produce less severe increases in postprandial blood glucose are preferred. Nutrient modifications that can help in this regard include an avoidance of RDCs, use of complex carbohydrates and dietary fiber, and use of protein instead of carbohydrates.

Complex carbohydrates include fiber or bran along with the starch, such as might be provided by whole grains. These are digested more slowly than the RDCs from sugars, flours, or polished grains, resulting in a delayed release of glucose into the bloodstream. Alternatively, fibrous ingredients or purified fiber sources can be incorporated into complete pet foods to provide a similar effect—a reduction in postprandial glucose [97–99]. The net effect of providing fiber in the diet is a slowing of carbohydrate absorption from the intestinal tract, a dampening of the postprandial glycemic effects of a meal, and beneficial modifications in blood lipids [100].

Several studies have evaluated fiber-enriched diets in dogs with diabetes. When dogs with well-regulated naturally occurring DM were fed canned diets supplemented with 20 g of wheat bran (a predominantly insoluble fiber source) or 20 g of guar gum (a purified soluble fiber source), reductions in postprandial hyperglycemia were noted [97]. The effect was most pronounced with the guar gum. In a similar study using dogs with alloxan-induced DM, significant reductions in the mean 24-hour blood glucose concentration and 24-hour urine glucose excretion were observed when dogs were fed diets supplemented with 15% (dry matter basis) cellulose (purified insoluble fiber) or pectin (purified soluble fiber) [98]. The cellulose-supplemented diet also caused a reduction in glycosylated hemoglobin. Total dietary fiber (TDF) in these diets was approximately 5.5 to 7.0 g per 420 kJ [101]. Kimmel et al [102] reported better results in insulin-dependent canine diabetics with an insoluble fiber diet, using TDF levels of 7.3 g and 5.6 g of TDF per 420 kJ for the insoluble and soluble fiber diets, respectively. A further study in dogs with naturally occurring DM demonstrated enhanced glycemic control when fiber from pea fiber and guar gum was included at 5.3% of a wet diet, or approximately 5.65 g of TDF per 420 kJ diet [99].

That dietary fiber can be beneficial in managing glycemic control seems to be well documented. What remains controversial is the appropriate amount of fiber needed for this purpose. Problems associated with excess fiber can include increased stool volume and undesirable calorie dilution. Little work has been done to compare a wide range of fiber levels in dogs. No differences were observed between diets when well-controlled diabetic dogs were fed 6.0 or 9.0 g of TDF per 420 kJ (J.W. Bartges, DVM, PhD, unpublished data) An evaluation of several moderate-fiber commercial diets (3.5–5.0 g of TDF per 420 kJ) showed no difference among these diets with regard to insulin or glucose measures [103], but no comparison was made with higher fiber levels. Lower levels of fiber, such as those evaluated in human diabetics, have not been investigated for use in canine diabetics. Based on the data available, diets that provide between 6 and 9 g of TDF per 420 kJ may be appropriate for overweight diabetic dogs, whereas 3 to 6 g of TDF per 420 kJ may be appropriate for diabetic dogs in ideal or thin body condition.

Fewer studies have evaluated fiber-supplemented diets for diabetic cats. Nelson et al [104] reported a significant improvement in serum glucose concentrations in insulin-treated diabetic cats fed a diet containing 12% cellulose (dry matter basis) compared with a low-fiber diet. Another study reported a decrease in insulin requirements in cats switched to a commercial high-fiber diet [105]. Conversely, cats improved significantly more when switched from a high-fiber diet to a high-protein and low-carbohydrate diet [105,106].

Increased dietary protein seems to be beneficial in patients with type II diabetes. In human beings with well-controlled type II diabetes, ingestion of higher protein and lower carbohydrate diets resulted in improved glycemic control as measured by reduced glycosylated hemoglobin or decreased blood glucose on the higher protein diets [107–109]. Similar benefits have been observed in feline diabetics, with decreased insulin requirements or enhanced glycemic control when cats were fed a high-protein diet [105,106,110]. Further, consumption of a high-protein and low-carbohydrate diet resulted in increased insulin sensitivity in diabetic cats [105].

Most studies evaluating higher protein diets have balanced the dietary change on carbohydrates, resulting in high-protein and low-carbohydrate diets. One study maintained a constant protein level (as percentage of energy), however, and varied carbohydrates with fat [111]. Measures of glycemic control and insulin dose were unchanged with the low-carbohydrate diet, indicating that protein is the responsible beneficial nutrient in type II diabetics. This hypothesis is further supported by evidence that inadequate dietary protein has a negative impact on insulin secretion and insulin activity [112].

These findings suggest that diets high in protein may be beneficial in patients with disturbed glucose metabolism. In human patients with insulin-dependent type I diabetes, however, increased protein intake was associated with an increased glucose response and increased exogenous insulin requirement [113,114]. This may reflect a difference between type I and type II diabetes. Conversely, protein requirements seem to be increased in type I diabetes due to increased protein catabolism.

Not only is insulin necessary for the efficient cellular uptake of glucose, but it is required for fat and protein metabolism as well. Insulin inhibits catabolism of proteins and gluconeogenesis from amino acids and promotes the uptake of amino acids and synthesis of new proteins. Abnormalities in serum insulin concentrations result in disruptions in protein metabolism. Glucagon, which is increased when insulin levels fall, decreases cellular protein synthesis and increases protein catabolism and gluconeogenesis. Even in well-controlled diabetics, protein catabolism seems to occur at significantly higher rates, leading to protein loss [115]. To avoid depletion of LBM and protein reserves from increased skeletal muscle catabolism, it is important to ensure adequate protein intake in diabetic patients.

Osteoarthritis

OA, also called degenerative joint disease, is the most prevalent joint disorder in dogs, affecting as many as 20% of adult dogs [116]. OA is associated with inflammation and increased degradation or loss of proteoglycans from the extracellular matrix, resulting in a morphologic breakdown in articular cartilage [117]. Obesity is recognized as a risk factor for OA, and preventing obesity can help to reduce the incidence and severity of OA [45,118,119]. In a recently completed 14-year study on food restriction in dogs, those dogs fed to maintain a lean body condition throughout their lifetime exhibited a delayed need for treatment and reduced severity of OA in the hips and other joints compared with their heavier siblings [45]. One of the most compelling findings from this study was the observation that even a mild degree of excess body weight can adversely affect joint health. This is important, because more than 25% of dogs seen by veterinarians are overweight or obese [1].

The effect of obesity on OA may be more than just physical strain caused by weight bearing. Obesity is now recognized as an inflammatory condition; adipose tissue or associated macrophages produce inflammatory cytokines [47–49]. C-reactive protein, TNFα, IL-6, and other inflammatory mediators are elevated in the blood and adipose tissue of obese subjects and are thought to contribute to many complications associated with obesity, such as OA [47–50,120]. Obesity is also associated with an increase in oxidative stress, [52,53] another feature of OA.

Multiple studies have shown that weight loss helps to decrease lameness and pain and to increase joint mobility in patients with OA [118,121,122]. Overweight dogs with coxofemoral joint OA demonstrated decreased lameness and increased activity after weight reduction to ideal body condition.

A primary target of OA treatment is the inhibition of cyclooxygenase (COX) enzymes—especially the COX-2 enzyme—through the use of nonsteroidal anti-inflammatory drugs (NSAIDs) [123,124]. COX-2–selective inhibitors can decrease prostaglandin E_2 (PGE$_2$) concentrations and block inflammatory pathways involved in OA as well as reduce pain and lameness [123–126]. Blocking the COX and lipo-oxygenase (LOX) enzymes at the active sites of 5-LOX, COX-1, and COX-2 significantly reduces matrix metalloproteinases (MMPs), IL-1β, leukotriene (LT) B_4, and PGE$_2$, resulting in decreased tissue damage in arthritic joints [127].

Another means of reducing PGE$_2$ and other inflammatory eicosanoids is through the use of dietary long-chain omega-3 (n-3) polyunsaturated fatty acids, especially eicosapentaenoic acid. The primary omega-6 (n-6) fatty acid in cell membranes is arachidonic acid, which serves as the precursor for the production of the potent inflammatory eicosanoids in OA: PGE$_2$, thromboxane (TX) A_2, and LTB$_4$. If the diet is enriched with long-chain n-3 polyunsaturated fatty acids—specifically eicosapentaenoic acid and docosahexaenoic acid—part of the arachidonic acid in cell membranes is replaced by these n-3 fatty acids [128–130]. Eicosapentaenoic acid may then be used instead of arachidonic acid for the production of eicosanoids, resulting in a different and less inflammatory set of compounds (eg, PGE$_3$, TXA$_3$, and LTB$_5$ instead of PGE$_2$, TXA$_2$, and LTB$_4$) [128,129]. Dietary n-3 polyunsaturated fatty acids also suppress the proinflammatory mediators IL-1, IL-2, and TNF in cartilage tissue [131,132]. Thus, substituting n-3 for part of the n-6 fatty acids should reduce inflammation and benefit inflammatory conditions, including OA.

A review of studies in arthritic people indicated that most showed positive results from long-chain n-3 polyunsaturated fatty acid supplementation [133]. Recent research in dogs supports many of these earlier findings confirming the clinical benefits of dietary n-3 fatty acids in OA. Twenty-two dogs with OA of the hip were given a fatty acid supplement marketed for dogs with inflammatory skin conditions [134]. Thirteen of these dogs had noticeable improvement in their arthritic signs within 2 weeks. Another uncontrolled study evaluated dogs with naturally occurring OA of the elbow and used force-plate analysis before and after dogs were fed a diet enriched with n-3 polyunsaturated fatty acids. Improvements in vertical peak force were observed within 7 to 10 days on the diet (S.C. Budsberg, DVM, unpublished data, 2004). In yet another study, dogs fed a diet enriched with n-3 polyunsaturated fatty acids after corrective surgery for ruptured cruciate ligaments showed a significant decrease in synovial fluid PGE_2 [135]. Synovial fluid MMP-2 and MMP-9, enzymes that degrade structural proteins in cartilage, were also decreased in these dogs compared with dogs fed the control diet.

Glucosamine, an endogenously produced aminosugar, is another compound that may be beneficial in dogs with OA. A decrease in glucosamine synthesis by chondrocytes has been implicated in OA, whereas supplemental glucosamine has a stimulatory effect on chondrocytes [136]. Glucosamine is considered a chondroprotective agent and may minimize the progression of OA [136,137].

Several short- and long-term, double-blind, randomized trials evaluating glucosamine supplementation in people with OA of the knee were recently reviewed by meta-analysis [137]. These studies documented significant improvement in clinical signs of OA in patients consuming glucosamine at a dose of 1500 mg/d (approximately 21 mg/kg of ideal body weight). Two of these studies followed patients for 3 years and demonstrated that oral glucosamine inhibited the long-term progression of OA [137]. Clinical studies in dogs involving glucosamine alone are lacking.

Chondroitin sulfate, an endogenously produced polysaccharide found in the joint cartilage matrix, also has been shown to be beneficial in osteoarthritis. A number of placebo-controlled clinical trials in humans have shown a protective action of chondroitin sulfate against cartilage deterioration or a decrease in pain with supplementation [138–142].

Combinations of chondroitin sulfate and glucosamine also have been evaluated. In vitro research using bovine cartilage demonstrated a synergistic effect on glycosaminoglycan synthesis from a combination of glucosamine hydrochloride, manganese ascorbate, and chondroitin sulfate [143]. Synergistic effects also were noted for this combination in an in vivo rabbit model of arthritis [143]. Canine studies using a combination of glucosamine and chondroitin sulfate reported a benefit similar to that seen in other species [136,144].

OA is associated with an increase in oxidative stress and chondrocyte-produced reactive oxygen species and a reduction in antioxidant capacity [145–151]. The severity of arthritic lesions is increased in the face of decreased antioxidant capacity [148].

In vitro studies have shown that exposure of chondrocytes to reactive oxygen species inhibits proteoglycan and DNA synthesis and depletes intracellular ATP [149,150]. Reactive oxygen species contribute to cartilage degradation directly as well as by upregulating the genetic expression of MMPs and decreasing the production (or activity) of tissue inhibitors of MMPs [149,151]. In addition, oxidative stress induced chondrocyte senescence in vitro, with reduced glycosaminoglycan production and replicative lifespan—an effect that was reversible with antioxidant supplementation [148,152]. Physiologic concentrations of vitamin E inhibited lipid peroxidation in chondrocytes and minimized oxidation-induced cartilage degradation in vitro [151]. In a different model, vitamin C was effective at reducing premature chondrocyte senescence induced by reactive oxygen species [151].

Although limited in number, the published studies assessing in vivo benefits of antioxidants in OA support the in vitro findings. A 10-year prospective cohort study showed that intake of supplemental vitamin E ($P = 0.06$), vitamin C ($P = 0.08$), and zinc ($P = 0.03$) independently reduced the risk for developing rheumatoid arthritis in elderly women [153]. A 2-year clinical trial in people with existing knee OA evaluated the benefit of vitamin E supplementation on cartilage degradation [154]. No statistically significant differences were observed in cartilage loss, most likely because of the small sample size. Researchers detected directional differences, with cartilage loss reduced in the vitamin E group compared with the placebo group, however. A 1-year study in mice genetically predisposed to developing OA also showed a benefit from dietary antioxidants [155]. Glutathione peroxidase activity was significantly increased in the serum and synovium of mice fed a complete diet supplemented with pyridoxine; riboflavin; selenium; and vitamins E, C, and A, confirming an antioxidant effect. The incidence of OA in the antioxidant-supplemented mice was decreased by one third to one half [155]. Together, these various studies strongly suggest a benefit of dietary antioxidants for patients with OA.

In addition to nutrient modifications that may help in the dietary management of dogs with OA directly, dogs need appropriately balanced nutrition to support normal maintenance of joints and other tissues. Many people with OA seem to consume nutritionally imbalanced diets. Deficiencies in antioxidant nutrients, B vitamins, zinc, calcium, magnesium, and selenium are frequently reported [156,157]. Although it is not known how many of these deficiencies contribute to OA, these nutrients play a role in the normal maintenance of cartilage and other tissues. Therefore, it is important that dogs with OA receive diets that provide complete and balanced nutrition.

Summary

Before recommending a diet for a senior pet, a thorough nutritional evaluation should be completed. Although many middle-aged and older pets are overweight, a large percentage of geriatric cats and dogs have a low BCS. Approximately one third of cats older than 12 years of age may have a decreased ability to digest fat, whereas one in five may have a compromised ability to digest protein. Thus, appropriate diets for these two age groups may differ considerably. Mature (middle-aged) cats would likely benefit from a lower calorie food, whereas geriatric cats ($\geq$12 years of age) may need a highly digestible nutrient-dense diet.

More than 40% of dogs between the ages of 5 and 10 years are overweight or obese. Such dogs may benefit from diets with lower fat and calories. Senior dogs also have an increased need for dietary protein, however. Therefore, healthy older dogs may benefit from diets with an increased protein-to-calorie ratio, providing a minimum of 25% of calories from protein.

Common obesity-related conditions in dogs or cats include DM and OA. Diabetes differs between dogs and cats. Type I diabetes, common in dogs, seems to respond to fiber-enriched diets, whereas type II diabetes, common in cats, seems to benefit from high-protein and low-carbohydrate diets. OA, an inflammatory condition that occurs in approximately 20% of dogs, may benefit from weight management and nutrients that reduce the inflammatory responses, such as long-chain n-3 fatty acids.

References

[1] Lund EM, Armstrong PJ, Kirk CA, et al. Health status and population characteristics of dogs and cats examined at private veterinary practices in the United States. J Am Vet Med Assoc 1999;214:1336–41.
[2] Stratton-Phelps M. AAFP and AFM panel report of feline senior health care. Compend Contin Educ Pract Vet 1999;21:531–9.
[3] Kraft W. Geriatrics in canine and feline internal medicine. Eur J Med Res 1998;3: 31–41.
[4] Harper EJ. Changing perspectives on aging and energy requirements: aging and energy intakes in humans, dogs and cats. J Nutr 1998;128(Suppl):2623S–6S.
[5] Laflamme DP, Martineau B, Jones W, et al. Effect of age on maintenance energy requirements and apparent digestibility of canine diets [abstract]. Compend Contin Educ Pract Vet 2000;22(Suppl 9A):113.
[6] Kienzle E, Rainbird A. Maintenance energy requirement of dogs: what is the correct value for the calculation of metabolic body weight in dogs? J Nutr 1991;121(Suppl): S39–40.
[7] Laflamme DP, Ballam JM. Effect of age on maintenance energy requirements of adult cats. Compend Contin Edu Pract Vet 2002;24(Suppl 9A):82.
[8] Cupp C, Perez-Camargo G, Patil A, et al. Long-term food consumption and body weight changes in a controlled population of geriatric cats [abstract]. Compend Contin Educ Pract Vet 2004;26(Suppl 2A):60.
[9] Elia M. The inter-organ flux of substrates in fed and fasted man, an indicated by arterio-venous balance studies. Nutr Res Rev 1991;4:3–31.
[10] Kealy RD. Factors influencing lean body mass in aging dogs. Compend Contin Educ Pract Vet 1999;21(Suppl 11K):34–7.

[11] Perez-Camargo G. Cat nutrition: what's new in the old? Compend Contin Educ Pract Vet 2004;26(Suppl 2A):5–10.

[12] Armstrong PJ, Lund EM. Changes in body composition and energy balance with aging. Vet Clin Nutr 1996;3:83–7.

[13] Waldron MK. Influence of age on apparent digestive function and energy intake in cats [abstract]. Compend Contin Educ Pract Vet 2002;24(Suppl 9A):83.

[14] Finco DR. Effects of dietary protein and phosphorus on the kidney of dogs. In: Proceedings of the Waltham/OSU Symposium. Vernon, CA: Kal Kan Foods, Inc.; 1992. p. 39–41.

[15] Finco DR, Brown SA, Crowell WA, et al. Effects of aging and dietary protein intake on uninephrectomized geriatric dogs. Am J Vet Res 1994;55:1282–90.

[16] Finco DR. Effects of dietary protein intake on renal functions. Vet Forum 1999;16: 34–44.

[17] Bovee KC. Mythology of protein restriction for dogs with reduced renal function. Compend Contin Educ Pract Vet 1999;21(11 Suppl):15–20.

[18] Wannemacher RW, McCoy JR. Determination of optimal dietary protein requirements of young and old dogs. J Nutr 1966;88:66–74.

[19] Richardson A, Birchenall-Sparks MC. Age-related changes in protein synthesis. Rev Biol Res Aging 1983;1:255–73.

[20] McMurray DN. Effect of moderate protein deficiency on immune function. Compend Contin Educ Pract Vet 1999;21(11K):21–4.

[21] Yoshino K, Sakai K, Okada H, et al. IgE responses in mice fed moderate protein deficient and high protein diets. J Nutr Sci Vitaminol 2003;49:172–8.

[22] Williams CC, Cummins KA, Hayek MG, et al. Effects of dietary protein on whole-body protein turnover and endocrine function in young-adult and aging dogs. J Anim Sci 2001; 79:3128–36.

[23] Hannah SS, Laflamme DP. Effect of dietary protein on nitrogen balance and lean body mass in cats [abstract]. Vet Clin Nutr 1996;3:30.

[24] Perez-Camargo G, Young L. Nutrient digestibility in old versus young cats. Compend Cont Educ Pract Vet 2005, in press.

[25] Williams DA, Steiner JM, Ruaux CG. Older cats with gastrointestinal disease are more likely to be cobalamin deficient [abstract]. Compend Contin Educ Pract Vet 2004; 26(Suppl 2A):62.

[26] Packer L, Landvik S. Vitamin E: introduction to biochemistry and health benefits. Ann NY Acad Sci 1989;570:1–6.

[27] Harman D. Role of free radicals in aging and disease. Ann NY Acad Sci 1992;673:126–41.

[28] Jacob RA, Burri BJ. Oxidative damage and defense. Am J Clin Nutr 1996;63(Suppl): 985S–90S.

[29] Tiku ML, Shah R, Allison GT. Evidence linking chondrocyte lipid peroxidation to cartilage matrix protein degradation. J Biol Chem 2000;275:20069–76.

[30] Gare M, Mraovic B, Kehl F, et al. Reactive oxygen species contribute to contractile dysfunction following rapid ventricular pacing in dogs. Int J Cardiol 2002;83:125–31.

[31] Sato R, Inanami O, Syuto B, et al. The plasma superoxide scavenging activity in canine cancer and hepatic disease. J Vet Med Sci 2003;65:465–9.

[32] Skoumalova A, Rofina J, Schwippelova Z, et al. The role of free radicals in canine counterpart of senile dementia of the Alzheimer type. Exp Gerontol 2003;38:711–9.

[33] Wu G, Fang YZ, Yang S, et al. Glutathione metabolism and its implications for health. J Nutr 2004;134:489–92.

[34] Langweiler M, Schultz RD, Sheffy BE. Effect of vitamin E deficiency on the proliferative response of canine lymphocytes. Am J Vet Res 1981;42:1681–5.

[35] Tengerdy RP. Vitamin E, immune response, and disease resistance. Ann NY Acad Sci 1989; 570:335–44.

[36] De la Fuente M. Effects of antioxidants on immune system aging. Eur J Clin Nutr 2002; 56(Suppl 3):S5–8.

[37] Fettman MJ, Valerius KD, Ogilvie GK, et al. Effects of dietary cysteine on blood sulfur amino acid, glutathione, and malondialdehyde concentrations in cats. Am J Vet Res 1999; 60:328–33.

[38] Hill AS, Christopher MM, O'Neill S, et al. Antioxidant prevention and treatment of Heinz body formation and oxidative injury in cats [abstract]. Compend Contin Educ Pract Vet 2000;22(9A):90.

[39] Heaton PR, Reed CF, Mann SJ, et al. Role of dietary antioxidants to protect against DNA damage in adult dogs. J Nutr 2002;132(Suppl):1720S–4S.

[40] Wedekind KJ, Zicker S, Lowry S, et al. Antioxidant status of adult beagles is affected by dietary antioxidant intake. J Nutr 2002;132(Suppl):1658S–60S.

[41] Massimino S, Kearns RJ, Loos KM, et al. Effects of age and dietary beta-carotene on immunological variables in dogs. J Vet Intern Med 2003;17:835–42.

[42] Macy DW, Ralston SL. Cause and control of decreased appetite. In: Kirk RW, editor. Current veterinary therapy X. Philadelphia: WB Saunders; 1989. p. 18–24.

[43] Rangel-Captillo A, Avendano-Carrillo H, Reyes-Delgado F, et al. Immediate appetite stimulation of anorexic cats with midazolam [abstract]. Compend Contin Educ Pract Vet 2004;26(Suppl 2A):61.

[44] Avendano-Carrillo H, Rangel-Captillo A, Reyes-Delgado F, et al. Immediate appetite stimulation of anorexic dogs with propofol [abstract]. Compend Contin Educ Pract Vet 2004;26(Suppl 2A):64.

[45] Kealy RD, Lawler DF, Ballam JM, et al. Effects of diet restriction on life span and age-related changes in dogs. J Am Vet Med Assoc 2002;220:1315–20.

[46] Scarlett JM, Donoghue S. Associations between body condition and disease in cats. J Am Vet Med Assoc 1998;212:1725–31.

[47] Miller D, Bartges J, Cornelius L, et al. Tumor necrosis factor-α levels in adipose tissue of lean and obese cats. J Nutr 1998;128(Suppl):2751S–2S.

[48] Coppack SW. Pro-inflammatory cytokines and adipose tissue. Proc Nutr Soc 2001;60: 349–56.

[49] Nicklas BJ, Ambrosius W, Messier SP, et al. Diet-induced weight loss, exercise, and chronic inflammation in older, obese adults: a randomized controlled clinical trial. Am J Clin Nutr 2004;79:544–51.

[50] Gayet C, Bailhache E, Dumon H, et al. Insulin resistance and changes in plasma concentration of TNFα, IGF1, and NEFA in dogs during weight gain and obesity. J Anim Physiol Anim Nutr 2004;88:157–65.

[51] Sowers M, Jannausch M, Stein E, et al. C-reactive protein as a biomarker of emergent osteoarthritis. Osteoarthritis Cartilage 2002;10:595–601.

[52] Urakawa H, Katsuki A, Sumida Y, et al. Oxidative stress is associated with adiposity and insulin resistance in men. J Clin Endocrinol Metab 2003;88(10):4673–6.

[53] Sonta T, Inoguchi T, Tsubouchi H, et al. Evidence for contribution of vascular NAD(P)H oxidase to increased oxidative stress in animal models of diabetes and obesity. Free Radic Biol Med 2004;37:115–23.

[54] Root MV. Early spay-neuter in the cat: effect on development of obesity and metabolic rate. Vet Clin Nutr 1995;2:132–4.

[55] Fettman MJ, Stanton CA, Banks LL, et al. Effects of neutering on bodyweight, metabolic rate and glucose tolerance of domestic cats. Res Vet Sci 1997;62:131–6.

[56] Jeusette I, Detilleux J, Cuvelier C, et al. Ad libitum feeding following ovariectomy in female Beagle dogs: effect on maintenance energy requirement and on blood metabolites. J Anim Physiol Anim Nutr 2004;88:117–21.

[57] Harper EJ, Stack DM, Watson TDG, et al. Effects of feeding regimens on bodyweight, composition and condition score in cats following ovariohysterectomy. J Small Anim Pract 2001;42:433–8.

[58] Laflamme DP. Development and validation of a body condition score system for cats: a clinical tool. Feline Pract 1997;25:13–8.

[59] Laflamme DP. Development and validation of a body condition score system for dogs: a clinical tool. Canine Pract 1997;22:10–5.

[60] Mawby DI, Bartges JW, d'Avignon A, et al. Comparison of various methods for estimating body fat in dogs. J Am Anim Hosp Assoc 2004;40:109–14.

[61] Hays NP, Starling RD, Liu X, et al. Effects of an ad libitum low-fat, high-carbohydrate diet on body weight, body composition and fat distribution in older men and women: a randomized, controlled trial. Arch Intern Med 2004;164:210–7.

[62] Borne AT, Wolfsheimer KJ, Truett AA, et al. Differential metabolic effects of energy restriction in dogs using diets varying in fat and fiber content. Obes Res 1996;4: 337–45.

[63] Volek JS, Westman EC. Very-low-carbohydrate weight-loss diets revisited. Cleveland Clin J Med 2002;69:849–62.

[64] Foster GD, Wyatt HR, Hill JO, et al. A randomized trial of a low-carbohydrate diet for obesity. N Engl J Med 2003;348:2082–90.

[65] Samaha FF, Iqbal N, Seshadri P, et al. A low-carbohydrate as compared with a low-fat diet in severe obesity. N Engl J Med 2003;348:2074–81.

[66] Hannah SS, Laflamme DP. Increased dietary protein spares lean body mass during weight loss in dogs [abstract]. J Vet Intern Med 1998;12:224.

[67] Laflamme DP, Hannah SS. Effect of dietary protein on composition of weight loss in cats [abstract]. In: Proceedings of the British Small Animal Veterinary Association. Birmingham, England; 1998. p. 277.

[68] Skov AR, Toubro S, Ronn B, et al. Randomized trial on protein vs carbohydrate in ad libitum fat reduced diet for the treatment of obesity. Int J Obes 1999;23:528–36.

[69] Farnsworth E, Luscombe ND, Noakes M, et al. Effect of a high-protein, energy-restricted diet on body composition, glycemic control, and lipid concentrations in overweight and obese hyperinsulinemic men and women. Am J Clin Nutr 2003;78:31–9.

[70] Layman DK, Boileau RA, Erickson DJ, et al. A reduced ratio of dietary carbohydrate to protein improves body composition and blood lipid profiles during weight loss in adult women. J Nutr 2003;133:411–7.

[71] Johnston CS, Tjonn SL, Swan PD. High-protein, low-fat diets are effective for weight loss and favorably alter biomarkers in healthy adults. J Nutr 2004;134:586–91.

[72] Karst H, Steiniger J, Noack R, et al. Diet-induced thermogenesis in man: thermic effects of single proteins, carbohydrates and fats depending on their energy amount. Ann Nutr Metab 1984;28:245–52.

[73] Crovetti R, Porrini M, Santangelo A, Testolin G. The influence of thermic effect of food on satiety. Eur J Clin Nutr 1997;52:482–8.

[74] Westerterp-Plantenga MS. The significance of protein in food intake and body weight. Curr Opin Clin Nutr Metab Care 2003;6:635–8.

[75] Westerterp-Plantenga MS, Lejeune MP, Nijs I, et al. High protein intake sustains weight maintenance after body weight loss in humans. Int J Obes 2004;28:57–64.

[76] Armstrong PJ, Hardie EM, Cullen JM, et al. l-carnitine reduced hepatic fat accumulation during rapid weight loss in cats. J Vet Int Med 1992;6:127.

[77] Feng Y, Guo C, Wei J, et al. Necessity of carnitine supplementation in semistarved rats fed a high-fat diet. Nutrition 2001;17:628–31.

[78] Davis AT, Davis PG, Phinney SD. Plasma and urinary carnitine of obese subjects on very-low-calorie diets. J Am Coll Nutr 1990;9:261–4.

[79] Dyck DJ. Dietary fat intake, supplements and weight loss. Can J Appl Physiol 2000;25: 495–523.

[80] Villani RG, Gannon J, Self M, et al. l-carnitine supplementation combined with aerobic training does not promote weight loss in moderately obese women. Int J Sport Nutr Exerc Metab 2000;10:199–207.

[81] Brandsch C, Eder K. Effect of l-carnitine on weight loss and body composition of rats fed a hypocaloric diet. Ann Nutr Metab 2002;46:205–10.

[82] Aoki MS, Almeida ALR, Navarro F, et al. Carnitine supplementation fails to maximize fat mass loss induced by endurance training in rats. Ann Nutr Metab 2004;48:90–4.

[83] Gross KL, Wedekind KJ, Kirk CA, et al. Effect of dietary carnitine or chromium on weight loss and body composition of obese dogs [abstract]. J Anim Sci 1998;76(Suppl 1):175.

[84] Sunvold GD, Vickers RJ, Kelley RL, et al. Effect of dietary carnitine during energy restriction in the canine [abstract 226.2]. FASEB J 1999;13:A268.

[85] Center SA, Harte J, Watrous D, et al. The clinical and metabolic effects of rapid weight loss in obese pet cats and the influence of supplemental oral L-carnitine. J Vet Intern Med 2000; 14:598–608.

[86] Laflamme DP, Kuhlman G. The effect of weight loss regimen on subsequent weight maintenance in dogs. Nutr Res 1995;15:1019–28.

[87] Panciera DL, Thomas CB, Eicker SW, et al. Epizootiologic patterns of diabetes mellitus in cats: 333 cases (1980 – 1986). J Am Vet Med Assoc 1990;197:1504–8.

[88] Prahl A, Glickman L, Guptill L, et al. Time trends and risk factors for diabetes mellitus in cats [abstract]. J Vet Intern Med 2003;17.434.

[89] Nelson RW, Himsel CA, Feldman ED, et al. Glucose tolerance and insulin response in normal-weight and obese cats. Am J Vet Res 1990;51:1357–62.

[90] Appleton DJ, Rand JS, Sunvold GD. Insulin sensitivity decreases with obesity, and lean cats with low insulin sensitivity are at greatest risk of glucose intolerance with weight gain. J Feline Med Surg 2001;3:211–28.

[91] Mingrone G, Rosa G, DiRocco R, et al. Skeletal muscle triglycerides lowering is associated with net improvement of insulin sensitivity, TNF-α reduction and GLUT4 expression enhancement. Int J Obes 2002;26:1165–72.

[92] Brennan CL, Hoenig M, Ferguson DC. GLUT4 but not GLUT1 expression decreases early in the development of feline obesity. Domest Anim Endocrinol 2004;26:291–301.

[93] Rand JS, Farrow HA, Fleeman LM, et al. Diet in the prevention of diabetes and obesity in companion animals [abstract]. Asia Pac J Clin Nutr 2004;12:S6.

[94] Hoenig M. Comparative aspects of diabetes mellitus in dogs and cats. Mol Cell Endocrinol 2002;197:221–9.

[95] Rand JS, Appleton DJ, Fleeman LM, et al. The link between obesity and diabetes in cats and dogs. In: Proceedings of the North American Veterinary Conference, Orlando, FL, 2003. p. 292–3.

[96] Nelson RW. Dietary management of diabetes mellitus. J Small Anim Pract 1992;33:213–7.

[97] Blaxter AC, Cripps PJ, Gruffydd-Jones TJ. Dietary fiber and postprandial hyperglycemia in normal and diabetic dogs. J Small Anim Pract 1990;31:229–33.

[98] Nelson RW, Ihle SL, Lewis LD, et al. Effects of dietary fiber supplementation on glycemic control in dogs with alloxan-induced diabetes mellitus. Am J Vet Res 1991;52:2060–6.

[99] Graham PA, Maskell IE, Rawlings JM, et al. Influence of a high fiber diet on glycemic control and quality of life in dogs with diabetes mellitus. J Small Anim Nutr 2002;43:67–73.

[100] Hagander B, Asp NG, Efendic S, et al. Dietary fiber decreases fasting blood glucose levels and plasma LDL concentration in noninsulin-dependent diabetes mellitus patients. Am J Clin Nutr 1988;47:852–8.

[101] Nelson RW. The role of fiber in managing diabetes mellitus. Vet Med 1989;84:1156–60.

[102] Kimmel SE, Michel KE, Hess RS, et al. Effects of insoluble and soluble dietary fiber on glycemic control in dogs with naturally occurring insulin-dependent diabetes mellitus. J Am Vet Med Assoc 2000;216:1076–81.

[103] Fleeman LM, Rand JS, Markwell PJ. Diets with high fiber and moderate starch are not advantageous for dogs with stabilized diabetes compared to a commercial diet with moderate fiber and low starch. J Vet Intern Med 2003;17:433.

[104] Nelson RW, Scott-Moncrieff JC, Feldman EC, et al. Effect of dietary insoluble fiber on control of glycemia in cats with naturally acquired diabetes mellitus. J Am Vet Med Assoc 2000;216:1082–8.

[105] Frank G, Anderson WH, Pazak HE, et al. Use of a high protein diet in the management of feline diabetes mellitus. Vet Ther 2001;2:238–46.

[106] Bennett N, Greco DS, Peterson ME. Comparison of a low carbohydrate diet versus high fiber diet in cats with diabetes mellitus [abstract]. J Vet Intern Med 2001;15:297.

[107] Conn JW, Newburgh LH. The glycemic response to isoglucogenic quantities of protein and carbohydrate. J Clin Invest 1936;15:665–71.

[108] Gutierrez M, Akhavan M, Jovanovic L, et al. Utility of a short-term 25% carbohydrate diet on improving glycemic control in type 2 diabetes mellitus. J Am Coll Nutr 1998;17: 595–600.

[109] Gannon MC, Nuttall FQ, Saeed A, et al. An increase in dietary protein improves the blood glucose response in persons with Type 2 diabetes. Am J Clin Nutr 2003;78:734–41.

[110] Mazzaferro EM, Greco DS, Turner SJ, et al. Treatment of feline diabetes mellitus using an alpha-glucosidase inhibitor and a low-carbohydrate diet. J Feline Med Surg 2003;5: 183–9.

[111] Hollenbeck CG, Riddle MC, Connor WE, et al. The effects of subject-selected high carbohydrate, low fat diets on glycemic control in insulin dependent diabetes mellitus. Am J Clin Nutr 1985;41:293–8.

[112] Holness MJ. The impact of dietary protein restriction on insulin secretion and action. Proc Nutr Soc 1999;58:647–53.

[113] Linn T, Geyer R, Prassek S, et al. Effect of dietary protein intake on insulin secretion and glucose metabolism in insulin-dependent diabetes mellitus. J Clin Endrocrinol Metab 1996; 81:3938–43.

[114] Peters AL, Davidson MB. Protein and fat effects on glucose responses and insulin requirements in subjects with insulin-dependent diabetes mellitus. Am J Clin Nutr 1993;58: 555–60.

[115] Freyse EJ, Rebrin K, Schneider T, et al. Increased urea synthesis in insulin-dependent diabetic dogs maintained normoglycemic: effect of portal insulin administration and food protein content. Diabetes 1996;45:667–74.

[116] Roush JK, McLaughlin RM, Radlinsky MA. Understanding the pathophysiology of osteoarthritis. Vet Med 2002;97:108–12.

[117] Johnston SA. Osteoarthritis. Joint anatomy, physiology and pathobiology. Vet Clin N Am Small Anim Pract 1997;27(4):699–723.

[118] Foye PM, Stitik TP, Chen B, et al. Osteoarthritis and body weight. Nutr Res 2000;20: 899–903.

[119] Andersen RE, Crespo CJ, Bartlett SJ, et al. Relationship between body weight gain and significant knee, hip and back pain in older Americans. Obes Res 2003;11:1159–62.

[120] Sowers M, Jannausch M, Stein E, et al. C-reactive protein as a biomarker of emergent osteoarthritis. Osteoarthritis Cartilage 2002;10:595–601.

[121] Burkholder WJ, Taylor L, Hulse DA. Weight loss to optimal body condition increases ground reactive force in dogs with osteoarthritis [abstract]. Compend Contin Educ Pract Vet 2001;23:74.

[122] Impellizeri JA, Tetrick MA, Muir P. Effect of weight reduction on clinical signs of lameness in dogs with hip osteoarthritis. J Am Vet Med Assoc 2000;216:1089–91.

[123] Dvorak LD, Cook JL, Kreeger JM, et al. Effects of carprofen and dexamethasone on canine chondrocytes in a three-dimensional culture model of osteoarthritis. Am J Vet Res 2002;63: 1363–9.

[124] Millis DL, Weigel JP, Moyers T, et al. The effect of deracoxib, a new COX-2 inhibitor, on the prevention of lameness induced by chemical synovitis in dogs. Vet Ther 2002;3:7–18.

[125] Dionne RA, Khan AA, Gordon SM. Analgesia and COX-2 inhibition. Clin Exp Rheumatol 2001;19(Suppl 25):S63–70.

[126] Holtzsinger RN, Parker RB, Beale BS, et al. The therapeutic effect of carprofen (Rimadyl) in 209 clinical cases of canine degenerative joint disease. Vet Comp Orthop Traumatol 1992; 5:140–4.

[127] Laufer S. Role of eicosanoids in structural degradation in osteoarthritis. Curr Opin Rheumatol 2003;15:623–7.

[128] Drevon CA. Marine oils and their effects. Nutr Rev 1992;50:38–45.

[129] Schoenherr WD, Jewell DE. Nutritional modulation of inflammatory diseases. Semin Vet Med Surg 1997;12:212–22.

[130] Waldron MK, Spencer AL, Hannah SS, et al. Plasma and neutrophil phospholipid n-3 fatty acid composition is independent of the n-6/n-3 fatty acid ratio [abstract]. Compend Contin Educ Pract Vet 2000;22(Suppl 9A):99.

[131] Curtis CL, Rees SG, Little CG, et al. Pathologic indicators of degradation and inflammation in human osteoarthritic cartilage are abrogated by exposure to n-3 fatty acids. Arthritis Rheum 2002;46:1544–53.

[132] Watkins BA, Li Y, Lippmann HE, et al. Omega-3 polyunsaturated fatty acids and skeletal health. Exp Biol Med 2001;226:485–97.

[133] Richardson DC, Schoenherr WD, Zicker SC. Nutritional management of osteoarthritis. Vet Clin N Am Small Anim Pract 1997;27:883–911.

[134] Miller WH, Scott DW, Wellington JR. Treatment of dogs with hip arthritis with a fatty acid supplement. Canine Pract 1992;17:6–8.

[135] Hansen RA, Waldron MK, Allen KGD, et al. Long chain n-3 PUFA improve biochemical parameters associated with canine osteoarthritis. In: Proceedings of the American Oil Chemists Society Meeting, Cincinnati, OH, May 9–12, 2004. Champagne (IL): American Oil Chemists Society.

[136] Anderson MA. Oral chondroprotective agents. Part I Common compounds. Compend Contin Educ Pract Vet 1999;21:601–9.

[137] Richy F, Bruyere O, Ethgen O, et al. Structural and symptomatic efficacy of glucosamine and chondroitin in knee osteoarthritis. Arch Intern Med 2003;163:1514–22.

[138] Morreale P, Manopulo R, Galati M, et al. Comparison of the anti-inflammatory efficacy of chondroitin sulfate and diclofenac sodium in patients with knee osteoarthritis. J Rheumatology 1996;23:1385–91.

[139] Bucsi L, Poor G. Efficacy and tolerability of oral chondroitin sulfate as a symptomatic slow-acting drug for osteoarthritis (SYSADOA) in the treatment of knee osteoarthritis. Osteoarthritis and Cartilage 1998;6(3):31–6.

[140] Uebelhart D, Eugene JM, Thonar A, et al. Effects of oral chondroitin sulfate on the progression of knee osteoarthritis: a pilot study. Osteoarthritis and Cartilage 1998;6(Suppl A):39–46.

[141] Michel B, Stucki G, Frey D, et al. Condroitins 4 and 6 sulphate in osteoarthritis of the knee: a randomized, controlled trial. Arthritis Rheum 2005;52:779–86.

[142] Verbruggen G, Goemaere S, Veys EM. Systems to assess the progression of finger joint osteoarthritis and the effects of disease modifying osteoarthritic drugs. Clin Rheumatol 2002;21(3):231–43.

[143] Lippiello L, Woodward J, Karpman R, et al. In vivo chondroprotection and metabolic synergy of glucosamine and chondroitin sulfate. Clin Orth Rel Res 2000; 381:229–40.

[144] Canapp SO, McLaughlin RM, Hoskinson JJ, et al. Scintigraphic evaluation of dogs with acute synovitis after treatment with glucosamine hydrochloride and chondroitin sulfate. Am J Vet Res 1999;60(12):1552–7.

[145] Chen JR, Takahashi M, Suzuki M, et al. Comparison of the concentrations of pentosidine in the synovial fluid, serum and urine of patients with rheumatoid arthritis and osteoarthritis. Rheumatology 1999;38:1275–8.

[146] Hay CW, Chu Q, Budsberg SC, et al. Synovial fluid interleukin 6, tumor necrosis factor, and nitric oxide values in dogs with osteoarthritis secondary to cranial cruciate ligament rupture. Am J Vet Res 1997;58:1027–32.

[147] Lunec J, Halloran SP, White AG, et al. Free-radical oxidation (peroxidation) products in serum and synovial fluid in rheumatoid arthritis. J Rheumatol 1981;8:233–45.

[148] Yudoh K, van Trieu N, Matsuno H, et al. Oxidative stress induces chondrocyte telomere instability and chondrocyte dysfunctions in osteoarthritis [abstract]. Arthritis Res Ther 2003;5(Suppl):164.

[149] Henrotin YE, Bruckner P, Pujol JPL. The role of reactive oxygen species in homeostasis and degradation of cartilage. Osteoarthritis Cartilage 2003;11:747–55.

[150] Johnson K, Svensson CL, Etten DV, et al. Mediation of spontaneous knee osteoarthritis by progressive chondrocyte ATP depletion in Hartley guinea pigs. Arthritis Rheum 2004;50: 1216–25.

[151] Tiku ML, Shah R, Allison GT. Evidence linking chondrocyte lipid peroxidation to cartilage matrix protein degradation. Possible role in cartilage aging and the pathogenesis of osteoarthritis. J Biol Chem 2000;275:20069–76.

[152] Martin JA, Klingelhutz AJ, Moussavi-Harami F, et al. Effects of oxidative damage and telomerase activity on human articular cartilage chondrocyte senescence. J Gerontol 2004; 59:324–36.

[153] Cerhan JR, Saag KG, Merlino LA, et al. Antioxidant micronutrients and risk of rheumatoid arthritis in a cohort of older women. Am J Epidemiol 2003;157:345–54.

[154] Wluka AE, Stuckey S, Brand C, et al. Supplementary vitamin E does not affect the loss of cartilage volume in knee osteoarthritis: a 2 year double blind randomized placebo controlled study. J Rheumatol 2002;29:2585–91.

[155] Kurz B, Jost B, Schanke M. Dietary vitamins and selenium diminish the development of mechanically induced osteoarthritis and increase the expression of antioxidative enzymes in the knee joint of STR/1N mice. Osteoarthritis Cartilage 2002;10:119–26.

[156] Kremer JM, Bigaouette J. Nutrient intake of patients with rheumatoid arthritis is deficient in pyridoxine, zinc, copper, and magnesium. J Rheumatol 1996;23(6):990–4.

[157] Stone J, Doube A, Dudson D, et al. Inadequate calcium, folic acid, vitamin E, zinc, and selenium intake in rheumatoid arthritis patients: results of a dietary survey. Semin Arthritis Rheum 1998;27:180–5.

ELSEVIER
SAUNDERS

Vet Clin Small Anim
35 (2005) 743–753

VETERINARY
CLINICS
Small Animal Practice

Senior and Geriatric Care Programs for Veterinarians

Fred L. Metzger, DVM

Metzger Animal Hospital, 1044 Benner Pike, State College, PA 16801, USA

Senior and geriatric veterinary medicine represents the basic mission of veterinarians and veterinary technicians—detecting diseases earlier so that intervention can help to improve the quality of life for older dogs, cats, and their owners. Complete diagnostic efforts are critical, because senior pets frequently have abnormalities in multiple body systems and frequently receive long-term medications for chronic diseases or conditions related to aging.

Owners are critical components of the successful senior program. Comprehensive histories are especially critical in senior medicine. Owners should be instructed to note changes in water consumption, decreased or increased appetite, alterations in body weight, decreased or increased activity level, the appearance or variations in skin masses, and, especially, modifications in behavior. Owners are in the unique position to note subtle changes in daily routines. Behavior changes should not be discounted as "senility" without our best diagnostic efforts.

Veterinarians and their hospital team are vital components and should be vocal advocates for older patients. Older patients should receive more frequent physical examinations (twice yearly or more frequently) depending on health status, current medication history, and preexisting health problems.

Routine monitoring of clinicopathologic data is a critical component in the management of older patients, because blood and urine testing allows the veterinarian to monitor trends in laboratory parameters that may be the earliest indicators of disease. For example, monitoring older patients for changes in blood urea nitrogen (BUN) and creatinine levels (ie, BUN and creatinine doubling from last year but within the normal reference range) may provide the earliest indicator of decreased renal function, because

E-mail address: FLMDVM@aol.com

doi:10.1016/j.cvsm.2004.12.005
vetsmall.theclinics.com

increases in these parameters may be significant even if these tests remain in the normal reference range [1].

Gaining owner compliance is often the most difficult component of veterinary medicine, and senior care is no different. Our practice earns compliance through a five-step process, which takes little time (usually 5 extra minutes) yet reaps rewards for the patient, the client, and the veterinary team. Finally, measuring compliance and rewarding your hospital staff are important components to any successful senior care program.

Defining the senior and geriatric pet

Clients and the entire veterinary staff must be aware of the practice's definition of the senior and geriatric pet for successful implementation of the program. Defining a senior or geriatric pet is somewhat arbitrary, because many factors influence aging, including genetics and nutrition as well as environmental factors like temperature, humidity, exposure to ultraviolet radiation, pollutants, and carcinogens. Economic factors, including the ability and willingness to seek quality veterinary care, also influence health and vary among patients and their owners.

The Metzger Animal Hospital age analogy chart (Fig. 1) is the critical education piece for our practice's entire senior and geriatric program because it defines the senior patient. The chart graphically educates clients by showing the pet's human age equivalent and then assigns a color code or risk to the pet. Clients can visually understand that senior pets are younger

AGE	Adult size in pounds			
	0-20	20-50	50-90	>90
6	40	42	45	49
7	44	47	50	56
8	48	51	55	64
9	52	56	61	71
10	56	60	66	78
11	60	65	72	86
12	64	69	77	93
13	68	74	82	101
14	72	78	88	108
15	76	83	93	115
16	80	87	99	123
17	84	92	104	
18	88	96	109	
19	92	101	115	
20	96	105	120	

SENIOR
GERIATRIC

Relative Age of Your Pet in Human Years

Fig. 1. Metzger Animal Hospital age analogy chart.

than geriatric pets; consequently, the chart recommends testing seniors and more vigorously advocates testing geriatrics. We also include a pet age calculator on our web site (http://www.metzgeranimal.com) under our Senior Care section. Clients can visit the calculator on-line to receive blood testing, nutritional, and vaccination recommendations specifically based on their pet's age. For example, according to Fig. 1 or the web site, an 80-lb Golden Retriever becomes a senior patient at 6 years of age and a geriatric patient at 10 years of age, thus emphasizing the distinction between senior and geriatric. This classification increases client discussions and, consequently, diagnostic opportunities, as owners become educated about senior and geriatric diseases and our early detection recommendations, including routine blood profiling on older healthy patients.

Physical, physiologic, metabolic, and immunologic effects of aging

Aging affects every body system. Owners may recognize many of the physical changes associated with aging, such as obesity, lameness, and skin changes. Skin becomes thickened, hyperpigmented, hyperkeratinized, and less elastic. Muscle, bone, and cartilage mass decreases. Dental tartar accumulates, calculus forms, and periodontal disease occurs, with resulting halitosis noticed by many owners [2]. The physical signs of aging are frequently less dramatic in senior cats, making diagnostic testing critical in older feline patients.

Physiologic effects of aging are medically important, and the urinary tract is an especially good example of the need for early diagnostic screening. Renal physiologic changes include decreased kidney weight, decreased glomerular filtration rate, and renal tubular atrophy. Fortunately for patients but unfortunately for diagnosticians, normal kidneys have huge functional reserves. For example, a healthy individual can relinquish an entire kidney, whether as a renal transplant donor or as a result of the kidney's destruction by disease, without notably altering ordinary indices of renal function. An additional perspective is gained by considering the amount of destruction and removal of renal tissue required to achieve "mild" azotemia (plasma creatinine concentrations of approximately 2–4 mg/dL) in initially healthy dogs (having plasma creatinine concentrations of approximately 1 mg/dL) so as to create the remnant kidney model of chronic kidney disease (CKD) in these animals [3]. To achieve this degree of azotemia after compensatory hypertrophy of the remaining renal tissue has occurred, investigators have to destroy 11/12 to 15/16 of one kidney and completely remove the other kidney [4]. From this perspective, one can appreciate that initial discovery of CKD that has already led to development of a plasma creatinine concentration on the order of 2 to 4 mg/dL despite compensatory changes, which can be presumed to have been exhausted during the course of a chronic disease process, does not constitute "early diagnosis" of renal disease. Indeed, this is a rather late stage in the course of any chronic progressive renal disease, leading to renal failure.

Hepatobiliary physiologic changes include decreased numbers of hepatocytes, increased hepatic fibrosis, and decreased detoxification capabilities. Cardiovascular physiologic changes include increased valvular fibrosis, resulting in valvular endocardiosis, and decreased cardiac output.

Aging results in a decrease in the basal metabolic rate. Older animals tend to have decreased activity levels, resulting in an increased body fat percentage. This is especially important, because increased body weight results in an increased incidence of diseases like diabetes; cardiovascular, respiratory, and orthopedic diseases; and, perhaps, neoplasia.

Immunologic effects include decreased phagocytic function and neutrophil chemotaxis, resulting in decreased immune competence despite normal numbers of lymphocytes. Aging is also associated with an increased incidence of immune-mediated diseases, such as immune-mediated hemolytic anemia and immune-mediated thrombocytopenia.

Pharmacologic effects of aging

Senior patients frequently require pharmacologic intervention for disease management. Aging affects the absorption, distribution, biotransformation, and elimination of most drugs; consequently, seniors have special pharmacologic concerns. [5]. Drug dosages may need to be adjusted for seniors, and many drugs should be avoided if organ function is compromised. Pharmaceutic agents biotransformed or eliminated by the liver and kidneys cause special concerns. Pharmaceutic agents with special concerns in geriatric patients include antibiotics, nonsteroidal anti-inflammatory drugs (NSAIDs), steroids, barbiturates, sedatives, analgesics, diuretics, angiotensin-converting enzyme (ACE) inhibitors, digitalis derivatives, chemotherapeutics, hormonal drugs, anesthetics, and many others [6]. Routine blood profiling increases the safety of drug administration by identifying underlying disease conditions that may preclude the use of certain pharmaceutic agents.

Senior diseases categorized by system

Diseases common to older pets are frequently the same diseases common to the pet's owners. Clients frequently recognize common senior diseases, such as diabetes, heart disease, hypothyroidism, and cancer. Educating clients about senior pet diseases also educates clients about diseases they might encounter themselves. In addition, elderly pet owners have many behaviors common to older dogs and cats, including more frequent doctor appointments; long-term medication administration, especially for degenerative joint disease and heart disease; and increased reliance on diagnostic testing to detect disease earlier.

Virtually every organ system is affected by aging and is prone to various disease processes. A brief review of several diseases by organ system is included for review.

The hepatobiliary system is especially susceptible to insult because of its position in relation to portal circulation and its important metabolic functions as well as detoxification, coagulation factor production, immune surveillance, and pharmaceutic biotransformation and elimination. Various diseases may affect the hepatobiliary tract, including inflammatory, infectious, metabolic, toxic, and neoplastic diseases among others. Several syndromes possible with liver disease include ascites, coagulopathy, icterus, hepatoencephalopathy, and cutaneous paraneoplastic syndrome [7].

Gastrointestinal diseases include dental and periodontal disease, inflammatory bowel disease, colitis and constipation, pancreatitis, exocrine pancreatic insufficiency, and, of course, neoplasia, especially lymphosarcoma.

Cardiovascular diseases are quite common in senior patients and include chronic mitral insufficiency, bacterial endocarditis, cardiomyopathy (especially hypertrophic cardiomyopathy in cats), pericardial effusion, cardiac arrhythmias, and cardiac neoplasia. Consequently, electrocardiography (ECG) and blood pressure measurements are important monitoring components of a complete senior program.

Urinary tract diseases include renal failure, renal cysts, pyelonephritis, renal tumors (carcinoma), prostatitis, prostatic tumors (adenocarcinoma), cystitis, incontinence, bladder tumors (transitional cell carcinoma), and urolithiasis. Chronic renal failure is an all too frequently diagnosed condition in seniors. Syndromes associated with chronic renal failure include anemia, hypertension, metabolic acidosis, hypokalemia, and hyperphosphatemia [8].

Endocrine diseases appear with greater frequently in senior pets and include diabetes mellitus (especially hyperosmolar nonketotic diabetes mellitus), hypothyroidism in dogs, hyperthyroidism in cats, insulinoma, and hyperadrenocorticism as well as occasional hypercalcemia, inborn errors of metabolism, and hypoadrenocorticism [9].

Comprehensive health screening is important in the early recognition and successful management of many of these diseases, and veterinarians should make diagnostic recommendations to owners when senior patients are encountered. Remember to institute a drug monitoring program when patients are receiving chronic or long-term medications, especially NSAIDs.

Defining the senior health program

Clients should become familiar with the definition of a senior or geriatric pet and understand the medical benefits of early disease detection. Recommend testing patients with the screening senior panel when they enter their senior years according to the age analogy chart (see Fig. 1). Many senior patients require anesthesia for dental or surgical procedures; this is an excellent time to recommend health profiling to improve anesthetic safety and establish baseline values. Explain in layman's terms the components of your program. Use analogies, because most clients are familiar with blood testing, urinalysis, ECG, and blood pressure testing through association with human medicine.

Senior screening panel

The minimum senior canine database, accessible to all practitioners, includes the complete blood cell count (CBC), biochemical profile with electrolytes, and complete urinalysis plus heartworm and tickborne disease testing in appropriate patients. The minimum senior feline database, accessible to all practitioners, includes the CBC, biochemical profile with electrolytes, complete urinalysis, total thyroxine (T_4), and feline leukemia virus (FeLV) and/or feline immunodeficiency virus (FIV) testing in appropriate patients [10].

Practices should include ECG, blood pressure measurement, and ocular tonometry screening if available. Fecal examination (by centrifugation), including *Giardia* antigen testing, should be considered in appropriate patients.

Specific senior panel

Primary senior profiling may reveal abnormalities that require further investigation. Laboratory tests, including renal testing (eg, urine protein/creatinine ratio, urine culture), thyroid confirmatory tests (eg, free T_4 by equilibrium dialysis, canine thyroid-stimulating hormone [TSH], thyroglobulin autoantibodies), adrenal profiling (eg, corticotropin stimulation, dexamethasone suppression, corticotropin assay, 17-hydroxyprogesterone analysis), hepatic function tests (eg, bile acids, ammonia tolerance), endocrine function tests (eg, serum fructosamine, glycosylated hemoglobin, insulin, ionized calcium, parathyroid hormone [PTH], PTH-like peptide), and blood gases among others. Other frequently performed senior procedures include imaging (eg, survey, contrast, and dental radiography; ultrasound; echocardiography; CT; MRI), cytology, histopathology, laparoscopy (especially hepatic biopsy), and endoscopy (eg, gastroduodenoscopy, colonoscopy, bronchoscopy).

Achieving client compliance: client materials

Yearly profiling should begin when the patient reaches the senior age threshold. Veterinarians may understand the recommendation, but how about our clients? Educational materials are critical if we expect clients to comply with our recommendations. Use questionnaires with specific senior questions to help clients tell you what is occurring at home. Report cards summarizing physical examination findings and our medical recommendations are helpful in increasing compliance. Define the senior pet by including age charts on your report card to help educate owners which pets are seniors. Specific brochures explaining the benefits, components, and costs of the senior program allow owners and other interested parties to continue the education process at home. A senior wall chart (a poster form of the age analogy chart) defines which pets are senior or geriatric, and thus educates owners who are waiting in the examination room. Metzger Animal Hospital uses a wall chart version of Fig. 1 in all examination rooms to emphasize the different recommendations based on the life stage of the patient. You can view the client education forms by visiting the web site (http://www. metzgeranimal.com) and accessing the Senior Care section.

Preanesthetic testing and drug monitoring screens set the table for senior profiling

Preanesthetic testing makes the transition to yearly blood profiling more logical as a patient ages. Baseline results obtained during preanesthetic testing for neutering, dental procedures, lumpectomies, or other anesthetic events provide valuable comparison data for interpretation later in life; in addition, owners become familiar with the procedure earlier in the pet's life, increasing compliance for future profiling.

Routine drug monitoring offers another avenue to senior testing. Many senior patients receive long-term medications and should routinely be monitored for changes in laboratory profiling. Senior patients routinely are prescribed NSAIDs, levothyroxine, methimazole, phenobarbital, potassium bromide, phenylpropanolamine, ACE inhibitors, insulin, nutraceuticals, chemotherapy drugs, glucocorticoids, and immunosuppressive medications; consequently, they should receive routine drug monitoring. Monitoring patients receiving long-term medication allows the veterinarian to monitor for drug side effects more closely and to detect coexisting diseases that may become evident. For example, feline hyperthyroid patients receiving methimazole should be closely monitored for renal disease, because treatment for hyperthyroidism may result in renal decompensation [11].

Achieving client compliance: use dentistry

Achieving increased client compliance can best be realistically accomplished by combining senior and geriatric blood profiling with ultrasonic dental scaling. Using the senior health profile as a preanesthetic test for dentistry procedures increases anesthetic safety and increases owner compliance by decreasing owner and veterinary anxiety. Most owners understand the need for dental scaling; however, owners of older pets may not comply with your recommendations because they fear anesthesia. A complete senior testing program helps to decrease anxiety by increasing safety, thus increasing the number of dental procedures and initiating the concept of yearly testing. Furthermore, most older patients require yearly dental scaling, setting the stage for yearly testing.

Annual reminder cards help to remind clients about vaccines, heartworm testing, and other recommended procedures—why not health screenings? Clients are familiar with reminder cards, so use them once the senior program has been initiated.

Use vaccines to increase compliance

Vaccinations are the number one reason why clients schedule appointments, and this holds true for senior pets. Vaccination guidelines are confusing and still being debated by academicians and practitioners. Vaccine titers seem to be an attractive alternative to annual vaccination; however, debate continues on the duration of immunity, assessment of humoral and cell-mediated immunity, core versus noncore vaccines, and what vaccines are appropriate for senior patients. Little debate exists when it comes to the medical benefits of using laboratory profiles with history and physical examinations to screen for hidden conditions. Why not use vaccines to increase senior compliance?

Metzger Animal Hospital offers a vaccine incentive toward the senior program when senior pets are presented for their annual examination, which usually includes vaccination. The vaccine incentive increases our compliance for several reasons. First, the client can apply the vaccine credit and save an amount proportionate to the vaccines that were recommended. Secondly and more importantly, our staff members recommend the program more vigorously because we believe the patient benefits more from senior screening than from vaccination. Furthermore, the price of the senior program is determined by the practice; consequently, the practice should determine a fair but profitable program price anticipating the vaccine credit.

Follow the Metzger Animal Hospital five-step program

As previously mentioned, preanesthetic testing, routine drug monitoring, and dental health help to build the foundation for senior testing, but how do your staff members actually present the program? We use a five-step 5-minute approach that results in senior success.

Step 1: front office stage

Our front office team members are instrumental in the success of any new program, and senior care is no exception. Front office staff members actually play two important roles in the senior and geriatric program—as initiators and closers. Front office staff members start the senior care experience by identifying which patients are potential candidates for the program using the age analogy chart. Patients are greeted and then weighed in the reception area, thereby allowing the front office team member to determine the appropriate age group using the age analogy chart (see Fig. 1). Clients with senior or geriatric pets are given a copy of the age analogy chart and senior questionnaire (see web site) on a clipboard and asked to complete the form in the examination room. Step 1 is completed.

Step 2: technician and/or assistant stage

Veterinary technicians and/or veterinary assistants initiate step 2 by assisting clients in completing the age analogy form (if necessary) and reinforcing the concept that the pet is senior or geriatric. If possible, they should examine the teeth to determine if dental prophylaxis is required; most older pets have various stages of dental disease. Two senior pet populations exist: those with dental disease and those that will soon have dental disease.

For pets with obvious dental disease

Dental photographs increase client compliance by providing visual reinforcement for the doctor's recommendation. Technicians or assistants usually produce the dental pictures with the clients in the examination room or in the procedure area when trimming nails or cleaning ears, for example. Technicians and/or assistants end their senior assignment by informing the doctor about the patient's age and dental status and providing the dental photograph for the continuing education in step 3.

For pets without obvious dental disease or for clients who simply do not comply with dental recommendations

Pets with obvious dental disease have increased compliance, because owners can visualize dental calculus and the odor of halitosis. Our practice's proportion of nondental senior programs is dramatically increasing, however, thereby drastically increasing our senior profiling. Why? The answer lies in the fact that most of these patients had a dental procedure the year before and now do not need a dental examination or the owner does not wish to have another dental procedure performed yet understands the benefit of the blood testing; in addition, the owner wants to use the vaccine credit.

Step 3: doctor stage

Veterinarians continue the education process by emphasizing the importance of dental health. Let clients grade their pet's dental health by comparing the dental photograph with a dental wall chart or dental pamphlet available through companies selling take-home dental products. Clients must understand that dental disease can contribute to serious medical problems, especially in older pets. Acknowledge the owner's fear of anesthetizing older pets and then help to dismiss those fears by explaining the benefits of your senior program in terms of increased anesthetic safety. Your senior program not only helps to improve anesthetic safety but allows the early detection of laboratory abnormalities, because early detection is the basis of the program. Give written recommendations using client dental education handouts, and then end the appointment. Hand the client the completed age analogy chart, give the doctor-completed recommendation form with the dental photograph to your front office staff, and begin step 4.

Step 4: schedule, schedule, schedule

Your front office staff members are the most important component ensuring the success of the senior program—they start it and end it. Receptionists must ask to schedule the senior or geriatric dental examination, or compliance decreases. If clients need more time or are not interested, simply send a reminder card in 1 or 2 months.

Measuring compliance increases compliance

Compliance must be measured if program success is to be achieved and a fair staff reward system is to be created. Compliance can be manually measured or automatically calculated using newer computer software programs [12]. Our practice rewards staff members as a group instead of individually, creating a true team effort.

Step 5: rewards

Successful teams share their rewards, so start sharing. You can use movie tickets, dinners, or other staff perks, but money is the most universally accepted motivational tool. You may also choose individually based rewards; however, our practice currently uses a team reward system that encompasses two teams: reception and technician. In our practice, doctors are compensated using production-based percentages; thus, they do not require a group reward system because their compensation increases with each senior program instituted. Part-time staff members receive 50% less than full-time staff members. If we employ two full-time and two part-time receptionists (three full-time equivalents) and our practice generated 200 senior profiles for the year, $1000 would be divided by 3, paying each full-time receptionist $330 and each part-time receptionist $165. Technicians and assistants are similarly compensated using the "pool" reward-based system.

Financial benefits of the senior health program

Senior testing is better medically for our patients because it allows earlier detection of diseases. Senior pets represent 30% to 40% of our patients, and this number is likely to increase as technology and education progresses. Senior medicine is likely to become an increasingly important profit center for veterinarians. Increased income results from increased laboratory testing, reflex testing, increased use of veterinary-recommended diets, increased numbers of dental procedures, and increased pharmaceutic income from diseases diagnosed.

Summary: senior health program benefits

Earlier detection allows earlier intervention, and thus improved treatment success. Senior profiling improves anesthetic safety by identifying hidden existing diseases and permitting the postponement of anesthesia or altering the anesthetic plan. Furthermore, pharmaceutic safety is increased through the detection of underlying diseases that may preclude the use of certain drugs or suggest new alternative treatments. Many dietary recommendations are based on disease diagnosis, making senior profiling an important dietary database. Finally, earlier disease management by means of improved anesthetic, pharmaceutic, and dietary recommendations offers our patients and clients the best medical management possible.

References

[1] Metzger FL. Help clients see geriatrics. Veterinary Economics Magazine 1997;38.
[2] Hoskins JD, Fortney WF. Geriatrics and aging. In: Geriatrics and gerontology of the dog and cat. 2nd edition. Philadelphia: WB Saunders; 2004. p. 1–4.
[3] Lees GE. Early diagnosis of renal disease. Vet Clin North Am Small Anim Pract 2004;34: 871–2.
[4] Finco DR, Brown SA, Brown CA, et al. Progression of chronic renal disease in the dog. J Vet Intern Med 1999;13(6):516–28.
[5] Plumb DC. Drug considerations in the geriatric patient. Proc Vet Med Forum 1999;17:14–7.
[6] Hoskins JD. Cancer and therapeutics. In: Geriatrics and gerontology of the dog and cat. 2nd edition. Philadelphia: WB Saunders; 2004. p. 44–9.
[7] Turek MM. Cutaneous paraneoplastic syndromes in dogs and cats: a review of literature. Vet Dermatol 2003;14(6):279–81.
[8] Polzin DJ, Osborne CA, Jacob F. Chronic renal failure. In: Ettinger SJ, Feldman EC, editors. Textbook of veterinary internal medicine. 5th edition. Philadelphia: WB Saunders; 2000. p. 1634–61.
[9] Hoskins JD, Chastain CB. The endocrine and metabolic systems. In: Geriatrics and gerontology of the dog and cat. 2nd edition. Philadelphia: WB Saunders; 2004. p. 271–302.
[10] Rebar A, Metzger F. CE advisor—interpreting the hemogram. Veterinary Medicine Magazine 2001;2:1–9.
[11] Becker TJ, Graves TK, Kruger JM, et al. Effects of methimazole on renal function in cats with hyperthyroidism [abstract]. J Am Anim Hosp Assoc 2000;36:215–23.
[12] Metzger FL. Report cards increase senior compliance. Trends magazine. J Am Anim Hosp Assoc 2004;24:8–12.

ELSEVIER
SAUNDERS

Vet Clin Small Anim
35 (2005) 755–762

VETERINARY
CLINICS
Small Animal Practice

Index

Note: Page numbers of article titles are in **boldface** type.

A

Aggression to humans
  by geriatric pets, 682–683

Aging
  effects on brain, 689–692
  immunologic effects of, 745–746
  in dogs and cats
    nutrition for, **713–741**. See also
      Geriatric pets, nutrition for.
  metabolic effects of, 745–746
  pharmacologic effects of, 746
  physical effects of, 745–746
  physiologic effects of, 745–746

Albuminuria
  implications of, 593–594
  in dogs and cats, 590–594
  β-Amyloid
    in cognitive decline, 690

Anesthesia/anesthetics
  for geriatric patients, **571–580**
    barbiturates in, 576–577
    dissociative anesthetic agents,
      577
    etomidate, 577
    halothane, 578
    inhalants, 577
    isoflurane, 578
    maintenance of, 578–579
    monitoring and support of, 579
    propofol, 577–578
    sevoflurane, 579

Anticholinergic agents
  in preanesthetic sedation of geriatric
    patients, 574–575

Anti-inflammatory drugs
  nonsteroidal
    for osteoarthritic pain in geriatric
      dogs and cats,
      658–660

Anxiety
  separation
    in geriatric pets,
      683–684

Auscultation
  in heart diseases in aging dogs,
    605–607

B

Barbiturate(s)
  for geriatric patients, 576–577

Behavior problems
  in geriatric pets, **675–698**
    aggression to humans, 682–683
    causes of, 677–680
    cognitive dysfunction syndrome,
      685–695
    compulsive disorders, 685
    diagnosis of, 680–681
    distribution of, 675–677
    excessive vocalization, 684–685
    fear, 683–684
    house soiling, 683
    medical conditions and, 678–679
    nocturnal restlessness, 684–685
    phobias, 683–684
    primary problems, 680
    repetitive disorders, 685
    separation anxiety, 683–684
    treatment of, 681–685

Biochemical testing
  of geriatric patients, **537–556**

Blood chemistry
  in heart diseases in aging dogs,
    613–614

Blood substitutes
  in biochemical testing of geriatric
    patients, 543

Bone graft(s)
  in fracture management in geriatric
    dogs and cats, 665

Brain
  aging effects on, 689–692

Breath sounds
  bronchial
    in heart diseases in aging dogs,
      607

Bronchial breath sounds
  in heart diseases in aging dogs, 607

C

Cancer
  in cats, 632
  in dogs, 628–629
  oral, 711

Canine hypothyroidism, 641–649
  clinical features of, 643–645
  described, 641–642
  diagnosis of, 645–647
  primary, 642–643
  prognosis of, 648–649
  secondary, 643
  treatment of, 647–648

Canine thyroid tumors, 649–651

Cardiovascular disease
  in geriatric patients
    pharmacology related to,
      563

Cardiovascular system
  biochemical testing of geriatric
    patients effects on, 555
  of geriatric patients
    physiology of, 572

Carprofen
  for osteoarthritic pain in geriatric dogs
    and cats, 658–659

Cat(s)
  aging
    nutrition for, **713–741.** See also
      Geriatric pets, nutrition for.
    liver diseases in, 629–632
      feline infectious peritonitis,
        631–632
      inflammatory liver disease,
        629–631
      neoplasia, 632
      pyogranulomatous hepatitis,
        631–632
      secondary hepatic lipidosis,
        632

Central nervous system (CNS)
  of geriatric patients
    physiology of, 573–574

Chondroprotective agents
  for osteoarthritic pain in geriatric dogs
    and cats, 661–662

Chronic infiltrative hepatopathies
  in dogs, 622

Chronic inflammatory hepatopathies
  in dogs, 617–621

Cirrhosis(es)
  hepatic
    in dogs, 621–622

CNS. See *Central nervous system (CNS).*

Cognitive decline
  β-amyloid and, 690
  reactive oxygen species effects on,
    690–692
  vascular insufficiency and, 692

Cognitive dysfunction syndrome
  described, 685–687
  in geriatric pets, 685–695
    behavioral changes due to,
      688–689
    diagnosis of, 689
    treatment of, 692–695
      dietary therapy, 692–693
      drug therapy, 693–695
      environmental enrichment in, 693
      nutritional therapy, 692–693

Compulsive disorders
  in geriatric pets, 685

Crackles
  in heart diseases in aging dogs, 607

D

Dentistry
  for geriatric pets
    client compliance in, 749–750

Deracoxib
  for osteoarthritic pain in geriatric dogs
    and cats, 659–660

Diabetes mellitus
  in geriatric patients
    nutrition related to, 728–731

Dietary therapy
  for cognitive dysfunction syndrome,
    692–693

Dissociative anesthetic agents
  for geriatric patients, 577

Dog(s)
  aging
    mitral regurgitation in
      heart diseases related to,
        599–603
    nutrition for, **713–741.** See also
      Geriatric pets, nutrition for.
  geriatric
    heart diseases in, **1–19.** See also
      *Heart diseases, geriatric, in
      dogs.*
    orthopedic problems in, **655–674.**

See also *Orthopedic problems, geriatric, in dogs and cats.*
  liver diseases in, 617–629
    chronic infiltrative hepatopathies, 622
    chronic inflammatory hepatopathies, 617–621
    hepatic cirrhosis, 621–622
    hepatic fibrosis, 621–622
    hepatocutaneous syndrome, 622–626
    hepatoencephalopathy, 627–628
    neoplasia, 628–629
    vascular diseases, 626–627

Drug(s)
  for cognitive dysfunction syndrome, 693–695

Drug monitoring
  for geriatric pets
    client compliance in, 749–750

Dyspnea
  in heart diseases in aging dogs, 607–608

E

ECG. See *Electrocardiography (ECG).*

Echocardiography
  in heart diseases in aging dogs, 613

Electrocardiography (ECG)
  in heart diseases in aging dogs, 611–613

Endocrine system
  biochemical testing of geriatric patients effects on, 552–554

Energy needs
  aging effects on, 714–716

Environmental enrichment
  for cognitive dysfunction syndrome, 693–695

Etodolac
  for osteoarthritic pain in geriatric dogs and cats, 660

Etomidate
  for geriatric patients, 577

Excessive vocalization
  in geriatric pets, 684–685

Exocrine pancreas
  biochemical testing of geriatric patients effects on, 549–550

F

Fear
  in geriatric pets, 683–684

Feline hyperthyroidism, 635–641
  clinical features of, 635–636
  described, 635
  diagnosis of, 636–638
  prognosis of, 641
  treatment of, 639–641

Feline infectious peritonitis, 631–632

Fibrosis(es)
  hepatic
    in dogs, 621–622

Fracture(s)
  in geriatric dogs and cats, 663–673
    management of
      bone grafts in, 665
      surgical approach to, 664–665
    stabilization of, 665–673
      external fixators in, 672–673
      interlocking nails in, 665–668
      plate-rod hybrid in, 668–672

Fractured teeth, 711

G

Gastrointestinal system
  in geriatric patients
    biochemical testing effects on, 550–552

Geriatric care programs
  benefits of, 753
  client compliance for, 748–749
  defining of, 747–748
  financial benefits of, 752–753
  for veterinarians, **743–753**
    benefits of, 753
  Metzger Animal Hospital five-step program, 750–752

Geriatric pets. See also *Aging.*
  anesthesia for, **571–580.** See also *Anesthesia/anesthetics, for geriatric patients.*
  behavior problems in, **675–698.** See also *Behavior problems, in geriatric pets.*
  biochemical testing of, **537–556**
    blood substitutes in, 543
    cardiovascular system–related, 555
    endocrine system–related, 552–554

Geriatric pets (*continued*)
    gastrointestinal system–related,
      550–552
    group-specific variables in, 540
    hemolysis in, 541–542
    hepatic system–related, 546–549
    hyperbilirubinemia in, 542
    icterus in, 542
    interfering substances in
      solutions to, 543–544
    laboratory methodology and
      substance interference in,
      540–541
    laboratory-specific variables in,
      539
    lipemia in, 541–542
    musculoskeletal system–related,
      554–555
    organ system–oriented
      biochemical profiling in, 544
    oxyglobin in, 543
    pancreas-related, 549–550
    reference intervals in
      establishment of, 538–539
    urinary system–related, 544–546
  clinical pathology in, **537–556**
  defining of, 744–745
  dentistry for
    client compliance in, 749–750
  diet-sensitive conditions in, 721–734
    diabetes mellitus, 728–731
    obesity, 724–728
    osteoarthritis, 731–734
    weight loss, 721–724
  diseases of
    systemic, 746–747
  drug monitoring screens for, 749
  heart diseases in
    dogs, **597–615**. See also *Heart
      diseases, geriatric, in dogs.*
  liver disease in, **617–634**
  medical conditions in
    behavior effects of, 678–679
  nutrition for, **713–741**
    evaluation of, 718–721
      dietary-related, 719–721
      feeding management–
        related, 721
      patient-related, 719
  orthopedic problems in
    dogs and cats, **655–674**. See also
      *Orthopedic problems,
      geriatric, in dogs and cats.*
  pharmacology related to, **557–569**.
    See also *Pharmacology, geriatric.*
  physiology of, 571–574
    cardiovascular system, 572
    CNS, 573–574
    hepatic system, 573
    pulmonary system, 572
    renal system, 573
  preanesthetic sedation of, 574–576
  preanesthetic testing for, 749
  preoperative assessment of, 574
  thyroid disorders in, **635–653**. See also
    *Thyroid disorders, in geriatric
    patients.*
  vaccines for
    for client compliance, 750
  veterinary dentistry in, **699–712**. See
    also *Veterinary dentistry, in
    geriatric patients.*

Glucocorticoid(s)
  for osteoarthritic pain in geriatric dogs
    and cats, 661

Group-specific variables
  in biochemical testing of geriatric
    patients, 540

H

Halothane
  in anesthesia maintenance in geriatric
    patients, 578

Heart diseases
  geriatric
    in dogs, **597–615**
      approach to, 604–605
      auscultation in, 605–607
      blood chemistry in, 613–614
      bronchial breath sounds in,
        607
      causes of, 598–599
      crackles in, 607
      dyspnea in, 607–608
      ECG in, 611–613
      echocardiography in, 613
      mitral regurgitation and,
        599–603
      percussion in, 608
      pharmacologic classification
        of, 603–604
      prevalence of, 598
      radiography in, 608–611
      tachypnea in, 607–608

Hemolysis
  in biochemical testing of geriatric
    patients, 541–542

Hepatic cirrhosis
  in dogs, 621–622

Hepatic diseases. See *Liver diseases.*

Hepatic failure
  in geriatric patients
    pharmacology related to,
      561–562

Hepatic fibrosis
    in dogs, 621–622

Hepatic insufficiency
    in geriatric patients
        pharmacology related to,
            561–562

Hepatic system
    biochemical testing of geriatric
        patients effects on, 546–549
    of geriatric patients
        physiology of, 573

Hepatitis
    pyogranulomatous
        in cats, 631–632

Hepatocutaneous syndrome
    in dogs, 622–626

Hepatoencephalopathy
    in dogs, 627–628

Hepatopathy(ies)
    chronic infiltrative
        in dogs, 622
    chronic inflammatory
        in dogs, 617–621

House soiling
    by geriatric pets, 683

Hyperbilirubinemia
    in biochemical testing of geriatric
        patients, 542

Hyperthyroidism
    feline, 635–641. See also *Feline
        hyperthyroidism.*

Hypothyroidism
    canine, 641–649. See also *Canine
        hypothyroidism.*

I

Icterus
    in biochemical testing of geriatric
        patients, 542

Inflammatory liver disease
    in cats, 629–631

Inhalant(s)
    for geriatric patients, 577

Isoflurane
    in anesthesia maintenance in geriatric
        patients, 578

J

Joint disorders
    in geriatric dogs and cats, 655–663. See

also specific disorder, e.g.,
    Osteoarthritis.

L

Laboratory-specific variables
    in biochemical testing of geriatric
        patients, 539

Lipemia
    in biochemical testing of geriatric
        patients, 541–542

Lipidosis
    secondary hepatic
        in cats, 632

Liver. See also under *Hepatic.*

Liver diseases
    in cats. See also specific disease and
        Cat(s), liver diseases in.
    in dogs. See also specific disease and
        Dog(s), liver diseases in.
    in geriatric pets, **617–634.** See also
        Geriatric pets, liver disease in.

Liver failure
    in geriatric patients
        pharmacology related to,
            561–562

M

Meloxicam
    for osteoarthritic pain in geriatric dogs
        and cats, 660

Metzger Animal Hospital five-step
    program, 750–752

Microalbuminuria
    in dogs and cats, 590–594
        causes of, 591–593

Mitral regurgitation
    in aging dogs
        heart diseases related to,
            599–603

Musculoskeletal system
    biochemical testing of geriatric
        patients effects on,
            554–555

N

Neoplasia
    in cats, 632
    in dogs, 628–629

Nocturnal restlessness
    in geriatric pets, 684–685

Nutraceutical(s)
    for osteoarthritic pain in geriatric dogs
      and cats, 662–663

Nutrient(s)
    aging effects on, 714–718

Nutrition
    aging effects on, 714–718
    for aging cats and dogs, **713–741**. See
      also *Geriatric pets, nutrition for.*

Nutritional therapy
    for cognitive dysfunction syndrome,
      692–693

O

Obesity
    in geriatric patients
      nutrition related to, 724–728

Opioid(s)
    in preanesthetic sedation of geriatric
      patients, 575

Oral neoplasia, 711

Organ system–oriented biochemical
    profiling
    in biochemical testing of geriatric
      patients, 544

Orthopedic problems
    geriatric
      in dogs and cats, **655–674**
        fractures, 663–673. See also
          Fracture(s), in
          geriatric dogs and cats.
        in postoperative period, 673
        joint-related disorders,
          655–663. See also
          specific disorder and
          Joint disorders, in
          geriatric dogs and cats.

Osteoarthritis
    in geriatric dogs and cats, 655
      diagnosis of, 655–656
      treatment of, 656–663
        carprofen in, 658–659
        chondroprotective agents
          in, 661–662
        deracoxib in, 659–660
        etodolac in, 660
        glucocorticoids in, 661
        goals for, 656
        meloxicam in, 660
        NSAIDs in, 658–660
        nutraceuticals in, 662–663
        nutrition in, 731–734
        steps in, 656
        tepoxalin in, 660

Oxyglobin
    in biochemical testing of geriatric
      patients, 543

P

Pancreas
    biochemical testing of geriatric
      patients effects on, 549–550
    exocrine
      biochemical testing of geriatric
        patients effects on, 549–550

Pancreatitis
    biochemical testing of geriatric
      patients and, 549–550

Percussion
    in heart diseases in aging dogs, 608

Periodontal disease
    treatment of, 709–711

Peritonitis
    infectious
      feline, 631–632

Pharmacology
    geriatric, **557–569**
      cardiovascular disease and, 563
      dosage adjustments, 563–566
      hepatic insufficiency and,
        561–562
      renal failure and, 560–561
      renal insufficiency and, 558–561

Phobia(s)
    in geriatric pets, 683–684

Preanesthetic testing
    for geriatric pets
      client compliance in, 749

Propofol
    for geriatric patients, 577–578

Protein needs
    aging effects on, 716–718

Proteinuria
    as diagnostic marker of early chronic
      renal disease, 589–590
    implications of, 593–594

Pulmonary system
    of geriatric patients
      physiology of, 572

Pyogranulomatous hepatitis
    in cats, 631–632

R

Radiography
    in heart diseases in aging dogs,
      608–611

Reactive oxygen species
  in cognitive decline, 690–692

Regurgitation
  mitral
    in aging dogs
      heart diseases related to,
        599–603

Renal damage
  acute
    in dogs and cats
      described, 581–583
      early detection of,
        581–587
      early recognition of,
        585–587
      risk factors for, 583–585
  early detection of
    in dogs and cats, **581–596**

Renal disease
  chronic
    early
      diagnostic markers of
        proteinuria as, 589–590
      in dogs and cats, 587–590
        described, 587–588
        early detection of,
          588–589
    in dogs and cats
      albuminuria, 590–594
      early detection of, **581–596**
      microalbuminuria, 590–594

Renal failure
  in geriatric patients
    hepatic metabolism in, 560
    metabolic balance in, 560–561

Renal insufficiency
  in geriatric patients, 558–561
    absorption in, 559
    bioavailability in, 559
    drug distribution and, 559–560
    renal clearance of drugs in,
      558–559

Renal system
  of geriatric patients
    physiology of, 573

Repetitive disorders
  in geriatric pets, 685

Restlessness
  nocturnal
    in geriatric pets, 684–685

S

Secondary hepatic lipidosis
  in cats, 632

Sedative(s)
  in preanesthetic sedation of geriatric
    patients, 575–576

Senior pets. See *Geriatric pets.*

Separation anxiety
  in geriatric pets, 683–684

Sevoflurane
  in anesthesia maintenance in geriatric
    patients, 579

Sound(s)
  breath
    bronchial
      in heart diseases in aging
        dogs, 607

T

Tachypnea
  in heart diseases in aging dogs,
    607–608

Tepoxalin
  for osteoarthritic pain in geriatric dogs
    and cats, 660

Thyroid disorders
  in geriatric patients, **635–653.** See also
    specific disorder, e.g., *Feline
    hyperthyroidism.*
    canine hypothyroidism, 641–649
    canine thyroid tumors, 649–651
    feline hyperthyroidism, 635–641

Thyroid tumors
  canine, 649–651

Tooth (teeth)
  fractured, 711

Tranquilizer(s)
  in preanesthetic sedation of geriatric
    patients, 575–576

Tumor(s)
  thyroid
    canine, 649–651

U

Urinary system
  biochemical testing of geriatric
    patients effects on, 544–546

V

Vaccine(s)
  for client compliance in geriatric pets,
    750

Variable(s)
  group-specific

Variable(s) (*continued*)
    in biochemical testing of geriatric
        patients, 540
    laboratory-specific
        in biochemical testing of geriatric
          patients, 539

Vascular diseases
    in dogs, 606–607

Vascular insufficiency
    in cognitive decline, 692

Veterinarian(s)
    geriatric care programs for, **743–753.**
        See also *Geriatric care programs,*
        for veterinarians.

Veterinary dentistry
    in geriatric patients, **699–712**
        client education related to,
          701–702

        complete prophylaxis in,
          705–709
        dental procedure in, 704–705
        fractured teeth, 711
        introducing of, 699–701
        oral neoplasia, 711
        periodontal disease treatment,
          709–711
        preprocedure evaluation in,
          702–704

Vocalization
    excessive
        in geriatric pets, 684–685

W

Weight loss
    in geriatric patients
        nutrition related to, 721–724

Changing Your Address?

Make sure your subscription changes too! When you notify us of your new address, you can help make our job easier by including an exact copy of your Clinics label number with your old address (see illustration below.) This number identifies you to our computer system and will speed the processing of your address change. Please be sure this label number accompanies your old address and your corrected address—you can send an old Clinics label with your number on it or just copy it exactly and send it to the address listed below.

We appreciate your help in our attempt to give you continuous coverage. Thank you.

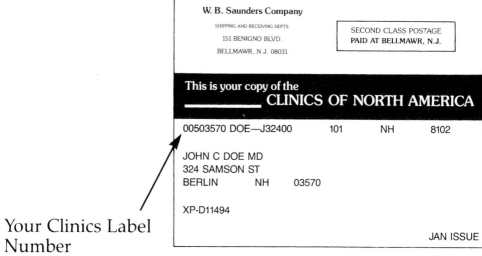

Your Clinics Label Number
Copy it exactly or send your label along with your address to:
W.B. Saunders Company, Customer Service
Orlando, FL 32887-4800
Call Toll Free 1-800-654-2452

Please allow four to six weeks for delivery of new subscriptions and for processing address changes.

8 Ways To Expand Your Practice
Step 1: Return this card.

Elsevier Clinics and Journals offer you that rare combination of up-to-date scholarly data, step-by-step techniques and authoritative insights...information you can easily apply to the situations you encounter in daily practice. You'll be better able to diagnose and treat a wider range of veterinary problems and broaden your client base.

Just indicate your choice(s) on the card below, fill out the rest of the card and drop it in the mail.

Your satisfaction is guaranteed. If you do not find that the periodical meets your expectations, write *cancel* on the invoice and return it within 30 days. You are under no further obligation.

SUBSCRIBE TODAY!
DETACH AND MAIL THIS NO-RISK CARD TODAY!

YES! Please start my subscription to the periodicals checked below with the ❑ first issue of the calendar year or ❑ current issues. If not completely satisfied with my first issue, I may write "cancel" on the invoice and return it within 30 days at no further obligation

Please Print:

Name_____

Address _____

_____

City_____ State_____

ZIP _____

Method of Payment

❑ Check (payable to **Elsevier**; add the applicable sales tax for your area)

❑ VISA   ❑ MasterCard   ❑ AmEx   ❑ Bill me

Card number _____

Exp. date _____

Signature _____

Staple this to your purchase order to expedite delivery

*To receive in-training rate, orders must be accompanied by the name of affiliated institution, dates of residency and signature of coordinator on institution letterhead. Orders will be billed at the individual rate until proof of resident status is received.

This is not a renewal notice. Professional references may be tax-deductible.
© **Elsevier 2005.** Offer valid in U.S. only. Prices subject to change without notice. **MO 10806 DF4169**

❑ **Clinical Techniques in Equine Practice**
Volume 4 (4 issues)
Individuals $124; Institutions $209; In-training $62*

❑ **Clinical Techniques in Small Animal Practice**
Volume 10 (4 issues)
Individuals $134; Institutions $220; In-training $67*

❑ **Journal of Equine Veterinary Science**
Volume 22 (12 issues)
Individuals $171; Institutions $242; In-training $54*

❑ **Seminars in Avian and Exotic Pet Medicine**
Volume 4 (4 issues)
Individuals $116; Institutions $220; In-training $54*

❑ **Veterinary Clinics-Equine Practice**
Volume 21 (3 issues)
Individuals $145; Institutions $230

❑ **Veterinary Clinics-Exotic Animal Practice**
Volume 8 (3 issues)
Individuals $130; Institutions $215

❑ **Veterinary Clinics-Food Animal Practice**
Volume 21 (3 issues)
Individuals $115; Institutions $182

❑ **Veterinary Clinics-Small Animal Practice**
Volume 35 (6 issues)
Individuals $170; Institutions $260

Elsevier, the premier publisher in veterinary medicine, keeps you current with the latest developments in your field to help you achieve optimal patient care. Subscribe today to any of the publications listed below and save considerably over the single issue price.

Clinical Techniques in Equine Practice
Clinical Techniques in Small Animal Practice
Journal of Equine Veterinary Science
Seminars in Avian and Exotic Pet Medicine
Veterinary Clinics – Equine Practice
Veterinary Clinics – Exotic Animal Practice
Veterinary Clinics – Food Animal Practice
Veterinary Clinics – Small Animal Practice

Just fill out the card on the reverse and drop it in the mail.
YOUR SATISFACTION IS GUARANTEED.

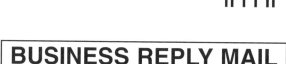

NO POSTAGE
NECESSARY
IF MAILED
IN THE
UNITED STATES

BUSINESS REPLY MAIL
FIRST-CLASS MAIL   PERMIT NO 7135   ORLANDO FL

POSTAGE WILL BE PAID BY ADDRESSEE

PERIODICALS ORDER FULFILLMENT DEPT
ELSEVIER
6277 SEA HARBOR DR
ORLANDO FL 32821-9816